Macular Edema

Developments in Ophthalmology

Vol. 47

Series Editors

F. Bandello Milan
W. Behrens-Baumann Magdeburg

Macular Edema

A Practical Approach

Volume Editor

Gabriel Coscas Créteil, Paris

Co-Editors

José Cunha-Vaz Coimbra
Anat Loewenstein Tel Aviv
Gisèle Soubrane Créteil, Paris

115 figures, 77 in color, and 8 tables, 2010

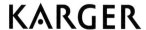

Basel · Freiburg · Paris · London · New York · Bangalore ·
Bangkok · Shanghai · Singapore · Tokyo · Sydney

Gabriel Coscas
Hôpital Intercommunal de Créteil
Service d'Ophthalmologie
Université Paris – XII
40, Avenue de Verdun
FR–94010 Créteil (France)

This book was generously supported by ALLERGAN *ophthalmology*

Library of Congress Cataloging-in-Publication Data

Macular edema : a practical approach / volume editor, G. Coscas ;
co-editors, J. Cunha-Vaz, A. Loewenstein, G. Soubrane.
     p. ; cm. -- (Developments in ophthalmology, ISSN 0250-3751 ; v. 47)
  Includes bibliographical references and index.
  ISBN 978-3-8055-9434-9 (hard cover : alk. paper) -- ISBN 978-3-8055-9435-6
(e-ISBN)
  1. Macula lutea--Diseases. 2. Edema. I. Coscas, Gabriel. II. Series:
Developments in ophthalmology ; v. 47. 0250-3751
  [DNLM: 1. Macular Edema--diagnosis. 2. Macular Edema--etiology. 3.
Macular Edema--therapy. W1 DE998NG v.47 2010 / WW 270 M1761 2010]
  RE661.M3M335 2010
  617.7'42--dc22
                                                        2010024216

Bibliographic Indices. This publication is listed in bibliographic services, including Current Contents® and Index Medicus.

© Copyright 2010 by S. Karger AG, P.O. Box, CH–4009 Basel (Switzerland)
www.karger.com
Printed in Switzerland on acid-free and non-aging paper (ISO 9706) by Reinhardt Druck, Basel
ISSN 0250–3751
ISBN 978–3–8055–9434–9
e-ISBN 978–3–8055–9435–6

Contents

V

List of Contributors

Albert Augustin, Prof.
Moltkestrasse 90
DE–76133 Karlsruhe (Germany)
E-Mail albertjaugustin@googlemail.com

Francesco Bandello, Prof.
Department of Ophthalmology
University Vita-Salute
Scientific Institute San Raffaele
Via Olgettina, 60
IT–20132 Milano (Italy)
E-Mail bandello.francesco@hsr.it

Maurizio Battaglia Parodi, Dr.
Department of Ophthalmology
University Vita-Salute
Scientific Institute San Raffaele
Via Olgettina, 60
IT–20132 Milano (Italy)
E-Mail battagliaparodi.maurizio@hsr.it

Sébastien Bonnel, Dr.
Department of Ophthalmology
Foundation Rothschild
25, rue Manin
FR–75019 Paris (France)
E-Mail bonneloph@gmail.com

Gabriel Coscas, Prof.
Hôpital Intercommunal de Créteil
Service d'Ophthalmologie
Université Paris – XII
40, Avenue de Verdun
FR–94010 Créteil (France)
E-Mail gabriel.coscas@gmail.com

Catherine Creuzot-Garcher, Prof.
Service d'Ophtalmologie
Centre Hospitalier Universitaire Dijon
FR–21000 Dijon (France)
E-Mail catherine.creuzot-garcher@
chu-dijon.fr

José Cunha-Vaz, Prof.
AIBILI
Azinhaga de Santa Comba
Celas
PT–3040 Coimbra (Portugal)
E-Mail cunhavaz@aibili.pt

Laura de Polo, Dr.
Eye Clinic
Department of Clinical Science "Luigi Sacco"
Sacco Hospital
Via G.B Grassi 74
IT–20157 Milan (Italy)
E-Mail lauradepolo@libero.it

Marc D. de Smet, Prof.
Department of Ophthalmology
University of Amsterdam
NL–1012 WX Amsterdam (The Netherlands)
E-Mail mddesmet1@mac.com

Agnès Glacet-Bernard, Dr.
Hôpital Intercommunal de Créteil
Service d'Ophthalmologie
Université Paris – XII
40, Avenue de Verdun
FR–94010 Créteil (France)
E-Mail Agnes.Glacet@chicreteil.fr

Zdenek J. Gregor, Dr.
Moorfields Eye Hospital
162 City Road
London EC1V 2PD (UK)
E-Mail zdenek.gregor@moorfields.nhs.uk

Alessandro Invernizzi, Dr.
Eye Clinic
Department of Clinical Science "Luigi Sacco"
Sacco Hospital
Via G.B Grassi 74
IT–20157 Milan (Italy)
E-Mail alessandro.invernizzi@gmail.com

Jost Jonas, Prof.
Department of Ophthalmology
Faculty of Clinical Medicine Mannheim
University of Heidelberg
DE–68167 Mannheim (Germany)
E-Mail Jost.Jonas@umm.de

Baruch D. Kuppermann, Dr.
UC Irvine Medical Center
Ophthalmology Clinic
101 The City Drive South
Irvine, CA 92697 (USA)
E-Mail bdkupper@uci.edu

Paolo Lanzetta, Prof.
University of Udine
Department of Ophthalmology
Piazzale S. Maria della Misericordia
IT–33100 Udine (Italy)
E-Mail paolo.lanzetta@uniud.it

Anat Loewenstein, Prof.
Department of Ophthalmology
Tel Aviv Medical Center
Sackler Faculty of Medicine
Tel Aviv University
6 Weizmann St.
Tel Aviv 64239 (Israel)
E-Mail anatl@tasmc.health.gov.il

Pascale Massin, Prof.
Department of Ophthalmology
Lariboisiere Hospital
2, rue Ambroise-Paré
FR–75475 Paris Cedex 10 (France)
E-Mail p.massin@lrb.ap-hop-paris.fr

Francesca Menchini, Dr.
University of Udine
Department of Ophthalmology
Piazzale S. Maria della Misericordia
IT–33100 Udine (Italy)
E-Mail francescamenchini@gmail.com

Jordi Monés, Dr.
Institut de la Màcula i de la Retina
Centro Médico Teknon
Vilana 12
ES–08022 Barcelona (Spain)
E-Mail jmones@institutmacularetina.com

Sarah Mrejen, Dr.
Department of Ophthalmology
Quinze-Vingts Hospital and the Vision Institute
Pierre et Marie Curie University
28, rue de Charenton
FR–75012 Paris (France)
E-Mail mrejen_sarah@yahoo.fr

Annabelle A. Okada, Prof.
Department of Ophthalmology
Kyorin University School of Medicine
6-20-2 Shinkawa, Mitaka
Tokyo 181–8611 (Japan)
E-Mail aokada@e23.jp

Michel Paques, Prof.
Quinze-Vingts Hospital and Vision Institute
Paris VI University
28, rue de Charenton
FR–75012 Paris (France)
E-Mail michel.paques@gmail.com

Marco Pellegrini, Dr.
Eye Clinic
Department of Clinical Science "Luigi Sacco"
Sacco Hospital
Via G.B Grassi 74
IT–20157 Milan (Italy)
E-Mail mar.pellegrini@gmail.com

José Sahel, Prof.
Department of Ophthalmology
Quinze-Vingts Hospital and the Vision Institute
Pierre et Marie Curie University
28, rue de Charenton
FR–75012 Paris (France)
E-Mail j.sahel@gmail.com

Gisèle Soubrane, Prof.
Hôpital Intercommunal de Créteil
Service d'Ophthalmologie
Université Paris – XII
40, Avenue de Verdun
FR–94010 Créteil (France)
E-Mail gisele.soubrane@chicreteil.fr

Giovanni Staurenghi, Prof.
Eye Clinic
Department of Clinical Science "Luigi Sacco"
Sacco Hospital
Via G.B Grassi 74
IT–20157 Milan (Italy)
E-Mail giovanni.staurenghi@unimi.it

Daniele Veritti, Dr.
University of Udine
Department of Ophthalmology
Piazzale S. Maria della Misericordia
IT–33100 Udine (Italy)
E-Mail verittidaniele@gmail.com

Sebastian Wolf, Prof.
Universitätsklinik für Augenheilkunde
Inselspital
University of Bern
CH–3010 Bern
E-Mail sebastian.wolf@insel.ch

Thomas J. Wolfensberger, Dr.
Vitreoretinal Department
Jules Gonin Eye Hospital
University of Lausanne
Ave de France 15
CH–1000 Lausanne 7 (Switzerland)
E-Mail Thomas.Wolfensberger@fa2.ch

Dinah Zur, Dr.
Department of Ophthalmology
Tel Aviv Medical Center
Sackler Faculty of Medicine
Tel Aviv University
6 Weizmann St.
Tel Aviv 64239 (Israel)
E-Mail dinahgelernter@gmail.com

Preface

Macular edema has for a long time been one of the most important issues in retinal pathologies, as damage to the macula has an immediate effect on central visual acuity and may substantially affect a patient's quality of life.

For more than 40 years, clinicians have attempted to identify macular edema in its initial state and to define its various etiologies. Diagnosing macular edema with certitude at an early stage has proven difficult despite the progress in contact lens biomicroscopy.

Fluorescein angiography has been critical for detecting macular edema and currently remains the 'gold standard' for the diagnosis, identifying the characteristic stellar pattern of cystoid macular edema. Fluorescein angiography also provides a qualitative assessment of vascular leakage, which is essential for identifying treatable lesions. However, it is only since the use of laser photocoagulation that it became possible to offer an effective modality of treatment for macular edema, despite the destructive localized laser scars.

During the last decade, the clinical diagnosis of macular edema and its treatment have been greatly improved due to multiple and remarkable advances of modern imaging technologies, which allow recognition of the main etiologies of this complication. By correlating results from fluorescein angiography, optical coherence tomography, and especially spectral domain optical coherence tomography, fluid accumulation within and under the sensory retina can be confirmed and located. This fluid accumulation, frequently associated with subretinal fluid and serous retinal detachment, may not otherwise be clinically detected.

Moreover, spectral domain optical coherence tomography can characterize the presence and integrity of the external limiting membrane and the photoreceptor inner and outer segments, which is useful information for prognosis as well as a guide for treatment. The diagnosis of macular edema and its clinical forms is now based primarily on the correlation of these imaging techniques.

One of the most important innovations in the field of macular edema has been the advent of intravitreal drug delivery approaches for the treatment of posterior segment pathologies. These emerging modalities treat posterior eye disease or restore the permeability of the blood-retinal barrier by delivering drug compounds either systemically, locally, or intravitreally with anti-inflammatory or anti-vascular endothelial growth factor drugs.

Multicenter controlled clinical trials testing these new compounds as well as biologic delivery systems and treatment strategies have already been completed or are currently under way. From this research, the care of macular edema will soon be more efficient and effective due to increased target specificity, noninvasive drug administration routes, and sustained-release compounds that will allow sufficient levels of therapeutic efficacy for longer durations.

Macular Edema: A Practical Approach describes the different patterns and etiologies of macular edema and the importance of preserving the photoreceptors at the early stage in order to retain central visual acuity. The book was designed to bring together the most recent data and evidence-based medicine while also including the multiple areas still unknown and debated.

Macular Edema: A Practical Approach presents the pathophysiological basis of macular edema and the different approaches of drug delivery to the posterior segment. Recommendations for treatment procedures or different therapies have been carefully analyzed and considered prior to inclusion.

The authors bring their personal experience and full teaching acumen to each chapter, culminating in a single book that brings to the forefront the importance of macular edema.

Macular Edema: A Practical Approach provides the ophthalmologist with a synthesis of knowledge to diagnose, determines the etiology, and offers viable treatment options for the benefit of all our patients.

Gabriel Coscas

Chapter 1

Coscas G (ed): Macular Edema.
Dev Ophthalmol. Basel, Karger, 2010, vol 47, pp 1–9

Macular Edema: Definition and Basic Concepts

Gabriel Coscas[a] · José Cunha-Vaz[b] · Gisèle Soubrane[a]

[a]Hôpital Intercommunal de Créteil, Service Universitaire d'Ophtalmologie, Créteil, Paris, France; [b]AIBILI, Coimbra, Portugal

Abstract

Macular edema is the result of an accumulation of fluid in the retinal layers around the fovea. It contributes to vision loss by altering the functional cell relationship in the retina and promoting an inflammatory reparative response. Macular edema may be intracellular or extracellular. Intracellular accumulation of fluid, also called cytotoxic edema, is an alteration of the cellular ionic distribution. Extracellular accumulation of fluid, which is more frequent and clinically more relevant, is directly associated with an alteration of the blood-retinal barrier (BRB). The following parameters are relevant for clinical evaluation of macular edema: extent of the macular edema (i.e., the area that shows increased retinal thickness); distribution of the edema in the macular area (i.e., focal versus diffuse macular edema); central foveal involvement (central area 500 μm); fluorescein leakage (evidence of alteration of the BRB or 'open barrier') and intraretinal cysts; signs of ischemia (broken perifoveolar capillary arcade and/or areas of capillary closure); presence or absence of vitreous traction; increase in retinal thickness and cysts in the retina (inner or outer), and chronicity of the edema (i.e., time elapsed since initial diagnosis and response to therapy). It is essential to establish associations and correlations of all the different images obtained, regardless of whether the same or different modalities are used.

Macular edema is the result of an accumulation of fluid in the retinal layers around the fovea. It contributes to vision loss by altering the functional cell relationship in the retina and promoting an inflammatory reparative response.

Macular edema is a *nonspecific sign of ocular disease* and not a specific entity. It should be viewed as a special and clinically relevant type of macular response to an altered retinal environment. In most cases, it is associated with an alteration of the blood-retinal barrier (BRB).

Macular edema may occur in a wide variety of ocular situations including uveitis, trauma, intraocular surgery, vascular retinopathies, vitreoretinal adhesions, hereditary dystrophies, diabetes, and age-related macular degeneration.

The *histopathological picture* of this condition is an accumulation of fluid in the outer plexiform (Henle's) and inner nuclear and plexiform layers of the retina (fig. 1). The increase in water content of the retinal tissue characterizing macular edema may be *intracellular* or *extracellular*. Intracellular accumulation of fluid, also called cytotoxic edema, is an alteration of the cellular ionic distribution. Extracellular accumulation of fluid, which is more frequent and clinically more relevant, is directly associated with an alteration of the BRB.

Intracellular Edema

Intracellular edema in the retina may occur when there is an intact BRB and the retinal cells are swollen due to an alteration of the cellular ionic

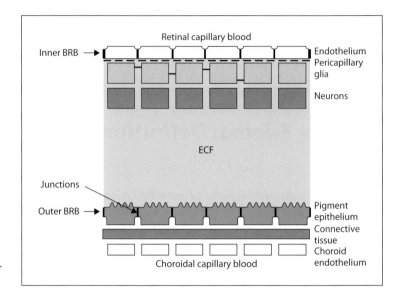

Fig. 1. Schematic presentation of the inner and outer BRBs and their relative location. ECF = Extracellular fluid.

distribution, resulting in excessive accumulation of sodium ions (Na^+) inside the cells.

This is known as cytotoxic edema. It may be induced by accumulation of excitatory neurotransmitters, such as glutamate, or excessive accumulation of lactic acid, or it may be the immediate result of *ischemia*, trauma, or toxic cell damage.

Extracellular Edema

Extracellular edema is directly associated with an open BRB (i.e., it is caused by a breakdown of the inner or outer BRB). The increase in tissue volume is due to an increase in the retinal extracellular space.

Breakdown of the BRB is identified by *fluorescein leakage*, which can be detected in a clinical environment by fluorescein angiography (FA) or vitreous fluorometry measurements. Starling's law[a], which governs the movements of fluids, applies in this type of edema (Cunha-Vaz et al., 1984)[1].

After a breakdown of the BRB, the progression of retinal edema depends directly on the hydrostatic pressure difference (ΔP) and osmotic pressure difference ($\Delta \pi$) gradients. In these conditions, tissue compliance becomes more important, directly influencing the rate of edema progression. Thus, in the presence of retinal edema, it is essential to recognize whether the edema has arisen due to an intact or open BRB.

[a] Starling's law: In extracellular edema, the 'force' driving water across the capillary wall is the result of a hydrostatic pressure difference (ΔP) and an effective osmotic pressure difference ($\Delta \pi$). The equation regulating fluid movements across the BRB is: driving force = L_p [($P_{plasma} - P_{tissue}$) – σ ($\pi_{plasma} - \pi_{tissue}$)], where L_p is the membrane permeability of the BRB; σ is an osmotic reflection coefficient; P_{plasma} is blood pressure, and P_{tissue} is the retinal tissue osmotic pressure. An increase in ΔP, contributing to retinal edema, may be due to an increase in P_{plasma} and/or a decrease in P_{tissue}. An increase in P_{plasma} due to increased systemic blood pressure contributes to retinal edema formation only after loss of autoregulation of retinal blood flow and alteration of the characteristics of the BRB. A decrease in P_{tissue} is an important component that has previously not been given sufficient attention. Any loss in the cohesiveness of the retinal tissue due to pathologies, such as cyst formation, vitreous traction, or pulling at the inner limiting membrane, will lead to a decrease in P_{tissue}.

A decrease in P_{tissue} (i.e., increased retinal tissue compliance) may lead to fluid accumulation, edema formation, and an increase in retinal thickness. A decrease in $\Delta \pi$ contributing to retinal edema may occur due to increased protein accumulation in the retina after breakdown of the BRB. Extravasation of proteins will draw more water into the retina. This is the main factor provoking a decrease in $\Delta \pi$, as a reduction in plasma osmolarity high enough to contribute to edema formation is an extremely rare event.

BRB breakdown leading to macular edema may be mediated by locally released cytokines, and it induces an inflammatory reparative response creating the conditions for further release of cytokines and growth factors. The BRB cells, retinal endothelial cells, and retinal pigment epithelium (RPE) cells are both the target and producer of eicosanoids, growth factors, and cytokines.

Macular edema is one of the most serious consequences of inflammation in the retinal tissue. Inflammatory cells can alter the permeability of the tight junctions that maintain the inner and outer BRB. Cell migration may occur primarily through splitting of the junctional complexes or through the formation of channels or pores across the junctional complexes.

Clinical Evaluation of Macular Edema

The clinical evaluation of macular edema has been difficult to characterize, but evaluation has become more precise with the help of modern imaging such as FA and optical coherence tomography (OCT).

The following parameters are relevant for clinical evaluation of macular edema: extent of the macular edema (i.e., the area that shows increased retinal thickness); distribution of the edema in the macular area (i.e., focal versus diffuse macular edema); central fovea involvement (central area 500 μm); fluorescein leakage (evidence of alteration of BRB or 'open barrier') and intraretinal cysts; signs of ischemia (broken perifoveolar capillary arcade and/or areas of capillary closure); presence or absence of vitreous traction; increase in retinal thickness and cysts in the retina (inner or outer), and chronicity of the edema (i.e., time elapsed since first diagnosis and response to therapy).

Direct and Indirect Ophthalmoscopy
Direct and indirect ophthalmoscopy may show only an alteration of the foveal reflexes. Slit lamp biomicroscopy and stereoscopic fundus photography have played an important role in

demonstrating changes in retinal volume in the macular area, but they are dependent on the observer's experience, and the results do not offer a reproducible measurement of the volume change (Gonzalez et al., 1995)[2].

The Early Treatment Diabetic Retinopathy Study specified the following characteristics as indicating clinically significant macular edema: (1) thickening of the retina (as seen by slit lamp biomicroscopy or stereoscopic fundus photography) at or within 500 μm of the center of the macula; (2) hard exudates at or within 500 μm of the center of the macula associated with thickening of the adjacent retina (but not residual hard exudates remaining after disappearance of retinal thickening), and (3) a zone or zones of retinal thickening 1 disk in area or larger in size, any part of which is within 1 disk diameter of the center of the macula. This definition of macular edema specifically takes into consideration the involvement of the center of the macula and its relationship to visual loss.

Fluorescein Angiography
FA documents if there is fluorescein leakage, which in turn determines whether a barrier is classified as open or intact. Clinical use of FA has contributed significantly to the present understanding of retinal disease, and it is considered the 'gold standard'.

The dye used in FA is sodium fluorescein, a small molecule that diffuses freely through the choriocapillaris and Bruch's membrane but does not diffuse through the tight junctions of the retinal endothelial cells and the RPE, which are the inner and outer BRBs. Understanding these barriers is the key to understanding and interpreting a fluorescein angiogram (Cunha-Vaz et al., 1984)[1].

FA also fundamentally contributes to our understanding of vascular retinopathy. FA will help for the identification of areas of capillary leakage and/ or capillary closure or capillary dropout. Capillary closure and fluorescein leakage were first clinically identified with FA, and they are accepted as the

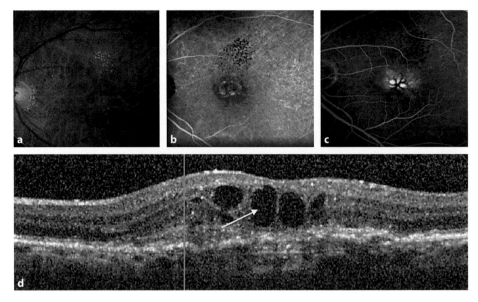

Fig. 2. CME. **a** Color photo. **b, c** FA (early and late stage); capillary dilation and leakage; fluorescein dye pools in cystoid spaces located in the outer plexiform layer (Henle's layer) and arranged radially from the fovea. **d** Spectral domain OCT (Spectralis): typical image of cystoid spaces. OCT imaging allows precise analysis of large cystoid spaces, and their location, the extent of an area of increased thickness, and the extent of the involvement of the central macula are essential in determining the presence of macular edema. Moreover, the analysis of the outer retinal layers could give valuable prognostic indications.

determinant alterations occurring in the diabetic retina, retinal vein occlusion, and other retinal vasculopathies identifying the progression of retinopathy (Kohner et al., 1970; Coscas et al., 1978)[3,4].

Intravenous injection of sodium fluorescein is generally safe and easy to perform. It is routinely used in ophthalmological clinics despite severe anaphylactic reactions that may occur on rare occasions (1 in 200,000) (Yannuzzi et al., 1986)[5].

FA is an indispensable imaging tool in determining the definitive diagnosis of macular edema (Gass, 1997)[6]. The angiographic definition distinguishes between noncystoid and cystoid macular edema (CME) (Richard et al., 1998)[7].

The noncystoid form of macular edema is characterized by diffuse abnormal permeability of the retinal capillary bed with diffuse leakage and intraretinal fluid accumulation that has not accumulated in cystoid spaces but may still do so in the later course of the disease. It is displayed as a diffusely outlined and ill-delimited area of hyperfluorescence.

In CME, early capillary dilation and leakage can be detected. In the late phase of the angiogram, fluorescein pools in cystoid spaces located in the outer plexiform layer (Henle's layer) displayed as the classic petaloid staining pattern (Guyer et al., 1999)[8]. These cystoid spaces are usually arranged radially from the fovea (fig. 2). In long-standing CME, the cystoid spaces enlarge and may merge, representing irreversible damage of the retina.

The extent of dye leakage alone does not completely correlate with functional damage and visual acuity. Duration of the edema and associated changes (RPE and the degree of ischemia) must also be taken into account.

Presence or predominance of the ischemic component needs to be analyzed with the help of FA and must be considered when signs of capillary dropout predominate in the central macular area.

Fundus imaging using *indocyanine green dye*, particularly with the scanning laser, may provide additional direct signs for macular edema but also for the precise analysis of RPE alterations and for the detection and delimitation of cystoid spaces progressively filled with the dye. Analogous to the Rosetta Stone, the key to interpretation is correlation of the data acquired from the different imaging systems.

Optical Coherence Tomography
OCT provides images of retinal structures that could not previously be obtained by any other noninvasive, noncontact, transpupillary diagnostic method. OCT allows assessment and detection of subretinal and intraretinal fluid related to changes in the inner and outer BRBs and abnormal exudation from the retinal capillary bed.

OCT provides anteroposterior images by measuring the echo time and intensity of reflected or backscattered light from intraretinal microstructures. These anteroposterior 2-dimensional or B-scan images (analogous to those of ultrasound) were demonstrated for the first time in 1991 by Huang (Huang et al., 1991)[9] and in the human retina in 1993 by Fercher (Fercher et al., 1993)[10] and Swanson (Swanson et al., 1993)[11]. These optical scans are based on the principle of low-coherence light interferometry (Puliafito et al., 1995; Schuman et al., 2004)[12,13].

Schematically, in conventional (time domain) OCT, the light beam emitted by a superluminescent diode is split into two beams by a beam splitter: an incident beam enters the ocular media and is reflected by the various layers of the fundus, while the other beam is reflected by a reference mirror. Displacement of the mirror placed on the path of the reference light beam allows analysis of structures situated at various depths during each light echo acquisition, forming an A-scan. The time necessary for this scanning and for the acquisition of these sections is the essential determinant of the quality of the signal, hence the name time domain OCT (TD-OCT).

Spectral-Domain OCT (SD-OCT), a method based on the famous Fourier transform mathematical equation (1807), eliminates the need for a moving mirror in the path of the reference beam, which allows for much more rapid image acquisition and provides excellent resolution (axial resolution of <10 μm). This property enables spectral domain SD-OCT systems to capture a large number of high-resolution images: 50 times faster than standard time domain OCT and 100 times faster than the first ultrahigh-resolution OCT. As the examination can be performed simultaneously in various planes, real high-speed 3-dimensional reconstructions can be obtained with hundreds of images per second.

Rapid scanning allows an increased number and density of scans of the retina to be obtained in a very short time, with a marked reduction of artifacts related to patient movements (eye and respiratory movements) during the examination. The use of image processing systems based on *real-time averaging* reduces the signal-to-noise ratio and increases image definition and image quality.

OCT has rapidly become a noninvasive optical imaging modality for medical diagnosis in ophthalmology, allowing in vivo visualization of the internal microstructures of the retina on these sections and evaluation of variations of *retinal thickness*. Images are obtained in 2 or 3 dimensions and represent variations of these reflections (and backscatter) of light either in a plane of section or in a volume of tissue. This anteroposterior dimension of OCT provides a spectacular complement to angiographic data.

OCT scans can visualize exudative reactions with fluid accumulation (intraretinal and/or subretinal). Comparative quantitative evaluation of these images during the course of the disease is particularly useful. OCT may allow discovery at a stage often difficult to assess by other imaging methods, considerably enhancing the ability to

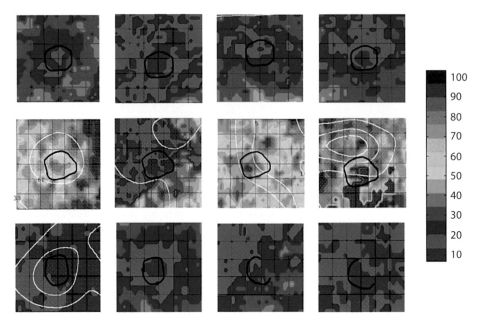

Fig. 3. Multimodal images from 3 patients (rows 1, 2, and 3) from visits 0, 12, 24, and 36 months showing the foveal avascular zone contour, retinal leakage analyzer results, and retinal thickness analyzer results. The retinal leakage analyzer color-coded maps of the BRB permeability indexes are shown. Retinal thickness analyzer views show white dot density maps of the percentage increases in retinal thickness. Patterns a, b, and c are shown on rows 1, 2, and 3, respectively.

diagnose and follow macular edema. Assessment and mapping of retinal thickness with the time domain OCT-3 Stratus has been the standard for many years and has been used in clinical studies.

After introduction of new spectral domain OCT (SD-OCT) instruments, studies have been published comparing retinal thickness measurements. These studies have demonstrated that retinal thickness measurements are dependent on the segmentation of the inner and outer retinal borders. The new spectral domain OCT systems image the outer retinal layers as 3 hyper-reflective bands: the external limiting membrane, the junction (or interface) of the photoreceptor outer and inner segments, and the RPE.

The *outer layers of the retina* can now be analyzed due to these recent technological progresses allowing high-definition, high-speed volume imaging. This allows analysis of structural changes particularly affecting photoreceptors and the IS/OS interface, thereby providing functional information on these tissues. The possibility of integrated structural imaging and functional imaging will play an increasingly important role in clinical applications (Coscas, 2009)[14].

Real-time images of the microscopic retinal tissues have been termed 'optical biopsy' and closely reflect histological sections of the macula and fovea.

Increasingly, they resemble a real anatomical representation, especially with the development of ultrahigh-resolution techniques and the upcoming combination with adaptive optics (Soubrane, 2009)[15].

In macular edema, the process begins with diffuse swelling of the outer retinal layers, advancing

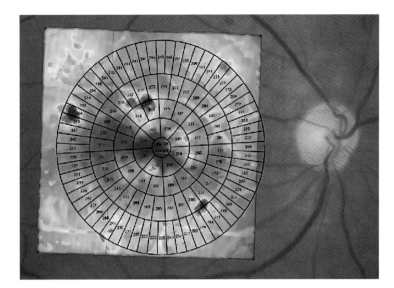

Fig. 4. Multimodal image composed of a color photograph of the eye fundus (morphology reference), a color-coded leakage map (BRB functional information), and a map of retinal thickness with average values for the earmarked areas. This image allows simultaneous correlation of both leakage and thickness in the eye fundus.

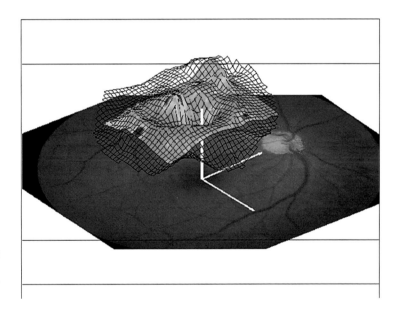

Fig. 5. The same information presented in figure 2 is now shown 3-dimensionally. The differences in the information presented is significant. Although the shape of the thickness is now clear, it occurs at the expense of having fewer details on the leakage itself and the location of both the thickness and leakage within the macular area.

to the typical image of cystoid spaces. Later, the large cystoid spaces can extend from the RPE to the internal limiting membrane and even rupture, causing macular holes. Hence, OCT is becoming a very efficient tool for following the distribution, evolution, and location of macular edema.

The extent of an area of increased thickness and the involvement of the central macula are essential to describe a clinical case of macular edema and predict visual loss. The presence of cysts and vitreous traction are particularly well documented using OCT. The analysis of the outer

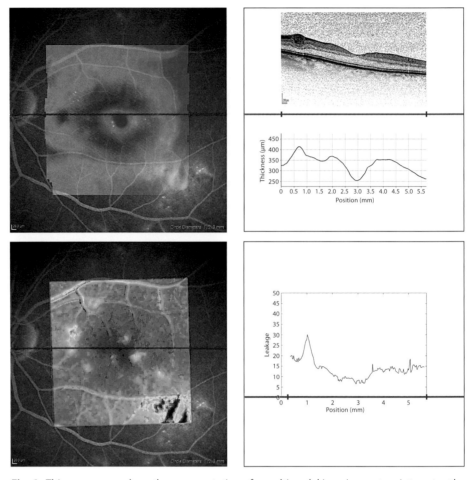

Fig. 6. This new approach on the representation of a multimodal imaging system integrates the fundus reference (left column), the color-coded thickness, and leakage maps (left column, top and bottom rows, respectively). A selected location (marked as a red horizontal line on the left column images) allows choosing the location where details are to be shown on the right. On the top right image, the detailed structure of the retina and the respective thickness profile is shown. On the bottom right image, the plotted profile of the leakage information for the same location is shown, allowing correlation of the structure, thickness, and leakage at the local level.

retinal layers may provide valuable prognostic indications (fig. 2).

To *establish a correlation between different images*, either from the same or from different modalities, it is essential to associate and to correlate them all. Multimodal macula mapping, for example, uses a variety of diagnostic tools and techniques to obtain additional information (fig. 3–6)

(Lobo et al., 2004; Bernardes et al., 2002; Cunha-Vaz, 2006)[16–18].

Spectral domain OCT facilitates correlations with clinical data, angiographies, and functional investigations.

These imaging techniques are essential to guide the indications for current treatment and to assess the response to treatment.

References

1 Cunha-Vaz JG, Travassos A: Breakdown of the blood-retinal barriers and cystoid macular edema. Surv Ophthalmol 1984; 28:485–492.

2 Gonzalez ME, Gonzalez C, Stern MP, Arredondo B, Martinez S, Mexico City Diabetes Study Retinopathy Group: Concordance in diagnosis of diabetic retinopathy by fundus photography between retina specialists and a standardized reading center. Arch Med Res 1995;26: 127–131.

3 Kohner EM, Henkind P: Correlation of fluorescein angiogram and retinal digest in diabetic retinopathy. Am J Ophthalmol 1970;69:403–414.

4 Coscas G, Dhermy P: Occlusions veineuses rétiniennes. Rapport Société Française d'Ophtalmologie. Paris, Masson, 1978.

5 Yannuzzi LA, Rohrer KJ, Tinder LJ, et al: Fluorescein angiography complications survey. Ophthalmology 1986;93,611–617.

6 Gass JD: Stereoscopic Atlas of Macular Disease – Diagnosis and Treatment, ed 4. St Louis, Mosby, 1997.

7 Richard G, Soubrane G, Yanuzzi L: Fluorescein and ICG Angiography: Textbook and Atlas, ed 2. New York, Thieme, 1998.

8 Guyer D, Yannuzzi LA, Chang S, Shields JA, Green WR: Retina-Vitreous-Macula, ed 1. Philadelphia, Saunders, 1999.

9 Huang D, Swanson E, Lin C, et al: Optical coherence tomography. Science 1991; 254:1178–1181.

10 Fercher AF, Hitzenberger CK, Drexler W, et al: In vivo optical coherence tomography. Am J Ophthalmol 1993;116:113–114.

11 Swanson EA, Izatt JA, Hee MR, et al: In vivo retinal imaging by optical coherence tomography. Opt Lett 1993;18: 1864–1866.

12 Puliafito CA, Hee MR, Lin CP, et al: Imaging of macular diseases with optical coherence tomography. Ophthalmology 1995;102:217–229.

13 Schuman JS, Puliafito CA, Fujimoto JG: Optical Coherence Tomography of Ocular Diseases, ed 2. Thorofare, Slack Incorporated, 2004.

14 Coscas G: Optical Coherence Tomography in Age-Related Macular Degeneration, ed 2. Berlin, Springer, 2009.

15 Soubrane G: (Personal communication, unpublished data).

16 Lobo CL, Bernardes RC, Figueira JP, de Abreu JR, Cunha-Vaz JG: Three-year follow-up study of blood-retinal barrier and retinal thickness alterations in patients with type 2 diabetes mellitus and mild nonproliferative diabetic retinopathy. Arch Ophthalmol 2004;122:211–217.

17 Bernardes R, Lobo C, Cunha-Vaz JG: Multimodal macula mapping: a new approach to study diseases of the macula. Surv Ophthalmol 2002;47:580–589.

18 Cunha-Vaz JG: Clinical characterization of diabetic macular edema. Int Ophthalmol 2006;1:99–100.

Prof. Gabriel Coscas
Hôpital Intercommunal de Créteil, Service Universitaire d'Ophtalmologie
40, avenue de Verdun
FR–94010 Créteil (France)
E-Mail gabriel.coscas@gmail.com

Chapter 2

Coscas G (ed): Macular Edema.
Dev Ophthalmol. Basel, Karger, 2010, vol 47, pp 10–26

General Pathophysiology

Albert Augustin[a] · Anat Loewenstein[b] · Baruch D. Kuppermann[c]

[a]Augenklinik, Karlsruhe, Germany; [b]Department of Ophthalmology, Tel Aviv Medical Center, Sackler Faculty of Medicine, Tel Aviv University, Tel Aviv, Israel; [c]Department of Ophthalmology, University of California, Irvine, Calif., USA

Abstract

Macular edema represents a common final pathway for many disease processes. Related ocular disorders include diabetic retinopathy, vascular occlusions, post surgical situations and inherited disorders. The pathophysiology includes breakdown of the blood ocular barrier, release of various cytokines and significant inflammations. These mechanisms may be complicated by ischemic processes. The various pathogenetic mechanisms and their contribution to the edema process are described in detail in this chapter.   Copyright © 2010 S. Karger AG, Basel

Macular edema represents a common final pathway of many intraocular and systemic diseases, which usually involve the retinal vessels.

It typically occurs with painless impairment of visual acuity in one eye but can also be bilateral, depending on the etiology. A macular edema is a nonspecific sign of many ocular disorders (Marmor, 1999; Tranos et al., 2004)[1, 2].

Usually the symptoms progress slowly. Nevertheless, while the progression of symptoms is usually slow, the patient may still experience a sudden onset, depending on the etiology.

Normal Retinal Anatomy and Physiology

Definition of Macular Edema

A macular edema is defined as an accumulation of fluid in the outer plexiform layer and the inner nuclear layer as well as a swelling of the Müller cells of the retina. It consists of a localized expansion of the retinal extracellular space (sometimes associated with the intracellular space) in the macular area.

The macular edema is caused by an abnormal permeability of the perifoveal retinal capillaries resulting in a thickening of the retinal tissue. A macular edema is considered chronic when persisting for more than 6 months.

Different manifestations can be observed: (fig. 1–3):
- perfused (nonischemic or associated with ischemic maculopathy);
- focal, diffuse or nonischemic (perfused).

A cystoid macular edema (CME) is a configuration with radially orientated, perifoveal cystic spaces (Rotsos and Moschos, 2008)[4]. The central fluid is more prominent in the outer plexiform layer (Henle's layer). The cysts are characterized by an altered light reflex with a decreased central reflex and a thin, highly reflective edge.

The pseudocysts are areas of the retina in which the cells have been displaced. They are more prominent and widely spread in the inner nuclear layer. Larger cysts are frequently surrounded by smaller peripheral cysts. Occasionally lamellar holes can form (the surface of the cyst elevates and lifts away).

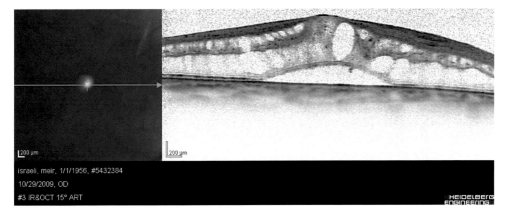

Fig. 1. Optical coherence tomography: cystoid macular edema.

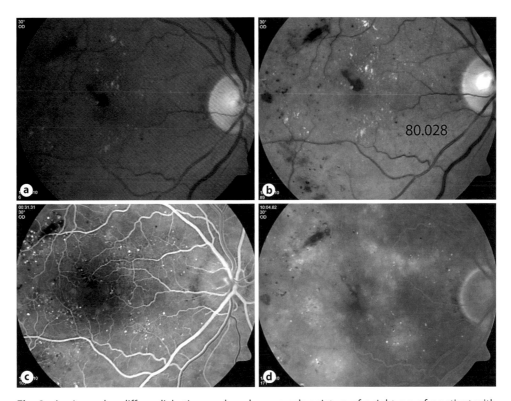

Fig. 2. Angiography: diffuse diabetic macular edema. **a** color picture of a right eye of a patient with moderate non proliferative diabetic retinopathy and diffuse macular edema. **b** Red free shows intraretinal dot and blot hemorrhages, intraretinal lipids. **c** Early phase of fluorescein angiogram shows perifoveal microaneurysms and some hypofluorescent areas caused by intra retinal hemorrhages. **d** Later phase of fluorescein angiogram shows leakage from these microaneurysms accumulating in a cystoid pattern.

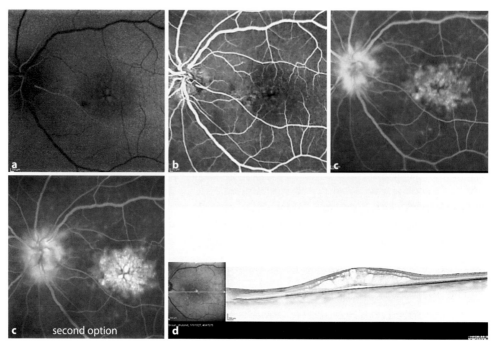

Fig. 3. Cystoid macular edema. **a** Red-free, fluorescein angiography. **b** Early phase. **c** Late phase. **d** Optical coherence tomography (Augustin et al., 2007)[3].

Macular edema is frequently associated with *relative ischemia* and a broken foveal capillary ring, which can be manifested by fluorescein angiography. The foveal avascular zone may become irregular and enlarged because of nonperfusion of the marginal capillaries. Closure of retinal arterioles may result in larger areas of nonperfusion and progressive ischemia. Evidence of enlargement of the foveal avascular zone greater than 1,000 μm generally indicates visual loss.

In some cases, mainly secondary to vascular occlusion, macular edema may be due to leakage of proteins through vascular walls following intracellular as well as extracellular hypertonic environment development following an ischemic event, similar to the development of brain ischemia (Finkelstein, 1992)[5].

The macular area of the retina is predisposed for the development of an edema due to its *unique anatomy*, which is characterized by the following facts:

- extremely high concentration of cells;
- high metabolic activity;
- the Henle fiber layer courses laterally away from the central fovea;
- potential reservoir for the accumulation of extravascular fluid due to the thickness and loose binding of inner connecting fibers in the outer plexiform layer;
- the central avascular zone creates a watershed arrangement between the choroidal and retinal circulation, thus decreasing resorption of extracellular fluid.

Related Ocular Disorders

Macular edema is a common cause of a sudden and/or chronic decrease in visual acuity occurring in many ophthalmic diseases.

Diabetic Macular Edema

Definition and Classification
Macular edema is the most important complication of diabetes mellitus leading to an impairment of visual acuity (Joussen et al., 2007)[6]. A diabetic macular edema is defined as a retinal thickening caused by the accumulation of intraretinal fluid and/or hard exudates within 2 disk diameters of the center of the macula, the fovea (fig. 4).

The incidence of diabetic macular edema is closely associated with the degree of diabetic retinopathy and the duration and type of the disease. The 25-year cumulative incidence in persons with type 1 diabetes mellitus is 29% for macular edema and 17% for clinically significant macular edema.

Further data show the incidence of diabetic macular edema for patients whose age at diagnosis was <30 years and who were taking insulin, varied from 0% in those who had diabetes <5 years to 29% in those whose duration of diabetes was 20 years or more.

For patients whose age at diagnosis was >30 years, the rates varied from 3% in those who had diabetes <5 years to 28% in those whose duration of diabetes was 20 years or more.

There are two subtypes of diabetic macular edema, a focal and a diffuse form (Girach and Lund-Andersen, 2007; Klein et al., 2009)[7, 8]. It also needs to be emphasized that there are slightly different definitions of these two subtypes in the international literature, which use different criteria. The correct classification is important, because the two subtypes have to be treated differently.

Focal macular edema refers to localized areas of retinal thickening, caused by foci of vascular

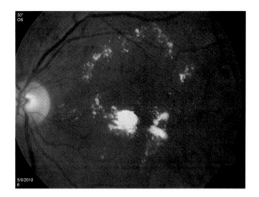

Fig. 4. Fundus photography of a patient with diabetic retinopathy and diabetic macular edema with exudates.

abnormalities, primarily microaneurysms, and less commonly intraretinal microvascular abnormalities. These have an increased tendency for fluid leakage, which is usually accompanied by hard exudates. The hard exudate pattern can be either focal or (often) ring-shaped.

Diffuse macular edema is caused by a general diffuse leakage from dilated retinal capillaries (and from microaneurysms and arterioles) throughout the posterior pole of the retina. It can usually be observed in both eyes with the degree of leakage being similar or extensively different.

There are also classifications for *ischemic and exudative macular edema*. In most cases, a hybrid type of these two can be observed.

A *clinically significant macular edema* is defined by the Early Treatment Diabetic Retinopathy Study to include any of the following features: (1) thickening of the retina at or within 500 μm of the center of the macula; (2) hard exudates at or within 500 μm of the center of the macula, if associated with thickening of the adjacent retina (not residual hard exudates remaining after the disappearance of retinal thickening); (3) a zone or zones of retinal thickening 1 disk area or larger, any part of which is within 1 disk diameter of the center of the macula.

Vascular Damage

Hyperglycemia is the distinguishing feature of diabetes mellitus, which leads to serious cellular damage. Endothelial cells are highly vulnerable to hyperglycemia, because the intracellular regulation of glucose levels is extremely difficult in this cell type. High doses of glucose can alter numerous cellular functions initiating a chain of metabolic reactions usually leading to serious damage of the cell.

Additional risk factors contributing to the pathogenesis of diabetic retinopathy/maculopathy with vascular disruption are hyperlipidemia and systemic hypertension.

Diabetic retinopathy is characterized by abnormal vascular flow, hyperpermeability (resulting in leakage) and/or closure or nonperfusion of capillaries.

The typical feature of early diabetic retinopathy is a change in the anatomical structure and cellular composition of the retinal microvasculature (arterioles, capillaries, and venules).

The following mechanisms are known to cause these changes:

- loss of pericytes (the earliest histologically detectable alteration); the interaction between pericytes and endothelial cells plays an important role in the maturation and maintenance of retinal vessels by initiating the secretion of growth factors and changes in the extracellular matrix;
- damage to vascular endothelial cells;
- thickening of the capillary basement membrane leading to abnormal autoregulation;
- deformation of the erythrocytes;
- increased aggregation of the platelets.

Several factors are known to cause and influence the development of diabetic macular edema due to damage of the retinal vasculature.

- Leukocytes mediate damage to endothelial cells by platelets binding to these cells and induce the expression of adhesion molecules (P-selectin, E-selectin, vascular cell adhesion molecule 1 and intercellular adhesion molecule 1).
- Leukocytes increase leukostasis, which is one of the first histological changes in diabetic retinopathy, with it occurring prior to any apparent clinical pathology; adherent leukocytes directly induce endothelial cell death in capillaries, causing vascular obstruction and vascular leakage.
- Angiogenic factors, mainly the vascular endothelial growth factor (VEGF) cause vascular hyperpermeability by leukocyte-mediated endothelial injury; this results in the opening of interendothelial junctions and induction of fenestrations as well as the formation of vesiculovacuolar organelles.
- Angiotensin II induces an inflammation in the vascular wall mainly by recruiting leukocytes and initiating their adhesion to the target tissue. Furthermore, this molecule leads to an increased vascular permeability.
- Advanced glycation end products are believed to enhance the oxidative stress level and induce an inflammatory response by hyperexpression of cytokines and lymphocyte adhesion molecules (vascular cell adhesion molecule 1) as well as vasoactive mediators.
- Sorbitol: hyperglycemia brings on elevated levels of sorbitol through the polyol pathway leading to:

buildup of intracellular sorbitol and fructose, disruption of osmotic balance in the cell, loss of integrity of the blood-retinal barrier (BRB), loss of pericytes due to their sensitivity to polyols and activation of protein kinase C.

- An enhanced production of reactive oxygen intermediates (oxidative stress) occurs due to an elevated oxidative stress level, which is induced by hyperglycemia; as a consequence, inflammation in vascular tissues occurs.
- Matrix changes affect the formation of diabetic macular edema. Matrix metalloproteinases cause a degradation and modulation of the extracellular matrix. They

belong to a family of zinc-binding, calcium-dependent enzymes.

It is likely that matrix metalloproteinases play an important role in various disease stages during the course of BRB dysfunction and breakdown. They cause changes of the endothelial cell resistance and have an influence on the formation and function of the intercellular junctions in the early stages of diabetic retinopathy/maculopathy. Furthermore they are actively involved in processes leading to cell death of both pericytes and endothelial cells.

In diabetes mellitus, early stages of vascular dysfunction are characterized by a breakdown of the BRB. The loss of endothelial cells in retinal vessel walls (inner BRB) is often responsible for the majority of the early BRB breakdown and is the initial site of the damage.

The development of macular edema has also been correlated with the presence of an attached posterior hyaloid. Patients with a posterior vitreous separation are much less likely to develop macular edema.

Venous Occlusive Disease

A central retinal vein occlusion or a branch retinal vein occlusion can cause macular edema, usually in cystoid form. In the latter, macular edema can be observed in cases of the occlusion involving a temporal vein and being located proximal to the venous drainage of the macula.

A leakage is caused by a disruption due to pressure transmitted to the perifoveal capillaries and by turbulent blood flow. An ischemic injury to the capillaries initiates the release of the VEGF, which causes an inflammatory response. This results in a breakdown of the inner BRB.

Two subtypes, ischemic and nonischemic (perfused) macular edema, can be differentiated. Regarding the prognosis for visual acuity, different studies with contradictory results exist (see above).

The Branch Retinal Vein Occlusion Study Group reported that 37% of the patients included in the study with nonischemic macular edema had an improvement of 2 or more lines after 3 years of follow-up.

The development of blood accumulation in central cystoid spaces is an important clinical finding in venous occlusive disease. It is common in patients suffering from retinal vein occlusion and less common with diabetic, aphakic or pseudophakic macular edema.

Pseudophakic/Aphakic Macular Edema (Irvine-Gass Syndrome)

A CME can develop following cataract surgery and is usually diagnosed 4–10 weeks after surgery. It is well known that damage to the blood-aqueous barrier leads to a release of prostaglandins causing the edema (Gulkilik et al., 2006)[9].

A surgical manipulation, which happens during the course of a cataract surgery, always causes an iris trauma. As a result, secondary inflammatory mediators can be liberated by the iris. Once the responsible stimulus (surgery) has been stopped, the physiological healing process is sufficient to suppress the inflammation slowly, but progressively.

In about 90% of macular edemas following cataract surgery, a spontaneous resolution of the edema with an improvement in visual acuity can be observed.

Although a massive leakage can lead to severe irreversible impairment of visual acuity, the patient may not even be aware of visual changes.

Often CME cannot be detected clinically, but the incidence of angiographically detectable CME is as high as 25% after phacoemulsification with no major intraoperative complications.

Another study (Mentes et al., 2003)[10] reported an incidence of 9.1%; however, only 1% of these patients experience a decrease in visual acuity. The fixation of the lens to the sulcus is also associated with a higher risk of CME.

The incidence of CME is significantly higher, up to 35.7%, after posterior capsule rupture.

In patients with diabetic retinopathy, cataract surgery may lead to a worsening of a preexisting macular edema, resulting in a poor visual outcome.

Prevention is possible if the fundus can be visualized and, if not, shortly afterwards. Thus, in patients with diabetes mellitus, an examination using fluorescein angiography and optical coherence tomography should be performed before cataract surgery.

Inflammatory Diseases
In uveitis, macular edema presents mostly in a cystoid form and is a common consequence of the disease. It often persists even after the uveitis has been successfully brought under control.

A macular edema is one of the most common vision-impairing complications of uveitis. It may occur in any type of ocular inflammation (Guex-Crosier, 1999)[11].

The forms of uveitis which are most commonly associated with macular edema are pars planitis, iridocyclitis, birdshot retinochoroidopathy, sarcoid uveitis and HLA-B27-associated uveitis.

CME can also be observed frequently in Behçet syndrome, Eales disease, Vogt-Koyanagi-Harada syndrome and ocular toxoplasmosis.

Although serous macular exudation has been observed in patients with AIDS-related cytomegalovirus retinitis, macular edema is rare.

Some patients with restored immune competence experience anterior segment and vitreous inflammatory reactions as well as a CME.

In ocular inflammation, an increased production and release of inflammatory mediators such as prostaglandins are the cause of an increased permeability of the parafoveal capillaries and exudation in the macular area.

Nonsteroidal anti-inflammatory drugs and steroids, targeting the arachidonic acid pathway in prostaglandin synthesis, are therefore successfully applied to treat this pathological condition.

Although it is still unknown what factors are responsible for most forms of uveitis, T-cell lymphocytes, the CD4+ subtype in particular, play a central role in this disease entity (Yeh et al., 2009)[12].

Experimental models of uveitis have shown that at the same time as T cells enter the eye, damage in the BRB can be observed.

It is also still unknown whether specific T-cell-secreted cytokines are directly responsible for this mechanism, but it is likely that many of these can damage and cause a breakdown of the BRB.

Phototraumatism
Phototraumatism of the retinal pigment epithelium (RPE) causing a breakdown of the outer BRB often leads to a CME following cataract surgery.

Three mechanisms of light damage can be differentiated:
– thermal lesions result from light absorption by the RPE during the course of the surgery;
– the use of the Q-switched mode of the Nd:YAG laser leads to a mechanical light damage;
– photochemical damage can be caused by the operating microscope when used for long periods during surgery.

A macular edema after Nd:YAG capsulotomy develops in 0–2.5% of all cases with the incidence increasing if the treatment is performed within the first 3 postoperative months.

Age-Related Macular Degeneration
Age-related macular degeneration can be subclassified into two major forms: the atrophic or dry form and the exudative or wet form.

Atrophic macular degeneration without exudative changes does not generally lead to macular edema.

The exudative form with choroidal neovascularization may cause a serous detachment of the overlying retina, resulting in CME.

The presence of CME is more likely if the serous detachment of the macula has been present for 3–6 months or if the choroidal neovascular membrane has involved the subfoveal region.

Retinal Telangiectasia, Coats Disease

Perifoveal retinal telangiectasia and Coats disease typically show irregularly dilated and incompetent retinal vessels.

These telangiectatic changes can occur at the level of the arterioles, venules or capillaries and cause a cystoid form of macular edema due to heavy leakage.

The closer the cysts are to the macula, the earlier the patient reports symptoms. Symptoms are mainly related to impairment of visual acuity.

Idiopathic juxtafoveal telangiectasia is a milder form of retinal telangiectasia and typically involves the temporal macula. CME is less common than in the previous disorders.

Radiation Retinopathy

Radiation retinopathy is caused by vascular damage from prior radiation treatment to the eye or orbit. A form of macular edema often develops that is quite similar to diabetic macular edema and may manifest as the cystoid form.

The largest study investigating radiation retinopathy included 218 patients treated by proton beam therapy for paramacular tumors. Within 3 years of treatment, 87% of the patients developed macular edema (Guyer et al., 1992)[13].

Inherited Dystrophies

The course of retinitis pigmentosa may be influenced by CME due to an increased permeability of the RPE and perifoveal capillaries (Fishman et al., 1977)[14]. An incidence of 28% has been reported (Sandberg et al., 2008)[15].

CME is usually more common in younger patients with minimal RPE disturbances. It can be treated successfully with oral acetazolamide.

Dominantly inherited CME has been described as a clinically distinct form of macular dystrophy usually beginning at approximately 30 years of age. A slow progression over the following decades can typically be observed (Notting and Pinckers, 1977; Hogewind et al., 2008)[16, 17].

Characteristics of this syndrome include an early onset and prolonged course of cystoid changes in the macula, followed by atrophy of the retinal tissue in later stages.

Some patients also show a leakage of fluorescein from the optic disk capillaries, a subnormal electrooculogram, an elevated rod dark adaptation threshold, red-green and blue-yellow color deficiencies, normal electroretinogram findings, hyperopia, peripheral pigmentary retinopathy and vitreous opacities.

Tumors

The cystoid form of macular edema can frequently be observed in patients with choroidal melanoma. Three main types of CME can be differentiated: direct, indirect and a combination of both.

Direct involvement may be observed when the melanoma is located subfoveally. An indirect involvement occurs due to subfoveal exudates when the melanoma is distant to the fovea. Indirect foveolar involvement appears without an associated subfoveal tumor or exudates.

The source of CME is at the level of the retinal capillary network and results from intraretinal microvascular abnormalities resembling endothelial cell proliferation.

Other tumors associated with CME are choroidal nevi and the capillary hemangioma.

Drug-Induced Macular Edema

Latanoprost, travoprost and bimotoprost are prostaglandin analogs, which may alter the blood-aqueous barrier in early postoperative pseudophakias or aphakias, thereby causing CME. This phenomenon occurs when these drugs are applied topically.

The drugs themselves are not known to have an influence on the permeability of blood vessels. It has been shown that they stimulate the endogenous synthesis of prostaglandins, which mediate inflammation, thus leading to the breakdown of the blood-aqueous barrier. CME typically resolves

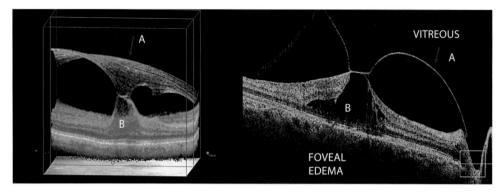

Fig. 5. Vitreomacular traction syndrome, optical coherence tomography. A = Vitreous traction is evident; B = causing foveal detachment.

after the drug has been discontinued (Schumer et al., 2000)[18].

Some systemic medications, such as nicotinic acid and docetaxel, may also cause a macular edema as well as long-term topical administration of epinephrine and dipivefrine.

Epiretinal Membrane
Epiretinal membranes can cause a surface wrinkling of the underlying retina resulting from contracture of the membrane.

CME is typically caused by a combination of several mechanisms:
- distortion and traction on the surrounding intraretinal vessels resulting in a leakage;
- disturbance of macular microcirculation resulting in a reduced capillary blood flow;
- loss of apposition between the retina and the RPE pump.

Vitreomacular Traction Syndrome
In the vitreomacular traction syndrome, a partial posterior vitreous detachment is combined with a persistent macular adherence and macular traction. A prolonged traction may cause macular edema (fig. 5). A complete vitreomacular separation allows a resolution of the cystoid changes and an improvement in visual acuity.

Acquired Immunodeficiency Syndrome, Immunocompetence
CME has been associated with cytomegalovirus retinitis in patients suffering from acquired immunodeficiency syndrome (AIDS) and immunocompetent patients. At times macular edema develops specifically while the cytomegalovirus retinitis resolves.

CME has also been observed in patients with inactive cytomegalovirus retinitis after immune recovery and improvement of their CD4 counts because of highly active antiretroviral therapy (Kersten et al., 1999)[19].

Vascular Components

The Blood-Retinal Barrier and the Role of Proteins
Different factors *prevent an accumulation* of extracellular intraretinal fluid and proteins by interacting to maintain a balance:
- osmotic forces;
- hydrostatic forces;
- capillary permeability;
- tissue compliance.

The result is that the rate of capillary filtration equals the rate of fluid removal from the

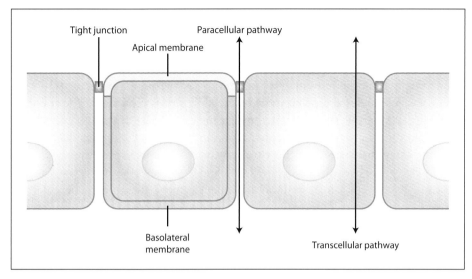

Fig. 6. Schematic presentation of a membrane on a cellular level. Apical and basolateral side and gap junctions are shown.

extracellular retinal tissue. Therefore, the interstitial spaces of the retina can be kept dry in physiological conditions.

The existence of a BRB formed by intercellular junctions is the precondition required to maintain this physiological status. These junctions are transmembrane molecules connecting cells with each other. They are linked to special cytoskeletal linker molecules. Furthermore, several regulatory molecules are present at the site, regulating the interaction with the cytoskeleton (fig. 6).

The role of the BRB is the separation of blood from the surrounding retinal tissue. In addition, this barrier has to control the protein and the cell passage from the blood into these tissues as well as the leukocyte extravasation when inflammation occurs.

In the inner retinal circulation, the BRB is formed by tight junctions (zonula occludens). Intercellular communication is realized by adherent junctions (zonula adherens) and gap junctions (macula communicans) joining the endothelium

of retinal capillaries. The molecular composition of these intercellular junctions is different along the vasculature of the retina.

In the outer retinal circulation, the tight junctions between the pigment epithelium cells maintain the BRB, as well as adherens junctions and desmosomes (macula adherens).

The BRB maintains the stability of the environment of ocular neurons and photoreceptors and ensures their physiological functions. Apart from these structures there are no other anatomical barriers to prevent water movement in the retina.

The interstitial pathway from the vitreous cavity to the subretinal space is long and ends with zonulae adherentes, forming the external limiting membrane (ELM). The internal limiting membrane (ILM) has, according to recent studies, probably no significant influence on water movement (Rotsos and Moschos, 2008)[4]. This means that surgical removal of the ILM would neither increase nor decrease fluid movement.

The zonulae adherentes between the photoreceptors and the Müller cells, forming the ELM, are not sealed like the zonulae occludentes of the RPE and retinal capillaries. As a consequence, they can only partially limit the movement of large molecules. Recent studies show that most of the albumins present at this site can pass through the ELM. The diffusion of fluoresceinated albumin from the subretinal space into the vitreous cavity and vice versa is easily possible (Rotsos and Moschos, 2008)[4]. The rate of albumin movement across the retina is significant and influences the development of macular edema. Large molecules cannot diffuse through the retina.

Protein that has already diffused into the retinal tissue remains for a certain period of time. To a limited extent it then diffuses into the vitreous cavity or the subretinal space. This protein amount has to be replaced by constant leakage, which is caused by the pathological conditions responsible for the development of macular edema. This ensures a constant amount of protein movement but also a constant accumulation of fluid in the retinal tissue.

These physiological phenomena show that more protein has to stay in the retina than diffusing away into the vitreous cavity or subretinal space to allow the development of edema. To the extent that protein is retained in the retina, fluid will also be retained by osmosis, this mechanism then causing a macular edema. The precondition for a higher amount of protein being retained in the retina than leaving the retina is a breakdown of the BRB.

In conclusion, all pathological conditions leading to a breakdown of the BRB cause a retention of proteins within the retinal tissue, resulting in the development of an edema due to consecutive water retention by osmosis.

Water Fluxes
Different forces, active and passive, work together moving water across the retina and out of the subretinal space.

Passive Forces
The intraocular pressure pushes water into the retina; however, this mechanism is limited in importance due to the flow resistance of the retina.

Osmotic pressure within the choroidal tissue draws the water to the choroid.

These passive forces are strong. Under physiological conditions they are sufficient to keep the subretinal space 'dry'.

Nevertheless, active forces are needed to remove the amount of water driven by intraocular pressure that diffuses through the retina. Furthermore, passive forces might be an additional safety mechanism to antagonize the accumulation of fluid in pathological conditions.

Active Forces
Active transport by the RPE pushes water out of the retina towards the choroid. The cells of the RPE are connected by tight junctions, forming the outer BRB and separating them into apical and basal regions. The RPE cells contain channels and transport systems. They are separately responsible for the apical and basal parts of the cell membranes. They move ions in an apical as well as basal direction. This *ionic movement* leads to a parallel movement of water due to resulting osmotic forces.

The net balance should always be towards the removal of water from the subretinal space in order to ensure a 'dry' environment for the retinal tissue.

Pathological disorders, leading to an accumulation of subretinal fluid, prevent water removal. It is not clearly known to what extent active RPE transport plays a role in the development of macular edema, which is caused by intraretinal fluid.

However, it is well established that the amount of intraretinal water diffusing to the subretinal space where the RPE may have access to it, is anatomically limited. As a consequence, active RPE transport can only remove a certain amount of water. When its capacity is exceeded, macular edema can develop more easily (fig. 7).

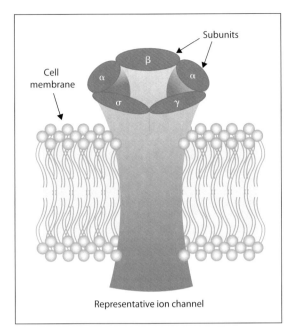

Fig. 7. Transmembrane channel.

Extracellular and Intracellular Edema
Generally, a macular edema can be caused by the accumulation of either extracellular or intracellular fluid. In many diseases it is likely that a hybrid type of fluid accumulation exists. Under physiological conditions every cell has membrane transport systems that maintain a constant balance of ionic and parallel water movement into and out of the cell.

Any metabolic insult (for example ischemia) can damage these ionic channels, causing a swelling of the cell (intracellular edema). Many disorders, causing the breakdown of the BRB, can also cause damage of the ionic channels. Intracellular decompensation can lead to the release of excitotoxins and free radicals, causing more pronounced damage of the BRB.

Extracellular swelling (extracellular edema) seems to be mainly caused by proteins. In case of a breakdown of the BRB, proteins such as albumin diffuse into the extracellular space driven by blood pressure and diffusion gradients. The proteins can leave the retina towards the vitreous cavity at the ILM. At the ELM level, however, they are retained and stay within the retinal tissue. Oncotic pressure develops, accumulating water in the extracellular space and causing extracellular edema.

The reason for proteins not retained in the subretinal space and causing a serous detachment in the RPE is that the capacity of the active transport systems is enough to keep the subretinal space 'dry' despite those oncotic effects.

It is likely that in most diseases with a breakdown of the BRB both the retinal capillaries and RPE are affected to a different degree.

As shown, macular edema usually contains extracellular and intracellular fluid accumulation of varying degrees. Whereas some diseases primarily cause extracellular edema, others cause intracellular edema.

It is not only proteins which can cause an accumulation of water in the intraretinal tissue. Larger molecules, whose clearance is limited by the ELM, urge an osmotic gradient leading to edema as well.

In diseases with choroidal neovascularization, exudation within the subretinal space is much stronger. As a consequence, a fluid pressure gradient as well as a diffusion gradient for proteins is created. The amount of proteins entering the retina is much higher as compared to diseases damaging the BRB only.

The result is an edema, which by far exceeds the intensity of an edema created by a breakdown of the BRB.

Inflammatory Components

An inflammation within the vascular wall plays a central role in the development of macular edema.

Several inflammatory mediators and inflammatory cells are present at the site and interact in

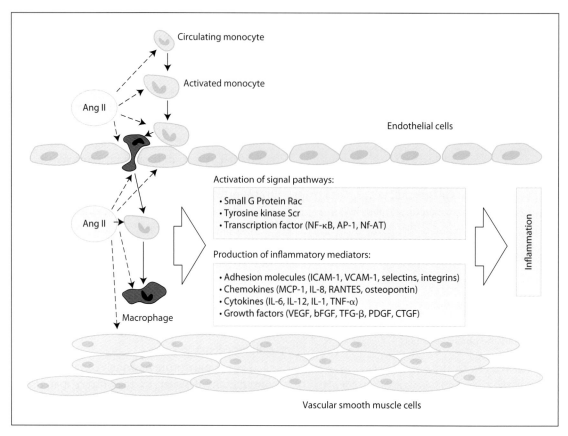

Fig. 8. Effects of angiotensin (Ang)-II-induced inflammatory response.

a complex chain of reactions, which has not yet been understood in every detail (Joussen et al., 2007; Pasqualetti et al., 2007)[6, 20].

The following inflammatory mediators play an important role in the pathogenesis of macular edema: angiotensin II; VEGF; prostaglandins; cytokines and chemokines; matrix metalloproteinases; interleukins; P-selectin, E-selectin; vascular cell adhesion molecule 1; intercellular adhesion molecule 1.

The following inflammatory cells play an important role in the pathogenesis of macular edema: macrophages and neutrophils.

Angiotensin II

Angiotensin is an oligopeptide in the blood that causes vasoconstriction, increased blood pressure and release of aldosterone from the adrenal cortex. It is a derivative of the precursor molecule angiotensinogen, which is a serum globulin.

Fundamental evidence exists that angiotensin II contributes to inflammation in the vasculature (Kersten et al., 1999)[19] (fig. 8). It is produced locally in the wall of an inflamed vessel via the renin-angiotensin system.

Angiotensin II leads to a breakdown of the BRB through blood-pressure-dependent and

-independent mechanisms. It plays a central role in the pathogenesis of different vascular diseases, including the development of macular edema.

Three major effects of angiotensin II as a key mediator of inflammation can be classified as follows.

Leukocyte Infiltration
A recruitment of leukocytes from the circulation to the perivascular space is initiated by the upregulation of adhesion molecules (selectins, immunglobulins, integrins). An adhesion of leukocytes to the target tissue is induced.

The upregulation of different chemokines and cytokines (monocyte chemoattractant protein 1, interleukins 1, 6, 8 and 12, tumor necrosis factor α) is leading to a transmigration of leukocytes into the target tissue.

Vascular Permeability Increase
A pressure-mediated mechanical injury to the endothelium, release of eicosanoids (leukotrienes, prostaglandins) and an upregulation of VEGF are leading to an increase in vascular permeability.

Extracellular Matrix Remodeling
Cell proliferation, hypertrophy and fibrosis are mediated by autocrine and paracrine growth factors (VEGF, platelet-derived growth factor, transforming growth factor β, basic fibroblast growth factor).

The overall effect of angiotensin II in vascular tissue is an endothelial dysfunction, the key pathophysiological step in macular edema development.

Angiogenic Factors: VEGF
VEGF is a disulfide-bound homodimer glycoprotein. It is one of the most important regulators of vasculogenesis and angiogenesis. VEGF has a selective mitogenic activity and is a survival factor for endothelial cells.

Under physiological conditions it is – among others – involved in the embryogenesis, wound healing and inflammation processes.

Under pathological conditions it plays a role in tumor growth, arthritis, cardiac disorders and several ocular disorders such as diabetic retinopathy, age-related macular degeneration and retinal vascular occlusive diseases.

The VEGF family includes 5 types: VEGF-A, VEGF-B, VEGF-C, VEGF-D and VEGF-E. VEGF-A is mainly involved in ocular pathological processes and is coresponsible for the development of macular edema.

Several different splicing isoforms exist: VEGF-121, VEGF-165, VEGF-189 and VEGF-206. VEGF-121 is freely diffusible. The other isoforms contain a heparin-binding site. VEGF-189 and VEGF-206 are strongly bound to the extracellular matrix, while VEGF-165 is moderately bound.

The key role of VEGF-A in vasculogenesis is shown by studies on embryonic development. A deletion of the gene in mice leads to the death of the embryo. This is caused by a failure of the development of the blood vessels (Ferrara et al., 1996)[21].

VEGF is primarily expressed in endothelial cells, as well as in pericytes, monocytes and neural cells. The effects are released when VEGF binds to its receptors on vessel endothelial cells.

Different receptors exist: VEGFR-1, VEGFR-2 and VEGFR-3. They are receptor tyrosine kinases that dimerize and become autophosphorylated upon VEGF binding. Activation of the receptors initiates multiple intracellular downstream signaling pathways that lead to the various effects of the growth factor.

VEGF is – among others – mainly induced, upregulated and released by:
- retinal ischemia/hypoxia: these are the most important inducers of VEGF-A; the expression is mediated by the activation of hypoxia-inducible factor 1, which binds to the VEGF gene;

- furthermore a VEGF-A (m)RNA half-life increase is induced by as much as threefold to fourfold;
- VEGF has several effects on different tissues in the human organism: angiogenesis; vasculogenesis; chemotaxis; inflammation; increase in vascular permeability; neuroprotection.

In patients suffering from diabetic macular edema, VEGF levels are elevated and correlate with the severity of the disease. The VEGF also contributes to the macular edema that goes along with age-related macular degeneration, retinal vein occlusion and uveitis. Two major effects leading to macular edema can be classified.

Inflammation

An inflammation-induced breakdown of the BRB is mediated by the VEGF via binding to leukocytes and inducing their recruitment to the site of the inflammation. An extensive leukostasis in the affected vascular tissue is initiated.

This is accompanied by an upregulation of intercellular adhesion molecule 1. VEGF receptors are present and active on all inflammatory cell subtypes, including platelets. Inflammatory cells also produce and release VEGF.

Vascular Permeability

VEGF is 50,000 times more potent than histamine in inducing vascular leakage. The increase in vascular permeability happens by a breakdown of the BRB initiated by different mechanisms:
- leukocyte-mediated (recruitment, adhesion, stasis) endothelial injury and cell death; the underlying pathomechanism needs further clarification;
- conformational changes and dissolution of tight junctions of endothelial cells by phosphorylation of the tight junction protein occludin;
- activation of protein kinase C;
- induction of fenestrations and vesiculovacuolar organelles.

Prostaglandins

A prostaglandin is a member of a group of lipid compounds that derives enzymatically from fatty acids. Every prostaglandin contains 20 carbon atoms, including a 5-carbon ring. They are mediators and have a variety of strong physiological effects.

The prostaglandins together with the thromboxanes and prostacyclins form the prostanoid class of fatty acid derivatives; the prostanoid class is a subclass of eicosanoids.

In the prostaglandin pathway, inflammation causes the enzyme phospholipase to release arachidonic acid from cell walls. Subsequently, arachidonic acid is converted into prostaglandins by the enzyme cyclooxygenase II and into leukotrienes by the enzyme 5-lipoxygenase (fig. 9).

In the pathophysiology of macular edema, prostaglandin E_1 causes a breakdown of the BRB via opening the tight junctions.

Ischemia

Glial Cell Swelling

Ischemic/hypoxic conditions play a central role in the development of macular edema. In neuronal cells, the rate of ATP synthesis is very high as compared to other cell types. This phenomenon results in excessive water production. The uptake of metabolic substrates such as glucose is related to an influx of water into the cells. This fluid has to be cleared from the cells.

Under physiological conditions, water leaves neuronal cells via an uptake by glial cells and is released into the blood or into the cerebrospinal fluid (brain)/the vitreous body (retina). The water release from the glial cells in the retina occurs through their perivascular endfeet, facing the vitreous. Aquaporin 4 water channels play a significant role in mediating these water fluxes.

In postischemic brain edema, the swelling of glial cell endfeet around blood vessels is thought to be enhanced by an altered expression of the

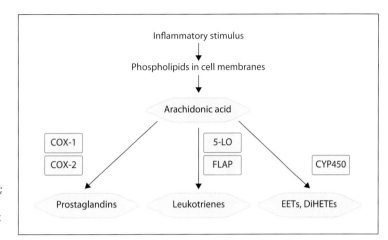

Fig. 9. Cyclooxygenase (COX) and 5-lipoxigenase (5-LO) pathway. FLAP = 5-Lipoxygenase-activating protein; CYP450 = cytochrome P450; EET = epoxyeicosatrienoic acid; DiHETE = dihydroxyeicosatetraenoic acid.

aquaporin 4 water channels in cell membranes (Pannicke et al., 2004)[22].

The water transport has been shown to be osmotically linked to K^+ currents in the membranes of the glial endfeet. The direction of the water fluxes through aquaporin 4 channels, driven by osmosis, may be determined by K^+ fluxes through specialized proteins, called the Kir4.1 channels. The main membrane conductance for glial cells is for K^+ ions. Therefore, K^+ may play a dominant role (Pannicke et al., 2004)[22].

It is well established that after ischemia the K^+ permeability of the glial plasma membranes is significantly decreased, meaning the cells cannot release K^+. As a consequence, the intracellular K^+ concentration increases. The concentration in the cells, however, has to stay at a constant high level producing a reversed osmotic gradient at the blood-glial cell interface. The relative osmolarity of the cytoplasma rises in relation to the hypotonic environment. Water can enter the cell, resulting in swelling of the respective cell (Pannicke et al., 2004)[22].

Macular edema is a *crucial complication* to various retinal diseases, participating in the degeneration of the photoreceptors and the death of neuronal cells. In the development of macular edema it is believed that the *swelling of the Müller cells* (glial cells) occurs before the formation of an extracellular edema. When macular edema is presenting in a cystoid form, the cysts are formed by swollen and dying Müller cells. Thus, intracellular edema occurs before extracellular edema.

Retinal glial cells progressively loose K^+ conductivity with increasing age. This fact may explain the higher incidence of macular edema under ischemic/hypoxic conditions in the elderly population.

It is hypothesized that another mechanism contributing to glial cell swelling may be mediated by Na^+ ions. Retinal injury caused by ischemia and reperfusion is induced by glutamate-evoked excitotoxicity. A prolonged glutamate exposure leads to glial cell swelling. The underlying mechanism is an intracellular accumulation of Na^+ ions with a resulting water influx leading to intracellular edema. These ions are transported by special glutamate uptake carriers (Widemann et al., 2004)[23]. It must be emphasized that despite the current knowledge of the aforementioned mechanisms of glial cell swelling, the complete pathogenesis is not yet understood in detail. It is likely that further types of ions or molecules may play an important role in retinal glial cell swelling.

Library and eLearning Centre
Gartnavel General Hospital

Scientific knowledge on the mechanisms underlying the development of macular edema has made a great leap forward in the last decade. Nevertheless, research is only at the edge of understanding the mechanisms on a molecular level, aiming to more specialized therapeutic strategies for the treatment of macular edema in the future.

References

1 Marmor MF: Mechanisms of fluid accumulation in retinal edema. Doc Ophthalmol 1999;97:239–249.
2 Tranos PG, Wickremasinghe SS, Stangos NT, Topouzis F, Tsinopoulos I, Pavesio CE: Macular edema. Surv Ophthalmol 2004;49:470–490.
3 Augustin AJ: Augenheilkunde, ed 3. Berlin, Springer, 2007.
4 Rotsos TG, Moschos MM: Cystoid macular edema. Clin Ophthalmol 2008;2:919–930.
5 Finkelstein D: Ischemic macular edema. recognition and favorable natural history in branch vein occlusion. Arch Ophthalmol 1992;110:1427–1434.
6 Joussen AM, Smyth N, Niessen C: Pathophysiology of diabetic macular edema. Dev Ophthalmol 2007;39:1–12.
7 Girach A, Lund-Andersen H: Diabetic macular oedema: a clinical overview. Int J Clin Pract 2007;61:88–97.
8 Klein R, Knudtson MD, Lee KE, Gangnon R, Klein BE: The Wisconsin Epidemiologic Study of Diabetic Retinopathy XXIII: the twenty-five-year incidence of macular edema in persons with type 1 diabetes. Ophthalmology 2009;116:497–503.
9 Gulkilik G, Kocabora S, Taskapili M, Engin G: Cystoid macular edema after phacoemulsification: risk factors and effect on visual acuity. Can J Ophthalmol 2006;41:699–703.

10 Mentes J, Erakgun T, Afrashi F, Kerci G: Incidence of cystoid macular edema after uncomplicated phacoemulsification. Ophthalmologica 2003;217:408–412.
11 Guex-Crosier Y: The pathogenesis and clinical presentation of macular edema in inflammatory diseases. Doc Ophthalmol 1999;97:297–309.
12 Yeh S, Li Z, Forooghian F, Hwang FS, Cunningham MA, Pantanelli S, Lew JC, Wroblewski KK, Vitale S, Nussenblatt RB: CD4+Foxp3+ T-regulatory cells in noninfectious uveitis. Arch Ophthalmol 2009;127:407–413.
13 Guyer DR, Mukai S, Egan KM, Seddon JM, Walsh SM, Gragoudas ES: Radiation maculopathy after proton beam irradiation for choroidal melanoma. Ophthalmology 1992;99:1278–1285.
14 Fishman GA, Fishman M, Maggiano J: Macular lesions associated with retinitis pigmentosa. Arch Ophthalmol 1977;95:798–803.
15 Sandberg MA, Brockhurst RJ, Gaudio AR, Berson EL: Visual acuity is related to parafoveal retinal thickness in patients with retinitis pigmentosa and macular cysts. Invest Ophthalmol Vis Sci 2008;49:4568–4572.
16 Notting JG, Pinckers JL: Dominant cystoid macular dystrophy. Am J Ophthalmol 1977;83:234–241.

17 Hogewind BF, Pieters G, Hoyng CB: Octreotide acetate in dominant cystoid macular dystrophy. Eur J Ophthalmol 2008;18:99–103.
18 Schumer RA, Camras CB, Mandahl AK: Latanoprost and cystoid macular edema: is there a causal relation? Curr Opin Ophthalmol 2000;11:94–100.
19 Kersten AJ, Althaus C, Best J, Sundmacher R: Cystoid macular edema following immune recovery and treatment with cidofovir for cytomegalovirus retinitis. Graefes Arch Clin Exp Ophthalmol 1999;237:893–896.
20 Pasqualetti G, Danesi R, Del Tacca M, Bocci G: Vascular endothelial growth factor pharmacogenetics: a new perspective for anti-angiogenic therapy. Pharmacogenomics 2007;8:49–66.
21 Ferrara N, Carver-Moore K, Chen H, Dowd M, Lu L, O'Shea KS, Powell-Braxton L, Hillan KJ, Moore MW: Heterozygous embryonic lethality induced by targeted inactivation of the VEGF gene. Nature 1996;380:439–442.
22 Pannicke T, Iandiev I, Uckermann O, Biedermann B, Kutzera F, Wiedemann P, Wolburg H, Reichenbach A, Bringmann A: A potassium channel linked mechanism of glial cell swelling in the postischemic retina. Mol Cell Neurosci 2004;26:493–502.
23 Widemann BC, Balis FM, Kempf-Bielack B, Bielack S, Pratt CB, Ferrari S, Bacci G, Craft AW, Adamson PC: High-dose methotrexate-induced nephrotoxicity in patients with osteosarcoma. Cancer 2004;100:2222–2232.

Prof. Anat Loewenstein
Department of Ophthalmology, Tel Aviv Medical Center
Sackler Faculty of Medicine, Tel Aviv University
6 Weizmann St.
Tel Aviv 64239 (Israel)
E-Mail anatl@tasmc.health.gov.il

Coscas G (ed): Macular Edema.
Dev Ophthalmol. Basel, Karger, 2010, vol 47, pp 27–48

Diagnosis and Detection

Giovanni Staurenghi · Alessandro Invernizzi · Laura de Polo · Marco Pellegrini

Eye Clinic, Department of Clinical Science "Luigi Sacco", Sacco Hospital, University of Milan, Milan, Italy

Abstract

The aim of the chapter is to provide a practical but exhaustive guide in detecting macular edema and to describe its features depending on the retinal condition which cause it. The most useful imaging techniques and tools (Biomicroscopy, retinography, Optical Coherence Tomography, Fluorescein/Indocyanine-Green Angiography) will be analysed in order to identify the best diagnostic algorithm in each pathology. At the end of the chapter a summary table synthesize what previously widely described.

Copyright © 2010 S. Karger AG, Basel

Introduction

Broadly defined, macular edema is an abnormal thickening of the macula associated with the accumulation of excess fluid in the extracellular space of the neurosensory retina. Intracellular edema involving Müller cells has also been observed histopathologically. The term 'cystoid macular edema' (CME) is applied when there is evidence by biomicroscopy, fluorescein angiography (FA) and/or optical coherence tomography (OCT) of fluid accumulation into multiple cyst-like spaces within the macula. Although the classical pathology of CME consists of large cystoid spaces in the outer plexiform layer of Henle, such fluid-filled spaces can be seen in various layers of the retina depending in part on the underlying etiology (Johnson, 2009)[1].

The standard clinical method for determining macular edema is the subjective assessment of the presence or absence of macular thickening by slit lamp fundus stereo biomicroscopy. The traditional methods of evaluating macular thickening, including slit lamp biomicroscopy and fundus photography, are useful for visualizing signs correlated with retinal thickness such as hard and soft exudates, hemorrhages and microaneurysms, but traditional evaluating methods are relatively insensitive to small changes in retinal thickness and are unable to detect specific anatomic details especially at the vitreomacular interface.

Observation of the fundus is obtained with the combined use of a slit lamp and a Goldmann contact lens or a 90- or 70-dpt noncontact lens. This is a complex psychomotor process that is highly dependent on the observer's skill and experience, the level of patient cooperation, the degree of pupillary dilation, the amount of media opacity, and the pattern and extent of retinal edema.

In diabetic retinopathy, macular edema is considered to be clinically significant if the following apply: (1) presence of any retinal thickening within 500 μm of the foveal center; (2) lipid exudates within 500 μm of the foveal center with adjacent thickening, and (3) an area of thickening >1 Macular Photocoagulation Study disk area (1 disk area = 1.767 mm^2) within 1 disk diameter

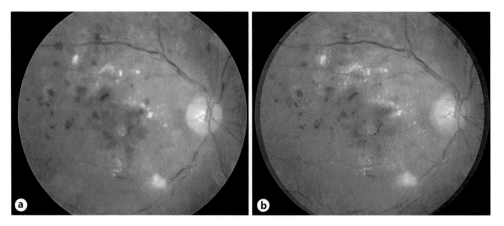

Fig. 1. Color pictures showing diabetic retinopathy. Macular edema and retinal thickness are better seen in a stereo image (wear red/cyan 3-dimensional goggles to visualize the stereo effect). **a** Single-frame image. **b** Stereo anaglyph image.

(1.5 mm) of the foveal center (Early Treatment Diabetic Retinopathy Study Research Group, 1985)[2].

Fundus photography is used mainly for follow-up. This type of fundus photography is commonly used for clinical trials and used less in clinical practice. Stereo images, rather than a single image, are necessary to identify macular edema and retinal thickening (fig. 1).

Variations in the amount of stereopsis present in paired stereo photographs or in the threshold for thickening adopted by the observer may further complicate the accurate and reproducible detection of areas of edema. The lack of sensitivity of the clinical examination for detection of mild edema has been demonstrated for eyes with a foveal center thickness between 201 and 300 μm (200 defined as the upper limit of normal). Only 14% of eyes were noted to have foveal edema by contact lens biomicroscopy. The term 'subclinical foveal edema' describes such cases (Brown et al., 2004)[3]. Although the system proposed by Brown et al. is useful for the identification of foveal edema, it is not likely to identify cases of nonfoveal clinically significant macular edema – that is,

if there was retinal thickening or hard exudates associated with adjacent retinal thickening observed within 500 ± 50 μm of the center of the foveal avascular zone or a zone or zones of retinal thickening 1 disk area or larger, any part of which was within 1 disk diameter of the center of the macula (Sadda et al., 2006)[4].

OCT is the criterion standard in the identification of CME. OCT is a noninvasive imaging modality that can determine the presence of CME by visualizing the fluid-filled spaces in the retina. The amount of CME can be monitored over time by quantifying the area of cystoid spaces on a cross-sectional image through the macula.

Studies have reported OCT to be comparable to FA in the evaluation of CME, especially with the newer, high-resolution OCT scanners. OCT is beneficial by quantifying the thickness of the retina and by allowing quantitative measurements of macular edema over time. This noninvasive method is especially useful in monitoring the response to treatment. Newer OCT software has increased imaging resolution, which has led to the identification of specific patterns of CME (fig. 2).

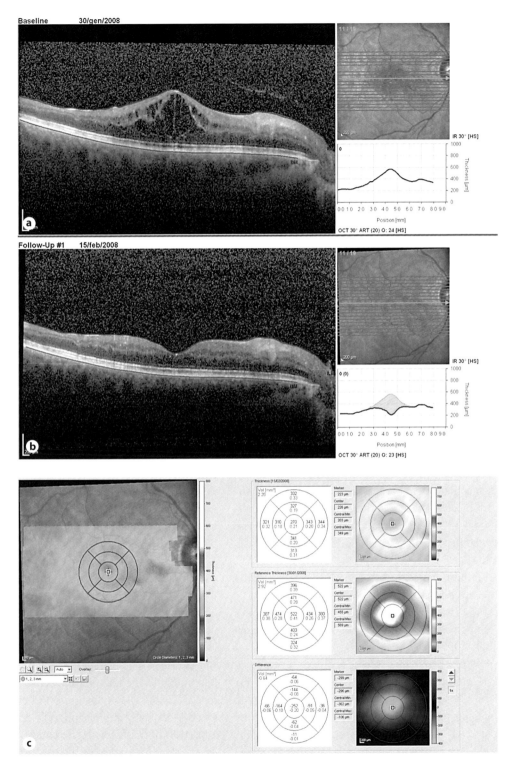

Fig. 2. OCT images of central vein occlusion with CME before (**a**) and after (**b**) treatment. The thickness map and differential thickness map (**c**) show resolution of the edema.

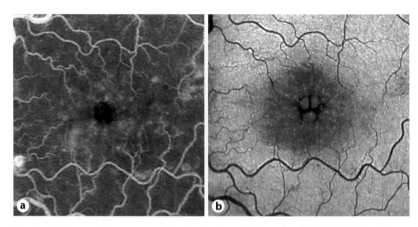

Fig. 3. CME secondary to central retinal vein occlusion visualized in FA (**a**) and 488-nm FAF (**b**).

Table 1. Excitation and barrier wavelength for acquiring with different instruments autofluorescence

	Heidelberg HRA	Topcon	Zeiss 450	Nidek F10	Canon CX-I	Optos
excitation wavelength (nm)	488	550–605	510–580	490	≅500	532
barrier filter (nm)	500	670–720	695–755	510	>600	>600

While OCT provides an objective evaluation of macular edema and is displacing conventional subjective methods, the older evaluation techniques still predominate, especially in the less developed world (Hee et al., 1998; Shahidi et al., 1994)[5, 6].

Fundus autofluorescence (FAF) is collecting the fluorescence emitted by fluorophores of the retina. In particular, to excite lipofuscin, excitation between 470 and 550 nm can be used (Delori et al., 1995)[7].

More than 1 instrument is able to acquire an FAF picture using different wavelengths (table 1).

For visualization of macular edema, however, macular pigment plays a major role. In a normal blue FAF image, the dark spot visible in the central fovea is due to the macular pigment's absorption of the blue light used to excite lipofuscin autofluorescence. In the case of CME, by using blue FAF, it is possible to visualize displacement of macular pigment and consequently the cysts (fig. 3). This tool could be used to evaluate changes during follow-up (fig. 4, 5).

Currently FA is the most common technique used for the diagnosis of macular edema, although it only provides a qualitative assessment of vascular leakage for this pathology. FA illustrates minute dots of fluorescence, which corresponds to leakage adjacent to the terminal macular vessels. In the case of macular edema, the fluorescence appears only in the late phase, becoming visible after 10–15 min. It appears around the fovea and extends centrally and peripherally, involving only a portion of the fovea. If the condition progresses into cyst formation at the macula, fluorescein can be seen to leak into the cysts. The edematous

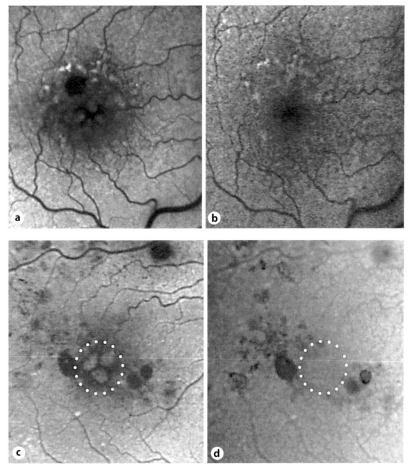

Fig. 4. CME secondary to Crohn disease, before (**a**) and after (**b**) treatment. The disappearance of CME restored the characteristic darker central area of the macular pigment. **c, d** Patient with diabetic retinopathy and CME. 488-nm FAF (**c**) and 550- to 605-nm FAF (**d**) show the importance of visualization of macular pigment and its displacement for indirect visualization of CME (dotted circles). The inability to visualize macular pigment with green or yellow FAF explains the nonvisualization of CME.

fluid accumulates in the outer plexiform layer of Henle over an area that is seldom more than 2 disk diameters.

Associated findings on FA may help determine the etiology of CME. If leaking microaneurysms are present in the setting of diabetic retinopathy, then diabetes is likely the cause. Vascular collaterals crossing the horizontal raphe on FA can help determine if the etiology of the edema (as well as retinal hemorrhages, if present) is likely due to a vascular occlusion.

Indocyanine green angiography (ICGA) is not considered an effective tool for detecting macular edema. In some cases, however, ICGA can be useful in assisting in or confirming a differential diagnosis.

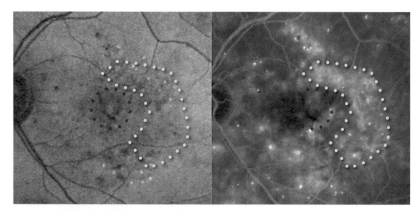

Fig. 5. Diabetic patient with diffuse macular edema and CME. As delimited by yellow dots, an area of diffuse edema is not clearly visible in 488-nm FAF (**a**). CME is visible in both images (red dotted circle). In contrast, diffuse edema is shown as a decrease in FAF intensity since the fluid under or inside the neurosensory retina is masking the fluorescence coming from the retinal pigment epithelium.

Considering Macular Edema Based on the Disease

Irvine-Gass Syndrome

The first identification of macular edema occurring after ocular surgery is attributed to Irvine (1953)[8] while its angiographic appearance was described by Gass (1997)[9] 13 years later. When CME develops following cataract surgery and its cause is thought to be directly related to the surgery, it is referred to as Irvine-Gass syndrome. Despite improvement of surgical techniques, this condition still represents one of the most frequent complications of cataract extraction.

When compared with normal postsurgical responses, the patient affected by postsurgical CME usually complains of blurred vision and reduced color perception and contrast sensibility.

The first set of images (fig. 6–13) shows a case of Irvine-Gass syndrome. At fundus examination, this condition usually appears as a blunted or irregular foveal light reflex with prominent cystic formations (fig. 6).

In autofluorescence (fig. 7), the cysts appear as hyperautofluorescent structures due to the shifting of the macular pigments that normally attenuate the autofluorescent signal in the macular region (Johnson, 2009)[1]. The appearance of the fundus alone is not usually enough to make an accurate diagnosis, so further examination is required.

The infrared retinography images (fig. 8) show a nonhomogeneous macular appearance while red-free images (fig. 9) often show bright irregular and almost round shapes in the macular region.

FA (fig. 10) still represents the 'gold standard' test to be performed in this pathology: in early and mid phases of the examination, a leakage from parafoveal retinal capillaries can be detected. In the late phases of the fluorescein angiogram, a progressive filling of the cystic spaces leads to a petaloid pattern of pooling in the macula. A leakage of the optic disk usually appears in late-phase angiography (fig. 11).

ICGA (fig. 12) does not show any alterations except for a pooling in very late phases (Ray and D'Amico, 2002)[10]. Sometimes the amount of fluorescein angiography leakage does not correlate well with visual acuity; as a result, an important distinction between angiographic and clinically significant CME has to be considered.

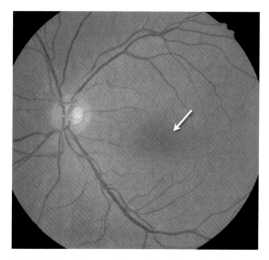

Fig. 6. Irvine-Gass syndrome. Fundus color photo. Arrow = CME.

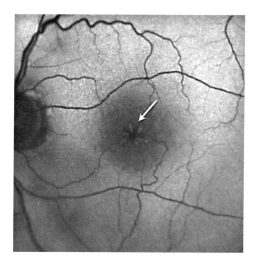

Fig. 7. Irvine-Gass syndrome. Autofluorescence. Arrow = CME.

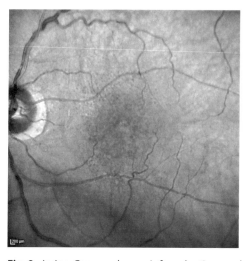

Fig. 8. Irvine-Gass syndrome. Infrared retinography.

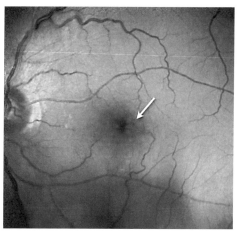

Fig. 9. Irvine-Gass syndrome. Red-free imaging. Arrow = CME.

Time domain OCT and more recently spectral domain OCT (fig. 13) have enabled this condition to be better defined and permit more accurate follow-up examinations. In addition, the presence of retinal thickening and cystoid spaces can be detected (usually in the foveal region of the outer retina and peripherally to the fovea in the inner retina). Sometimes a detachment of the neurosensory retina occurs which is easily visualized with OCT.

Irvine-Gass syndrome is often a self-limited pathology, and it can regress spontaneously. In some cases, postsurgical CME can persist for more than 6 months in a chronic form. In the chronic syndrome, cystic spaces can coalesce to develop a foveal macrocyst characterized by photoreceptor

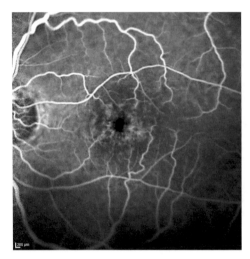

Fig. 10. Irvine-Gass syndrome. FA (early phases).

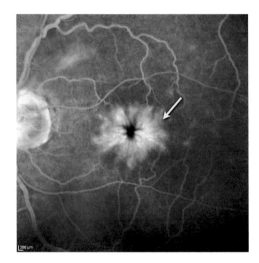

Fig. 11. Irvine-Gass syndrome. FA (late phases). Arrow = CME.

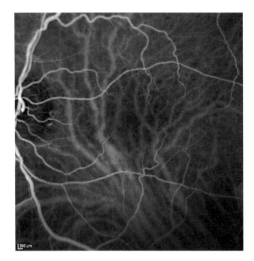

Fig. 12. Irvine-Gass syndrome. ICGA.

disruptions or even evolve with the formation of a lamellar macular hole.

Diabetic Macular Edema

Diabetic macular edema results from the inner blood-retinal barrier being compromised, which leads to leakage of plasma constituents in the surrounding retina. This condition represents the leading cause of legal blindness in the working age population of most developed countries.

In diabetic retinopathy, at fundus examination (fig. 14), diabetic edema can appear as a localized or diffuse macular thickening depending on the severity of retinopathy. The localization of macular edema can be guided by the presence of characteristic elements such as microaneurysms and hard exudates.

Except for autofluorescence, retinography is not useful for the diagnosis of diabetic macular edema: infrared (fig. 15) and red-free (fig. 16) images can show microaneurysms, hard exudates or hemorrhages; however, CME can sometimes be detected by infrared as hyperreflectant round areas. The autofluorescence (fig. 17) of cysts looks hyperautofluorescent because of the displacement of macular pigments that naturally attenuate the autofluorescent signal.

FA (fig. 18, 19) allows areas of focal versus diffuse edema to be distinguished: a focal edema consists of a well-defined, focal area of leakage from microaneurysms or dilated capillaries, whereas diffuse edema appears as a widespread zone of leakage from altered vascular structures. Diffuse cystoid edema can be detected by the presence of

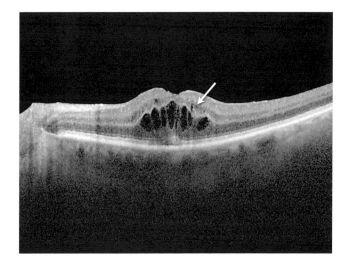

Fig. 13. Irvine-Gass syndrome. Spectral domain OCT. Arrow = CME.

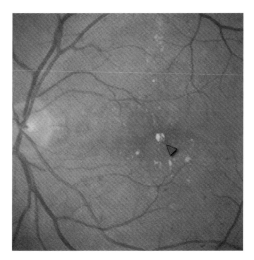

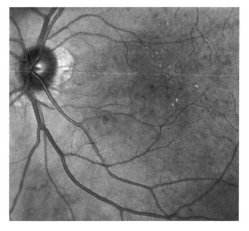

Fig. 15. Diabetic macular edema. Infrared imaging.

Fig. 14. Diabetic macular edema (arrowhead). Fundus examination.

diffuse macular leakage accompanied by pooling of dye in cystic spaces (Bhagat et al., 2009)[11].

ICGA cannot be used to detect diabetic macular edema but can reveal the presence and localization of a microaneurysm. Sometimes diabetic edema appears in ICGA, however, as diffuse hyperfluorescence due to a diabetic choroidopathy or due to a breakdown of the blood-retinal barrier (Weinberger et al., 1998)[12].

OCT represents an important tool, helpful both in the diagnosis and follow-up procedure. According to Kim et al. (2006)[13], macular edema can assume 5 different morphologic patterns at OCT evaluation:

Pattern I is a diffuse retinal thickening, which appears as increased retinal thickness with areas of reduced intraretinal reflectivity, especially in the outer retinal layers (fig. 20);

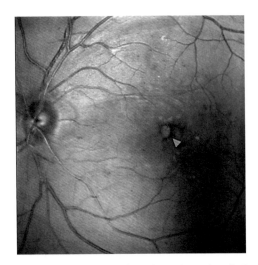

Fig. 16. Diabetic macular edema (arrowhead). Red-free imaging.

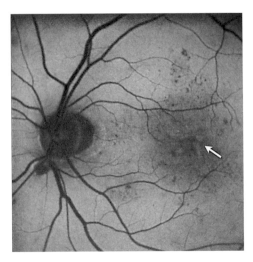

Fig. 17. Diabetic macular edema. Autofluorescence. Arrow = CME.

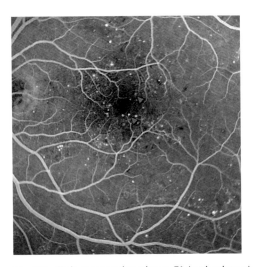

Fig. 18. Diabetic macular edema. FA (early phases). Blue arrowheads = Microaneurysms.

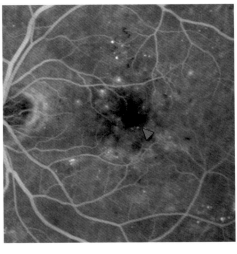

Fig. 19. Diabetic macular edema. FA (late phases). Red arrowhead = Hard exudates.

Pattern II is CME, which appears as oval, only slightly reflective intraretinal cavities, separated by highly reflective septa (fig. 21);

Pattern III shows posterior hyaloidal traction, which appears as a highly reflective band over the retinal surface (fig. 22);

Pattern IV exhibits serous retinal detachment not associated with posterior hyaloidal traction, which appears as a dark accumulation of subretinal fluid beneath a highly reflective and dome-like elevation of detached retina (fig. 23);

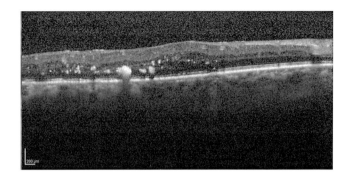

Fig. 20. Diabetic macular edema. Pattern I.

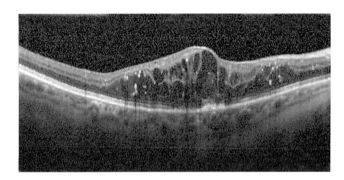

Fig. 21. Diabetic macular edema. Pattern II.

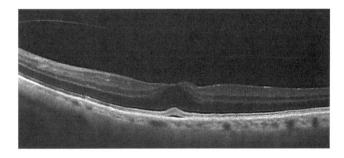

Fig. 22. Diabetic macular edema. Pattern III.

Pattern V shows posterior hyaloidal traction and tractional retinal detachment, which appear as a peak-shaped detachment with a highly reflective signal arising from the inner retinal surface and with an area of low signal beneath the highly reflective border of detached retina (fig. 24).

Retinal Vein Occlusions
Macular edema can also characterize retinal vein occlusions. The most important feature of CME in this condition is that its extension is related to the nonperfused area. Consequently during fundus examination an involvement of the entire posterior pole can occur during central retinal

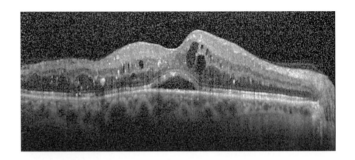

Fig. 23. Diabetic macular edema. Pattern IV.

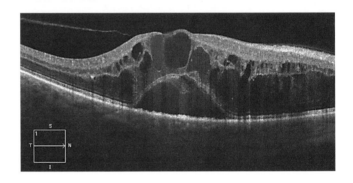

Fig. 24. Diabetic macular edema. Pattern V. S = Superior; N = nasal; I = inferior; T = temporal.

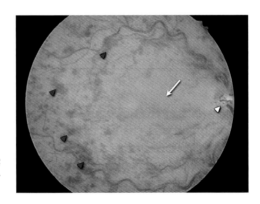

Fig. 25. Fundus CRVO. White arrow = CME; blue arrowheads = hemorrhages; white arrowhead = thrombotic vessel.

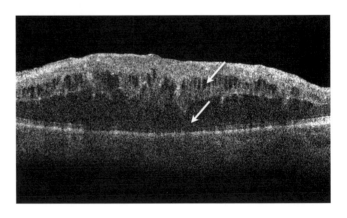

Fig. 26. OCT of CRVO. Arrows = CME.

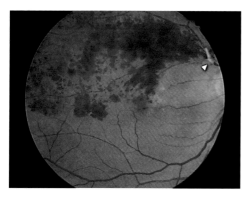

Fig. 27. Fundus BRVO. Arrowhead = Thrombotic vessel.

vein occlusion (CRVO; fig. 25, 26), while branch retinal vein occlusion (BRVO) usually involves a limited portion of the posterior pole (fig. 27).

In the late phases of the fluorescein angiogram, the pooling of dye into the cystic spaces is clearly visible. In CRVO in the mid to late phase there is papillary and vascular leakage (Tranos et al., 2004)[14].

OCT shows retinal thickening and/or CME involving 1 or more quadrants depending on the occlusion site and severity in BRVO (fig. 28) while it is diffuse in CRVO (fig. 26). CME consists of differently sized cysts affecting all the retinal layers and can sometimes be complicated by a neurosensory retinal detachment.

Uveitis

CME represents a common but not specific feature associated with uveitis, and it is the most frequent cause of vision loss in patients affected by this pathology. CME develops most commonly in pars planitis, birdshot retinochoroiditis, idiopathic acute iridocyclitis and retinal vasculitis.

CME also develops in anterior uveitis, HLA-B27-related uveitis and any chronic uveitis. Since CME is not specific to a typical category of uveitis, a global examination of the patient including FA and ICGA, inflammatory indexes

and immunohistochemical analysis should be required (Johnson, 2009)[1].

FA (fig. 29) and ICGA (fig. 30) are useful in order to characterize the vascular involvement and help to classify the vasculitic processes as either occlusive or nonocclusive.

OCT (fig. 31) is helpful to distinguish the retinal thickening and allows the presence of inflammatory epiretinal membranes, alterations in vitreoretinal interfaces and uveitic macular edema to be detected.

CME associated with uveitis can appear with 3 different patterns depending on its localization and extension (Roesel et al., 2009)[15]: (1) cysts involving the inner layers; (2) cysts involving the outer plexiform layer, and (3) cysts involving all the retinal thickness associated with a disruption or loss of the photoreceptors' inner-outer segment junction. In chronic CME, fluid accumulation is associated with thinning of the retina and fibrosis.

Vitreoretinal Tractional Conditions

Vitreoretinal tractional conditions can sometimes be characterized by a particular type of CME. At biomicroscopy examination, CME is difficult to detect since the posterior pole appearance is usually subverted by the epiretinal membrane. Retinography or FA does not provide further information about CME features, but both can be useful in visualizing epiretinal membrane traction lines or pooling of dye in the cystic spaces.

OCT represents the most helpful tool for the diagnosis and follow-up of these pathologies. OCT can show perifoveal vitreous detachment, a thickened hyperreflective posterior hyaloid and epiretinal membranes. CME can appear both as multiple cystic spaces (fig. 32) or with a typical pagoda-shaped profile, especially when the edema is caused by an incomplete vitreous detachment, such as a gull-wing posterior vitreous detachment (fig. 33). Sometimes a neurosensory retinal detachment occurs. The macular traction may resolve in the formation of a lamellar-macular hole (Tranos et al., 2004)[14].

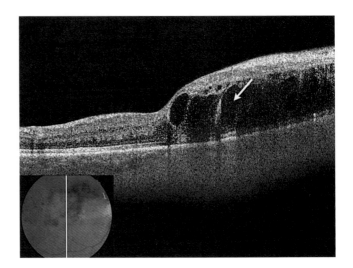

Fig. 28. OCT of BRVO. Arrow = CME. **Inset**
Plane of imaging.

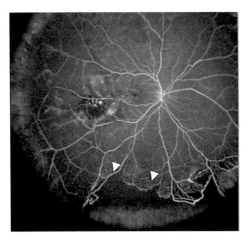

Fig. 29. Uveitis. FA, wide field. Red arrowhead = Vessel
abnormalities; white arrowheads = histochemical areas.

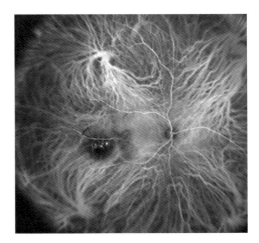

Fig. 30. Uveitis. ICGA, wide field. Red arrowhead =
Vessel abnormalities.

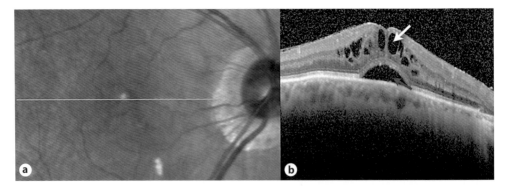

Fig. 31. Uveitis. **a** Site of imaging. **b** OCT. White arrow = CME; red arrow = neuroretinal detachment.

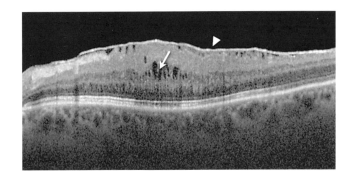

Fig. 32. Vitreoretinal tractional conditions. OCT. Arrow = CME; arrowhead = epiretinal membrane.

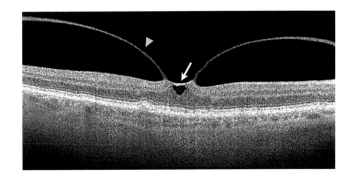

Fig. 33. Vitreoretinal tractional conditions. OCT. White arrow = CME; green arrowhead = gull-wing posterior vitreous detachment.

Idiopathic Macular Telangiectasias

Idiopathic macular telangiectasia is a retinal disorder characterized by the presence of dilated ectasias of retinal capillaries that can lead to chronic macular edema. A recent classification includes 2 different types of idiopathic macular telangiectasias (Charbel Issa et al., 2008)[16]:

Type 1 shows aneurysmal telangiectasia which is visible at fundus examination and affects men in their midlife; this variant usually has a monocular presentation;

Type 2 exhibits perifoveal telangiectasia which is not visible at fundus examination; this category is usually bilateral, without sex preference, and affects people between 50 and 60 years of age.

Important information can be acquired from retinal imaging. Regarding retinography, in infrared imaging (fig. 34), macular cystic spaces appear as hyporeflectant, almost round zones. In red-free/confocal blue reflectance imaging (Heidelberg HRA2, 488 nm; fig. 35), a focal or oval hyperreflectance pattern is usually detectable, and it usually appears larger than the hyperfluorescent area characterized in FA images, thus suggesting that the margins of the lesion go beyond the angiographically appearing leakage. Parafoveal deposits appear as spots with increased reflectance. A circle area of hyperreflectance around the macula (due to a lack of macular pigment) can be observed. A correspondence between areas of increased confocal blue reflectance and increased autofluorescence in the perifoveal area can be seen; areas of only increased confocal blue reflectance reveal a normal outer retina in OCT. In autofluorescence (fig. 36), macular cystic spaces appear as hyperautofluorescent almost

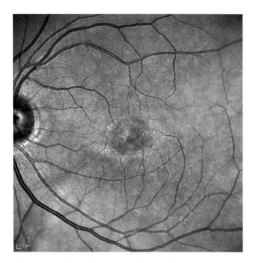

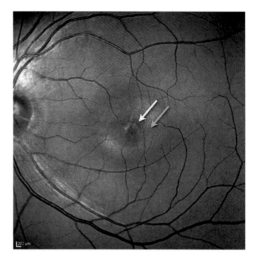

Fig. 34. Idiopathic macular telangiectasias. Infrared retinography.

Fig. 35. Idiopathic macular telangiectasias. Red-free imaging. White arrow = CME; orange arrow = areas of macular pigment loss.

round zones, and the highest central autofluorescence of longstanding cysts may suggest the loss of foveal macular pigments and photoreceptors. A correlation can be shown between areas of increased confocal blue reflectance and increased autofluorescence in the perifoveal region.

In FA (fig. 37, 38), parafoveal telangiectatic capillaries can be detected in the early angiographic phases (fig. 37). In the mid to late phases (fig. 38) of the examination, FA images reveal hyperfluorescent areas corresponding to zones of macular pigment loss in autofluorescence and of increased reflectance in red-free zones. The areas of late hyperfluorescence show abnormalities of the outer retina on OCT examination and do not correspond to intraretinal or subretinal fluid.

ICGA (fig. 39) usually shows no choroidal alterations (Bottoni et al., 2010)[17].

OCT (fig. 40) shows the presence of intraretinal foveal cysts localized in the outer retinal layers and abnormalities of the outer plexiform layer with a 'wrinkled' appearance suggesting Müller cell sufferance. One of the main features of idiopathic macular telangiectasias is that strangely

intraretinal cysts that can be observed in OCT scans do not appear hyperfluorescent in late phases of FA, while outer retina abnormalities correspond to the areas of late hyperfluorescence.

Age-Related Macular Degeneration

Macular edema represents a common finding in wet age-related macular degeneration (AMD) due to the exudation which characterizes this pathology.

In the early phases of the disease, cystic spaces usually appear small in size and are difficult to observe on biomicroscopic examination, while other features of the lesion-like drusen, such as macular hemorrhages, subretinal fluid and pigmented epithelium retinal detachments, are predominant.

FA (Macula Photocoagulation Study Group, 1991)[18] is still considered the 'gold standard' test for the diagnosis of wet AMD, and it usually enables detection of mid- to late-phase CME due to the pooling of dye inside the cysts. However, active lesions are characterized by an increase in dye leakage during the test, which causes a masking effect on the subretina. In contrast, old lesions

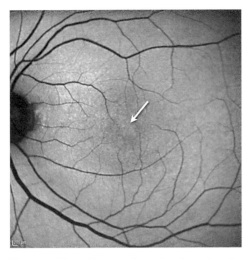

Fig. 36. Idiopathic macular telangiectasias. Autofluorescence. Arrow = CME.

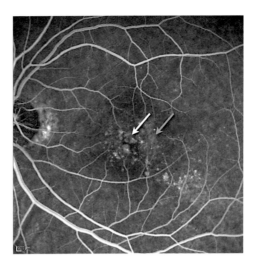

Fig. 37. Idiopathic macular telangiectasias. FA (early phases). White arrow = CME; orange arrow = areas of macular pigment loss.

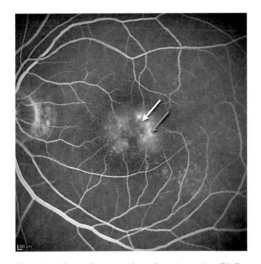

Fig. 38. Idiopathic macular telangiectasias. FA (late phases). White arrow = CME; orange arrow = areas of macular pigment loss.

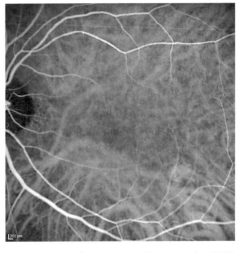

Fig. 39. Idiopathic macular telangiectasias. ICGA.

are characterized by a confluence of the cystic spaces and reduced leakage; as a consequence, CME becomes easier to observe both at fundus examination and with FA (fig. 41).

ICGA is a very useful examination to study AMD lesions, such as occult, polypoidal, chorioretinal anastomoses and choroidal neovascularization (CNV). However, ICGA is not as helpful in identifying CME.

Currently the most useful technique to detect and study CME in wet AMD is OCT. With the development of the spectral domain OCT

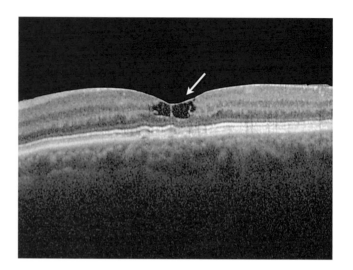

Fig. 40. Idiopathic macular telangiectasias. OCT. Arrow = CME.

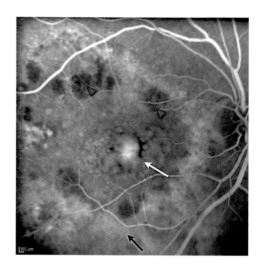

Fig. 41. AMD. FA, advanced CNV. White arrow = CME; red arrowhead = hard exudates; black arrow = retinal pigment epithelium detachment.

technology, OCTs are able to acquire high-definition images, which allow the operator to identify even extremely small cysts in the earliest phases of the disease and to describe their distribution into the different retinal layers.

Depending on lesion type and in the early phases of the disease, CME shows different patterns of localization: classical lesions usually present intraretinal fluid localized in small cystic spaces primarily disposed into the internal layers

(nuclear and plexiform; fig. 42). Occult CNVs are seldom characterized by a huge macular edema: in these lesions CME, when present, is typically represented by intraretinal small cystic spaces localized to the external retinal layers (nuclear and, more rarely, plexiform; fig. 43).

Retinal angiomatous proliferation lesions represent the type of CNV characterized by the larger amount of CME and often involve both external and internal retinal layers (fig. 44). The same cyst

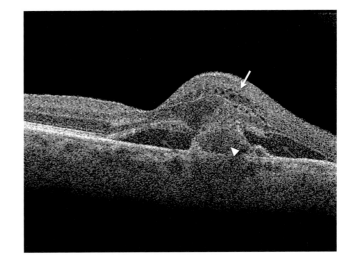

Fig. 42. AMD. OCT, classical lesion. White arrow = CME; white arrowhead = CNV complex; red arrows = neurosensory retinal detachment.

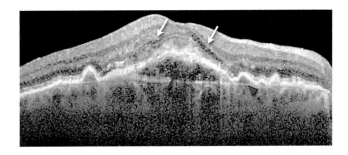

Fig. 43. AMD. OCT, occult lesion. White arrows = CME; red arrowhead = hard exudates; blue arrow = retinal pigment epithelium detachment.

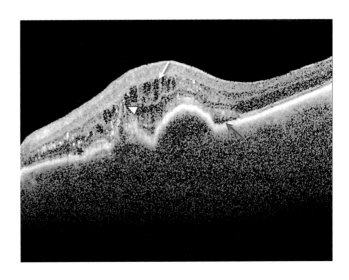

Fig. 44. AMD. OCT, retinal angiomatous proliferation lesion. White arrow = CME; white arrowhead = CNV complex; red arrow = neurosensory retinal detachment; blue arrows = retinal pigment epithelium detachment.

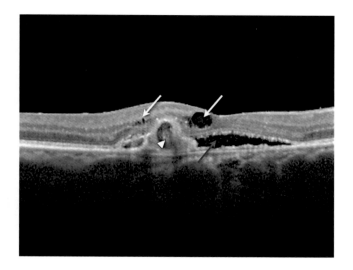

Fig. 45. AMD. OCT, polypoidal lesion. White arrows = CME; white arrowhead = CNV complex; red arrow = neurosensory retinal detachment.

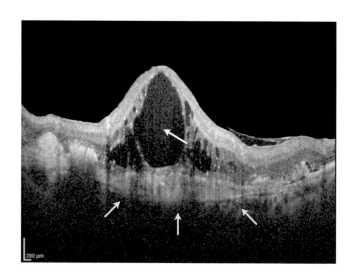

Fig. 46. AMD. OCT, advanced CNV. White arrow = CME; yellow arrows = fibrosis.

localization can be observed in polypoidal lesions (fig. 45).

In advanced CNV, CME is characterized by large cystic round spaces surrounded by hyperreflective boundaries; sometimes a single cyst can involve the entire neurosensory retina (fig. 41, 46). Small round/oval structures with circular midreflectant elements and a central brighter core, which can be observed surrounded by a crown of hyperreflectant spots, can be confused with CME. These formations, called a 'rosette' or 'outer retinal tubulation', represent a stability mark of the lesion (fig. 47) (Zweifel et al., 2009)[19].

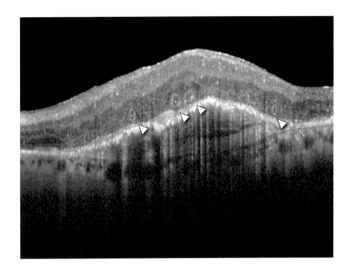

Fig. 47. AMD. OCT, advanced CNV.
Arrowheads = Outer retinal tubulations.

Table 2. Summary of examination methods

	Fundus photography	Retinography	FA	ICGA	OCT
Irvine-Gass syndrome	R	S	U	–	U
Diabetic retinopathy	U	U	U	R	U
Retinal vein occlusions	U	U	U	–	U
Uveitis	U	R	U	U	S
Vitreoretinal tractions	S	U	R	–	U
Idiopathic macular telangiectasias	S	U	S	R	U
AMD	S	S	U	U	U

ICGA = Indocyanine green angiography; AMD = age-related macular degeneration; R = rarely useful; S = sometimes useful; U = usually useful; – = usually not performed.

For these many reasons, OCT is extremely useful in both the diagnostic process and during follow-up examinations.

Table 2 resumes what previously described in the text and estimates the relevance of each di-agnostic technique in defining the aetiology of cystoid macular edema.

References

1 Johnson MW: Etiology and treatment of macular edema. Am J Ophthalmol 2009;147:11–21.
2 Early Treatment Diabetic Retinopathy Study Research Group: Photocoagulation for diabetic macular edema. Early Treatment Diabetic Retinopathy Study report No 1. Arch Ophthalmol 1985;103:1796–806.
3 Brown JC, Solomon SD, Bressler SB, Schachat AP, Di Bernardo C, Bressler NM: Detection of diabetic foveal edema: contact lens biomicroscopy compared with optical coherence tomography. Arch Ophthalmol 2004;122:330–335.
4 Sadda SR, Tan O, Walsh AC, Schuman JS, Varma R, Huang D: Automated detection of clinically significant macular edema by grid scanning optical coherence tomography. Ophthalmology 2006;113:1187e1–12.
5 Hee MR, Puliafito CA, Duker JS, Reichel E, Coker JG, Wilkins JR, Schuman JS, Swanson EA, Fujimoto JG: Topography of diabetic macular edema with optical coherence tomography. Ophthalmology 1998;105:360–370.
6 Shahidi M, Ogura Y, Blair NP, Zeimer R: Retinal thickness change after focal laser treatment of diabetic macular oedema. Br J Ophthalmol 1994;78:827–830.
7 Delori FC, Dorey CK, Staurenghi G, Arend O, Goger DG, Weiter JJ: In vivo fluorescence of the ocular fundus exhibits retinal pigment epithelium lipofuscin characteristics. Invest Ophthalmol Vis Sci 1995;36:718–729.
8 Irvine SR: A newly defined vitreous syndrome following cataract surgery, interpreted according to recent concepts of the structure of the vitreous. Am J Ophthalmol 1953;36:599–619.
9 Gass JDM: Stereoscopic Atlas of Macular Diseases: Diagnosis and Treatment, ed 4. St Louis, Mosby, 1997.
10 Ray S, D'Amico DJ: Pseudophakic cystoid macular edema. Semin Ophthalmol 2002;17:167–180.
11 Bhagat N, Grigorian RA, Tutela A, Zarbin MA: Diabetic macular edema: pathogenesis and treatment. Surv Ophthalmol 2009;54:1–32.
12 Weinberger D, Kramer M, Priel E, et al: Indocyanine green angiographic findings in nonproliferative diabetic retinopathy. Am J Ophthalmol 1998;126:238–247.
13 Kim BY, Smith SD, Kaiser PK: Optical coherence tomographic patterns of diabetic macular edema. Am J Ophthalmol 2006;142:405–412.
14 Tranos PG, Wickremasinghe SS, Stangos NT, Topouzis F, Tsinopoulos I, Pavesio CE: Macular edema. Surv Ophthalmol 2004;49:470–490.
15 Roesel M, Henschel A, Heinz C, Dietzel M, Spital G, Heiligenhaus A: Fundus autofluorescence and spectral domain optical coherence tomography in uveitic macular edema. Graefes Arch Clin Exp Ophthalmol 2009;247:1685–1689.
16 Charbel Issa P, Berendschot TT, Staurenghi G, Holz FG, Scholl HP: Confocal blue reflectance imaging in type 2 idiopathic macular telangiectasia. Invest Ophthalmol Vis Sci 2008;49:1172–1177.
17 Bottoni F, Eandi CM, Pedenovi S, Staurenghi G: Integrated clinical evaluation of type 2A idiopathic juxtafoveolar retinal telangiectasis. Retina 2010;30:317–326.
18 Macular Photocoagulation Study Group: Subfoveal neovascular lesions in age-related macular degeneration: guidelines for evaluation and treatment in the Macular Photocoagulation Study. Arch Ophthalmol 1991;109:1242–1257.
19 Zweifel SA, Engelbert M, Laud K, Margolis R, Spaide RF, Freund KB: Outer retinal tubulation: a novel optical coherence tomography finding. Arch Ophthalmol 2009;127:1596–1602.

Prof. Giovanni Staurenghi
Eye Clinic
Department of Clinical Science "Luigi Sacco"
Sacco Hospital
Via G.B Grassi 74
IT-20157 Milan (Italy)
E-Mail giovanni.staurenghi@unimi.it

Chapter 4

Coscas G (ed): Macular Edema.
Dev Ophthalmol. Basel, Karger, 2010, vol 47, pp 49–58

Macular Edema – Rationale for Therapy

Thomas J. Wolfensberger[a] · Zdenek J. Gregor[b]

[a]Jules Gonin Eye Hospital, Lausanne, Switzerland; [b]Moorfields Eye Hospital, London, UK

Abstract

Blood-retinal barrier breakdown with macular edema is caused by many diseases, which modulate – via different growth factors – the integrity of the tight junctions. Starling's law predicts furthermore that macular edema will develop if the hydrostatic pressure gradient between capillary and retinal tissue is increased, for example in the presence of elevated blood pressure, or if the osmotic pressure gradient is decreased, for example when protein accumulates excessively in the extracellular space within the retina. The rationale for clinical treatment of macular edema is based on the understanding and the inhibition of these pathophysiological mechanisms. On the medical side, nonsteroidal anti-inflammatory drugs inhibit the production of prostaglandins and leukotrienes, and modulate fluid movement coupled to chloride movement. Corticosteroids block cyclooxygenase and interleukin, downregulate vascular endothelial growth factor (VEGF) and decrease the phosphorylation of occludin, thereby increasing the tightness of the blood-retinal barrier. Carbonic anhydrase inhibitors are thought to modulate the polarized distribution of carbonic anhydrase at the level of the retinal pigment epithelium via extracellular pH gradients and thus the fluid resorption from the retina into the choroid. Anti-VEGF agents restore occludin proteins in the blood-retinal barrier and reduce protein kinase C activation. On the surgical side, the beneficial effect of vitrectomy with release of traction on the macula is explained by an increase in tissue pressure and a lowering of the hydrostatic pressure gradient, reducing the water flux from blood vessels into retinal tissue. The therapeutic action of vitrectomy in nontractional edema is thought to be based on two mechanisms: increased oxygen transport between the anterior and posterior segments of the eye and the removal of growth factors which are secreted in large amounts into the vitreous during proliferative vasculopathies.

Copyright © 2010 S. Karger AG, Basel

Macular edema occurs when the blood-retinal barrier breaks down. From a clinical and biological point of view this can be caused by many different vascular, inflammatory and other diseases, which modulate the integrity of the tight junctions between the retinal vascular endothelial cells as well as at the level of the retinal pigment epithelium (RPE) (fig. 1) and they are governed by a host of different growth factors (Tranos et al., 2004)[1].

Starling's law predicts that macular edema will develop if the hydrostatic pressure gradient between capillary and retinal tissue is increased, for example in the presence of elevated blood pressure, or if the osmotic pressure gradient is decreased, for example when protein accumulates excessively in the extracellular space within the retina (Stefánsson, 2009)[2].

The rationale for clinical treatment of macular edema is based on the understanding and the inhibition of these pathophysiological mechanisms.

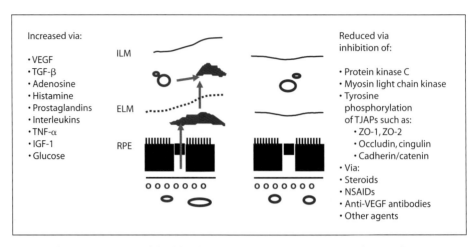

Fig. 1. Schematic diagram of the blood-retinal barrier showing on the left the different growth factors, whose upregulation can lead to a breakdown of the tight junctions in the retinal endothelial and/or RPE cells inducing macular edema. On the right-hand side of the diagram, the different possible therapies are listed, which can reduce the permeability of the blood-retinal barrier. TJAPs = Tight junction-associated proteins; ILM = internal limiting membrane; ELM = external limiting membrane.

Rationale for Medical Management

Systemic Medical Therapy

In many cases, macular edema is caused by a generalized health problem such as diabetes, high blood pressure or inflammatory conditions (Gillies et al., 1997; Gardner et al., 2009; Aiello et al., 2001)[3–5]. It is evident that these generalized diseases need to be treated first and foremost.

There have been several reports in the literature that such treatments – particularly in diabetes, high blood pressure and inflammatory diseases – can cure macular edema without any additional specific ocular treatment (Liew et al., 2009)[6].

Nonsteroidal Anti-Inflammatory Drugs

The action of nonsteroidal anti-inflammatory drugs (NSAIDs) is based on the inhibition of the enzyme cyclooxygenase, which in turn inhibits the production of prostaglandins, a degradation product of arachidonic acid in the eye (Colin, 2007)[7] (fig. 2).

Some NSAIDs also act on other mediators. Diclofenac sodium, for example, in high doses, inhibits the formation of leukotrienes, which amplify cellular infiltration during an inflammatory reaction (Ku et al., 1986)[8].

NSAIDs have also been shown to modulate chloride movement, and, as a consequence, fluid movement through the RPE (Bialek et al., 1996)[9] (fig. 3).

On the basis of these scientific findings, topical NSAIDs have become the mainstay in the treatment of inflammatory cystoid macular edema (CME) (Wolfensberger et al., 1999)[10]. The clinical efficacy of topical NSAIDs has been shown to be of value both in the prevention (Flach et al., 1990; Almeida et al., 2008; DeCroos et al., 2008; Rossetti et al., 1998)[11–14] and in the treatment (Nelson et al., 2003; Sivaprasad et al., 2005; Rojas et al., 1999)[15–17] of inflammatory CME, particularly when related to cataract surgery.

Two double-masked, placebo-controlled studies in which corticosteroids were not used

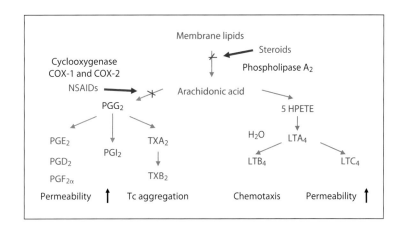

Fig. 2. Schematic diagram of the pharmacological action of corticosteroids and NSAIDs. Note the dual action of steroids both on the prostaglandin and the leukotriene production.

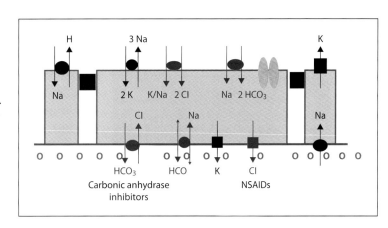

Fig. 3. Schematic diagram showing selected ion channels in the RPE. Note that carbonic anhydrase inhibitors act on the bicarbonate/chloride exchange channel in the basal membrane, and NSAIDs have been shown to act on the chloride channel in the basal membrane of the RPE. Both channels are associated with transcellular fluid transport.

demonstrated that ketorolac 0.5% ophthalmic solution, administered for up to 3 months, improves vision in some patients with chronic CME after cataract surgery (Flach et al., 1987; Flach et al., 1991)[18,19]. A meta-analysis of the results from several different randomized controlled trials suggests that NSAIDs are beneficial as a medical prophylaxis for aphakic and pseudophakic CME and as medical treatment for chronic CME (Rossetti et al., 1998)[14].

On the basis of these findings, it has been suggested to employ topical NSAIDs in the treatment of inflammatory CME especially when related to ocular surgery.

Corticosteroids
Corticosteroids have been used in many different ways such as topical, sub-Tenon and intravitreal administration. Corticosteroids have different potency levels depending on their chemical composition (Haynes et al., 1985)[20] and the newer synthetically produced compounds show an up to 25-fold increase in activity, as compared to cortisone. These new agents, such as triamcinolone, dexamethasone and fluocinolone acetonide, have fluor at the 9α position, which increases corticosteroid receptor binding.

Corticosteroids inhibit the enzyme cyclooxygenase (fig. 2), but they also have a multitude of

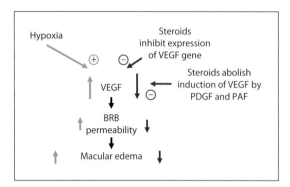

Fig. 4. Schematic diagram showing that hypoxia upregulates VEGF production, which increases blood-retinal barrier (BRB) permeability with the induction of macular edema. Steroids inhibit not only the expression of the VEGF gene but also abolish the induction of VEGF by platelet-derived growth factor (PDGF) and platelet-activating factor (PAF).

other anti-inflammatory effects by acting, among others, on interleukin (IL)-1 and by reducing vascular permeability (Nehmé et al., 2008)[21]. Their additive anti-inflammatory effect to NSAIDs has been shown to be useful in the treatment of various postoperative inflammatory conditions (Othenin-Girard et al., 1992)[22].

One potential mode of action is the increased resorption of fluid through the RPE, although the exact mechanism of this is not as yet clear. Another action of steroids is the downregulation of the production of the vascular endothelial growth factor (VEGF), which, in turn, renders the blood-retinal barrier tighter (fig. 4). Steroids also downregulate VEGF production (Edelmann et al., 2005)[23] specifically in the retina (Wang et al., 2008; Zhang et al., 2008)[24,25], and this explains the clinical observation that the application of steroids both intravitreally and into the sub-Tenon space can reduce macular edema considerably.

Cortisone has also been shown to decrease the phosphorylation of occludin, increasing the tightness of the blood-retinal barrier (Antonetti et al., 2002)[26].

Furthermore, steroids have been shown to prevent the induction of VEFG production by platelet-activating factor and platelet-derived growth factor (Nauck et al., 1997)[27] (fig. 4). Triamcinolone also inhibits IL-6- and VEGF-induced angiogenesis downstream of the IL-6 and VEGF receptors (Ebrahem et al., 2006)[28].

Leukocyte adhesion plays an important role in macular edema – particularly so in diabetic maculopathy. The endothelial damage resulting from this leukocyte adherence to vessel walls is mediated by nitric oxide, adhesion molecules, and other inflammatory mediators (Leal et al., 2007)[29]. Sub-Tenon triamcinolone inhibits leukocyte-endothelium interactions in the retina and downregulates adhesion molecules of retinal vascular endothelium (Mizuno et al., 2007)[30] and thus decreases the retinal thickness.

The *Müller cells* represent a further site of action of steroids (Reichenbach et al., 2007)[31]. Macular edema is thought to be partly linked to the downregulation of the Müller cell protein Kir4.1. The resultant increase in intracellular K^+ leads to the uptake of proteins and osmotic swelling of the Müller cells via aquaporin 4 channels. The administration of triamcinolone reduces the production of VEGF, arachidonic acid and prostaglandins, allowing the reactivation of fluid clearance by Müller cells via endogenous adenosine and the increase in TASK channels. These processes lead to an efflux of potassium thus correcting the downregulation of the Kir4.1 protein (Reichenbach et al., 2007)[31].

Carbonic Anhydrase Inhibitors
Carbonic anhydrase (CA) inhibitors have been used clinically for over 20 years in the treatment of macular edema. The initial observation on its therapeutic efficacy was reported in 1988 in a study of 41 patients with CME of various etiologies (Cox et al., 1988)[32]. It appears that CA inhibitors modulate the polarized distribution of CA at the level of the RPE and thus the fluid resorption from the retina into the choroid.

In the retina, CA is found in the cytoplasm of red/green cones (albeit not in rods) and especially inside Müller cells (Wistrand et al., 1986)[33]. The RPE, however, appears to contain almost exclusively the membrane-bound form of CA (Wolfensberger et al., 1999)[34]. The latter appears to regulate and modulate the extracellular pH gradients created by the metabolic activity of cells and may act as a bicarbonate channel (Wolfensberger et al., 1999; Miller et al., 1977)[35,36]. The CA activity in the RPE shows a clear-cut polarized distribution with a large amount of enzyme on the apical surface of the cell, whereas there is less CA activity on the basolateral portion of the cell membrane. Further immunohistochemical differentiation has shown that the isozyme IV is responsible for apical CA activity in the RPE (Wolfensberger et al., 1999)[34]. Under normal conditions, roughly 70% of the subretinal fluid is removed by metabolic transport to the choroid. In an in vivo rabbit model, it could be shown that this fluid transport (which is driven to a large extent by active ion transport through the RPE) can be enhanced by acetazolamide (Marmor et al., 1986; Wolfensberger et al., 2000)[37,38] (fig. 3). Furthermore, experiments in an animal model of iatrogenically induced retinal detachments showed that the disappearance of fluorescein through the RPE increased by 25% after intravenous injection of acetazolamide (Tsuboi et al., 1985)[39]. The same authors also observed a marked increase in resorption of subretinal fluid at a higher dosage of 50–65 mg/kg body weight. Further studies on the frog RPE demonstrated that active chloride and bicarbonate transport probably occurs at the basal surface, which faces the choroidal blood supply and it was postulated that subretinal fluid absorption occurs at this level (Miller et al., 1977)[36].

Intravenous injection of acetazolamide has been shown to decrease the pH in the subretinal space in both chicks and cats (Wolfensberger et al., 1999; Yamamoto et al., 1992)[35,40]. This acidification was followed immediately by a reduction of the subretinal volume, and it has been postulated that it is the acidification that induces changes in ion and consequent fluid transport through the RPE.

Anti-VEGF Agents

On a cellular level, VEGF has been implicated in many different mechanisms, which lead to macular edema. VEGF has, for example, been shown to decrease the occludin protein responsible for the tightness of the intracellular junctions (Antonetti et al., 1998)[41]. VEGF also induces rapid phosphorylation of the tight junction protein occludin and zonula occludens 1 resulting in the breakdown of the blood-retinal barrier (Antonetti et al., 1999)[42]. VEGF-induced blood-retinal barrier breakdown appears to be effected via nitric oxide (Laksminarayanan et al., 2000)[43]. VEGF also increases paracellular transport without altering the solvent drag reflection coefficient (DeMaio et al., 2004)[44]. Furthermore, VEGF activation of protein kinase C stimulates occludin phosphorylation and contributes to endothelial permeability (Harhaj et al., 2006)[45].

As discussed above, there are several reports, which support the notion that corticosteroids act as *indirect anti-VEGF agents* (fig. 4). However, more recently, directly acting anti-VEGF agents have come to the forefront as promising treatment options for macular edema of different origins (Cordero Coma et al., 2007; Mason et al., 2006; Rodriguez-Fontal et al., 2009; Spaide et al., 2009)[46–49]. Several direct antibody compounds, which interfere with the VEGF receptor, have been used clinically. Ranibizumab (Lucentis) and bevacizumab (Avastin) are antibodies with high affinity for VEGF, which bind to all VEGF isoforms. These and other drugs have been widely used in age-related macular degeneration for several years, but recently interest has arisen for using these agents in other vascular diseases as well. The VEGF aptamer pegaptanib (modified RNA oligonucleotide, which binds and inactivates VEGF165 only) has been shown in animal models to restore the blood-retinal barrier in diabetic retinopathy (Starita et al., 2007)[50]. Furthermore, it has been shown that intravitreal injection of bevacizumab potentially reduces not only VEGF but also stromal cell-derived factor 1α. This suggests that intravitreal bevacizumab may influence intraocular mediators other than VEGF (Arimura et al., 2009)[51].

Other Medical Treatments
Steroid-sparing immunosuppressive drugs are frequently used as additional, second-line agents particularly in patients with severe intraocular inflammation and CME (Tranos et al., 2004)[1]. The rationale for these treatments relies on the inhibition of several different proinflammatory cytokines, which are specifically involved in causing macular edema by breaking down the blood-retinal barrier in intraocular inflammatory disorders.

Apart from the well-known agents such as VEFG, prostaglandins and leukotrienes, these cytokines also include insulin-like growth factor 1, IL-6, stromal cell-derived factor 1, and the hepatocyte growth factor. Particularly elevated levels of intraocular VEGF and IL-6 have been correlated with the severity of uveitic macular edema (van Kooij et al., 2006; Curnow et al., 2006)[52,53] and treatments directed specifically against these factors have been proposed.

Promising results have also been reported using interferon α₂ (Deuter et al., 2006)[54] as a treatment for long-standing refractory CME in uveitis. In addition, a beneficial effect of interferon on inflammatory CME was noted in a retrospective study of patients with multiple sclerosis-associated intermediate uveitis (Becker et al., 2005)[55].

Others reported comparable efficacy of cyclosporine A to prednisolone in the treatment of macular edema in patients with endogenous uveitis (Nussenblatt et al., 1991)[56]. Anti-TNF therapy has also been demonstrated as a promising therapy for uveitic macular edema (Theodossiadis et al., 2007)[57].

Somatostatin analogues such as octreotide may also be effective in the treatment of CME by blocking the local and systemic production of growth hormone, insulin-like growth factor and VEGF (Rothova, 2007)[58]. Treatment with octreotide resulted in marked improvement or even complete resolution of CME in uveitic patients (Kafkala et al., 2006)[59].

Rationale for Surgical Management of Macular Edema by Vitrectomy

Although pars plana vitrectomy may be considered as a very simple surgical procedure, its manifold effects on a cellular level are becoming more and more understood (Stefánsson, 2009)[2].

Tractional Origin of Macular Edema
The initial rationale for using vitrectomy in cases of macular edema was entirely structural, i.e. aimed at the removal of vitreous traction on the macula (Fung et al., 1985; Lewis et al., 1992)[60,61]. The effect of traction on retinal structures becomes understandable by using Newton's third law: to any action there is always an equal reaction in the opposite direction. The force of vitreoretinal traction will thus be met by an equal and opposite force in the retina, resulting in the retinal tissues being pulled apart.

Eventually this results in the lowering of the tissue pressure within the retina, which in turn increases the difference between the hydrostatic pressure in the blood vessels and the tissue and contributes thus to edema formation (Starling's law). Releasing the traction will increase tissue pressure and lower the hydrostatic pressure gradient, reducing the water flux from blood vessels into retinal tissue (Stefánsson, 2009)[2].

Vitreoretinal traction associated with macular edema has been identified in diabetic retinopathy, following complicated cataract surgery

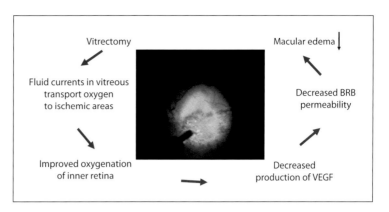

Fig. 5. Schematic diagram showing the effect of a pars plana vitrectomy on intraocular oxygen distribution. Fluid currents during the vitrectomy transport oxygen to the ischemic areas, which creates an improved oxygenation of the inner retina. This in turn reduces VEGF production and blood-retinal barrier (BRB) permeability resulting in a decrease in macular edema.

(Irvine-Gass syndrome) and in several other disease entities. The removal of such traction by vitreoretinal surgery has been found to be beneficial (Fung et al., 1985; Lewis et al., 1992; Margherio et al., 1989)[60–62].

Nontractional Origin of Macular Edema
Recent discoveries have shown that vitrectomy may not only be beneficial in the presence of macular traction, but also in cases where no particular deformation of the macula can be identified. This is particularly true for macular edema of vascular origin, such as diabetes or retinal vein occlusion.

The beneficial effect of vitrectomy is thought to be based – at least in part – on two mechanisms. Firstly, it has been found, for example, that oxygen transport between the anterior and posterior segments of the eye is increased in the vitrectomized-lentectomized eyes (Stefánsson et al., 1990; Holekamp et al., 2005)[63,64]. Others have shown that pharmacologic vitreolysis also improves oxygen diffusion within the vitreous cavity (Giblin

et al., 2009)[65]. This means that following vitrectomy and/or posterior vitreous detachment, the transport of molecules to and from the retina is increased (fig. 5).

Secondly, it has been shown that several growth factors such as VEGF, IL-6, platelet-derived growth factor, and others are secreted in large amounts into the vitreous during proliferative vasculopathies such as diabetic retinopathy or retinal vein occlusion (Noma et al., 2009; Praidou et al., 2009)[66,67] and it is conceivable that a complete vitrectomy will remove this excess of growth factors mechanically with the desired effect of a restitution of the blood-retinal barrier. The rapid clearance of VEGF and other cytokines may thus help to prevent macular edema and retinal neovascularization in ischemic retinopathies, such as diabetic retinopathy and retinal vein occlusions. Vitreous clearance of growth factors may indeed have the same effect as the presence of, for example, VEGF antibodies in the vitreous cavity (Stefánsson, 2001; Stefánsson, 2006; Stefánsson, 2009)[2,68,69].

References

1 Tranos PG, Wickremasinghe SS, Stangos NT, Topouzis F, Tsinopoulos I, Pavesio CE: Macular edema. Surv Ophthalmol 2004;49:470–490.

2 Stefánsson E: Physiology of vitreous surgery. Graefes Arch Clin Exp Ophthalmol 2009;247:147–163.

3 Gillies MC, Su T, Stayt J, Simpson JM, Naidoo D, Salonikas C: Effect of high glucose on permeability of retinal capillary endothelium in vitro. Invest Ophthalmol Vis Sci 1997;38:635–642.

4 Gardner TW, Gabbay RA: Diabetes and obesity: a challenge for every ophthalmologist. Arch Ophthalmol 2009;127:328–329.

5 Aiello LP, Cahill MT, Wong JS: Systemic considerations in the management of diabetic retinopathy. Am J Ophthalmol 2001;132:760–776.

6 Liew G, Mitchell P, Wong TY: Systemic management of diabetic retinopathy. BMJ 2009;338:b441.

7 Colin J: The role of NSAIDs in the management of postoperative ophthalmic inflammation. Drugs 2007;67:1291–308.

8 Ku EC, Lee W, Kothari HV, Scholer DW: Effect of diclofenac sodium on the arachidonic acid cascade. Am J Med 1986;80:18–23.

9 Bialek S, Quong JN, Yu K, Miller SS: Nonsteroidal anti-inflammatory drugs alter chloride and fluid transport in bovine retinal pigment epithelium. Am J Physiol 1996;270:C1175–C1189.

10 Wolfensberger TJ, Herbort CP: Treatment of cystoid macular edema with non-steroidal anti-inflammatory drugs and corticosteroids. Doc Ophthalmol 1999;97:381–386.

11 Flach AJ, Stegman RC, Graham J, Kruger LP: Prophylaxis of aphakic cystoid macular edema without corticosteroids. A paired-comparison, placebo-controlled double-masked study. Ophthalmology 1990;97:1253–1258.

12 Almeida DR, Johnson D, Hollands H, et al: Effect of prophylactic nonsteroidal antiinflammatory drugs on cystoid macular edema assessed using optical coherence tomography quantification of total macular volume after cataract surgery. J Cataract Refract Surg 2008;34:64–69.

13 DeCroos FC, Afshari NA: Perioperative antibiotics and anti-inflammatory agents in cataract surgery. Curr Opin Ophthalmol 2008;19:22–26.

14 Rossetti L, Chaudhuri J, Dickersin K: Medical prophylaxis and treatment of cystoid macular edema after cataract surgery. The results of a meta-analysis. Ophthalmology 1998;105:397–405.

15 Nelson ML, Martidis A: Managing cystoid macular edema after cataract surgery. Curr Opin Ophthalmol 2003;14:39–43.

16 Sivaprasad S, Bunce C, Patel N: Non-steroidal anti-inflammatory agents for treating cystoid macular oedema following cataract surgery. Cochrane Database Syst Rev 2005;1:CD004239.

17 Rojas B, Zafirakis P, Christen W, Markomichelakis NN, Foster CS: Medical treatment of macular edema in patients with uveitis. Doc Ophthalmol 1999;97:399–407.

18 Flach AJ, Dolan BJ, Irvine AR: Effectiveness of ketorolac tromethamine 0.5% ophthalmic solution for chronic aphakic and pseudophakic cystoid macular edema. Am J Ophthalmol 1987;103:479–486.

19 Flach AJ, Jampol LM, Weinberg D, et al: Improvement in visual acuity in chronic aphakic and pseudophakic cystoid macular edema after treatment with topical 0.5% ketorolac tromethamine. Am J Ophthalmol 1991;112:514–519.

20 Haynes RC Jr, Murad F: Adrenocorticotropic hormone: adrenocortical steroids and their synthetic analogs: inhibitors of adrenocortical steroid biosynthesis; in Gilman AG, Goodman LS, Rall TW, Murad F (eds): Goodman and Gilman's The Pharmacological Basis of Therapeutics. New York, Macmillan, 1985, pp 1459–1489.

21 Nehmé A, Edelman J: Dexamethasone inhibits high glucose-, TNF-α-, and IL-1β-induced secretion of inflammatory and angiogenic mediators from retinal microvascular pericytes. Invest Ophthalmol Vis Sci 2008;49:2030–2038.

22 Othenin-Girard P, Borruat X, Bovey E, Pittet N, Herbort CP: Diclofenac-dexamethasone combination in treatment of postoperative inflammation: prospective double-blind study. Klin Monatsbl Augenheilkd 1992;200:362–366.

23 Edelman JL, Lutz D, Castro MR: Corticosteroids inhibit VEGF-induced vascular leakage in a rabbit model of blood-retinal and blood-aqueous barrier breakdown. Exp Eye Res 2005;80:249–258.

24 Wang K, Wang Y, Gao L, Li X, Li M, Guo J: Dexamethasone inhibits leukocyte accumulation and vascular permeability in retina of streptozotocin-induced diabetic rats via reducing vascular endothelial growth factor and intercellular adhesion molecule-1 expression. Biol Pharm Bull 2008;31:1541–1546.

25 Zhang X, Bao S, Lai D, Rapkins RW, Gillies MC: Intravitreal triamcinolone acetonide inhibits breakdown of the blood-retinal barrier through differential regulation of VEGF-A and its receptors in early diabetic rat retinas. Diabetes 2008;57:1026–1033.

26 Antonetti DA, Wolpert EB, DeMaio L, Harhaj NS, Scaduto RC Jr: Hydrocortisone decreases retinal endothelial cell water and solute flux coincident with increased content and decreased phosphorylation of occludin. J Neurochem 2002;80:667–677.

27 Nauck M, Roth M, Tamm M, Eickelberg O, Wieland H, Stulz P, Perruchoud AP: Induction of vascular endothelial growth factor by platelet-activating factor and platelet-derived growth factor is downregulated by corticosteroids. Am J Respir Cell Mol Biol 1997;16:398–406.

28 Ebrahem Q, Minamoto A, Hoppe G, Anand-Apte B, Sears JE: Triamcinolone acetonide inhibits IL-6- and VEGF-induced angiogenesis downstream of the IL-6 and VEGF receptors. Invest Ophthalmol Vis Sci 2006;47:4935–4941.

29 Leal EC, Manivannan A, Hosoya K, Terasaki T, Cunha-Vaz J, Ambrosio AF, Forrester JV: Inducible nitric oxide synthase isoform is a key mediator of leukostasis and blood-retinal barrier breakdown in diabetic retinopathy. Invest Ophthalmol Vis Sci 2007;48:5257–5265.

30 Mizuno S, Nishiwaki A, Morita H, Miyake T, Ogura Y: Effects of periocular administration of triamcinolone acetonide on leukocyte-endothelium interactions in the ischemic retina. Invest Ophthalmol Vis Sci 2007;48:2831–2836.

31 Reichenbach A, Wurm A, Pannicke T, Iandiev I, Wiedemann P, Bringmann A: Müller cells as players in retinal degeneration and edema. Graefes Arch Clin Exp Ophthalmol 2007;245:627–636.

32 Cox SN, Hay E, Bird AC: Treatment of chronic macular edema with acetazolamide. Arch Ophthalmol 1988;106:1190–1195.

33 Wistrand PJ, Schenholm M, Lönnerholm G: Carbonic anhydrase isoenzymes C in the human eye. Invest Ophthalmol Vis Sci 1986;27:419–428.

34 Wolfensberger TJ, Mahieu I, Jarvis-Evans J, et al: Membrane-bound carbonic anhydrase in human retinal pigment epithelium. Invest Ophthalmol Vis Sci 1994;35:3401–3407.

35 Wolfensberger TJ, Dmitriev AV, Govardovskii VI: Inhibition of membrane-bound carbonic anhydrase decreases subretinal pH and volume. Doc Ophthalmol 1999;97:261–271.

36 Miller SS, Steinberg RH: Active transport of ions across frog retinal pigment epithelium. Exp Eye Res 1977;25:235.

37 Marmor MF, Negi A: Pharmacologic modification of subretinal fluid absorption in the rabbit eye. Arch Ophthalmol 1986;104:1674–1677.

38 Wolfensberger TJ, Chiang RK, Takeuchi A, Marmor MF: Inhibition of membrane-bound carbonic anhydrase enhances subretinal fluid absorption and retinal adhesiveness. Graefes Arch Clin Exp Ophthalmol 2000;238:76–80.

39 Tsuboi S, Pederson JE: Experimental retinal detachment. 10. Effect of acetazolamide on vitreous fluorescein disappearance. Arch Ophthalmol 1985;103:1557–1558.

40 Yamamoto F, Steinberg RH: Effects of intravenous acetazolamide on retinal pH in the cat. Exp Eye Res 1992;54:711–718.

41 Antonetti DA, Barber AJ, Khin S, Lieth E, Tarbell JM, Gardner TW: Vascular permeability in experimental diabetes is associated with reduced endothelial occludin content: vascular endothelial growth factor decreases occludin in retinal endothelial cells. Penn State Retina Research Group. Diabetes 1998;47:1953–1959.

42 Antonetti DA, Barber AJ, Hollinger LA, Wolpert EB, Gardner TW: Vascular endothelial growth factor induces rapid phosphorylation of tight junction proteins occludin and zonula occluden 1. J Biol Chem 1999;274:23463–23467.

43 Lakshminarayanan S, Antonetti DA, Gardner TW, Tarbell JM: Effect of VEGF on retinal microvascular endothelial hydraulic conductivity: the role of NO. Invest Ophthalmol Vis Sci 2000;41:4256–4261.

44 DeMaio L, Antonetti DA, Scaduto RC Jr, Gardner TW, Tarbell JM: VEGF increases paracellular transport without altering the solvent-drag reflection coefficient. Microvasc Res 2004;68:295–302.

45 Harhaj NS, Felinski EA, Wolpert EB, Sundstrom JM, Gardner TW, Antonetti DA: VEGF activation of protein kinase C stimulates occludin phosphorylation and contributes to endothelial permeability. Invest Ophthalmol Vis Sci 2006;47:5106–5115.

46 Cordero Coma M, Sobrin L, Onal S, Christen W, Foster CS: Intravitreal bevacizumab for treatment of uveitic macular edema. Ophthalmology 2007;114:1574–1579.

47 Mason JO 3rd, Albert MA Jr, Vail R: Intravitreal bevacizumab (Avastin) for refractory pseudophakic cystoid macular edema. Retina 2006;26:356–357.

48 Rodriguez-Fontal M, Alfaro V, Kerrison JB, Jablon EP: Ranibizumab for diabetic retinopathy. Curr Diabetes Rev 2009;5:47–51.

49 Spaide RF, Chang LK, Klancnik JM, Yannuzzi LA, Sorenson J, Slakter JS, Freund KB, Klein R: Prospective study of intravitreal ranibizumab as a treatment for decreased visual acuity secondary to central retinal vein occlusion. Am J Ophthalmol 2009;147:298–306.

50 Starita C, Patel M, Katz B, Adamis AP: Vascular endothelial growth factor and the potential therapeutic use of pegaptanib (macugen) in diabetic retinopathy. Dev Ophthalmol 2007;39:122–148.

51 Arimura N, Otsuka H, Yamakiri K, Sonoda Y, Nakao S, Noda Y, Hashiguchi T, Maruyama I, Sakamoto T: Vitreous mediators after intravitreal bevacizumab or triamcinolone acetonide in eyes with proliferative diabetic retinopathy. Ophthalmology 2009;116:921–926.

52 van Kooij B, Rothova A, Rijkers GT, de Groot-Mijnes JD: Distinct cytokine and chemokine profiles in the aqueous of patients with uveitis and cystoid macular edema. Am J Ophthalmol 2006;142:192–194.

53 Curnow SJ, Murray PI: Inflammatory mediators of uveitis: cytokines and chemokines. Curr Opin Ophthalmol 2006;17:532–537.

54 Deuter CM, Koetter I, Guenaydin I, Stuebiger N, Zierhut M: Interferon alfa-2a: a new treatment option for long lasting refractory cystoid macular edema in uveitis? A pilot study. Retina 2006;26:786–791.

55 Becker MD, Heiligenhaus A, Hudde T, et al: Interferon as a treatment for uveitis associated with multiple sclerosis. Br J Ophthalmol 2005;89:1254–1257.

56 Nussenblatt RB, Palestine AG, Chan CC, Stevens G Jr, Mellow SD, Green SB: Randomized, double-masked study of cyclosporine compared to prednisolone in the treatment of endogenous uveitis. Am J Ophthalmol 1991;112:138–146.

57 Theodossiadis PG, Markomichelakis NN, Sfikakis PP: Tumor necrosis factor antagonists: preliminary evidence for an emerging approach in the treatment of ocular inflammation. Retina 2007;27:399–413.

58 Rothova A: Inflammatory cystoid macular edema. Curr Opin Ophthalmol 2007;18:487–492.

59 Kafkala C, Choi JY, Choopong P, Foster CS: Octreotide as a treatment for uveitic cystoid macular edema. Arch Ophthalmol 2006;124:1353–1355.

60 Fung WE: Vitrectomy for chronic aphakic cystoid macular edema. Results of a national, collaborative, prospective, randomized investigation. Ophthalmology 1985;92:1102–1111.

61 Lewis H, Abrams GW, Blumenkranz MS, Campo RV: Vitrectomy for diabetic macular traction and edema associated with posterior hyaloidal traction. Ophthalmology 1992;99:753–759.

62 Margherio RR, Trese MT, Margherio AR, Cartright K: Surgical management of vitreomacular traction syndromes. Ophthalmology 1989;96:1437–1445.

63 Stefánsson E, Novack RL, Hatchell DL: Vitrectomy prevents retinal hypoxia in branch retinal vein occlusion. Invest Ophthalmol Vis Sci 1990;31:284–289.

64 Holekamp NM, Shui YB, Beebe DC: Vitrectomy surgery increases oxygen exposure to the lens: a possible mechanism for nuclear cataract formation. Am J Ophthalmol 2005;139:302–310.

65 Giblin FJ, Quiram PA, Leverenz VR, Baker RM, Dang L, Trese MT: Enzyme-induced posterior vitreous detachment in the rat produces increased lens nuclear pO_2 levels. Exp Eye Res 2009;88:286–292.

66 Noma H, Funatsu H, Mimura T, Harino S, Hori S: Vitreous levels of interleukin-6 and vascular endothelial growth factor in macular edema with central retinal vein occlusion. Ophthalmology 2009; 116:87–93.

67 Praidou A, Klangas I, Papakonstantinou E, Androudi S, Georgiadis N, Karakiulakis G, Dimitrakos S: Vitreous and serum levels of platelet-derived growth factor and their correlation in patients with proliferative diabetic retinopathy. Curr Eye Res 2009;34:152–161.

68 Stefánsson E: The therapeutic effects of retinal laser treatment and vitrectomy. A theory based on oxygen and vascular physiology. Acta Ophthalmol Scand 2001;79:435–440.

69 Stefánsson E: Ocular oxygenation and the treatment of diabetic retinopathy. Surv Ophthalmol 2006;4:364–380.

Thomas J. Wolfensberger, MD, PD, MER
Vitreoretinal Department, Jules Gonin Eye Hospital, University of Lausanne
Ave de France 15
CH–1000 Lausanne 7 (Switzerland)
E-Mail thomas.wolfensberger@fa2.ch

Chapter 5

Coscas G (ed): Macular Edema.
Dev Ophthalmol. Basel, Karger, 2010, vol 47, pp 59–72

Drug Delivery to the Posterior Segment of the Eye

Baruch D. Kuppermann[a] · Anat Loewenstein[b]

[a]Department of Ophthalmology, University of California, Irvine, Calif., USA; [b]Department of Ophthalmology, Tel Aviv Medical Center, Sackler Faculty of Medicine, Tel Aviv University, Tel Aviv, Israel

Abstract

Drug delivery into the posterior segment of the eye is complicated by the existence of the blood-ocular barrier. Strategies for delivering drugs to the posterior segment include systemic administration, modification of the barrier, and local drug delivery (including transcorneal, transscleral, and intravitreal). Recently, new topical treatments have emerged for the treatment of posterior eye disease. Iontophoretic, juxtascleral, and intravitreal routes can be used to achieve therapeutic levels in the posterior segment. Extended-release intravitreal drug delivery systems can achieve sustained therapeutic levels with the goal of providing a prolonged clinical benefit.

Copyright © 2010 S. Karger AG, Basel

The Posterior Segment of the Eye and the Blood-Ocular Barrier

The blood-ocular barrier has three key functions: it maintains tissue/fluid composition, produces aqueous humor, and keeps pathogens out of the eye. The barrier consists of tight junctions at the level of the iris vascular epithelium and nonpigmented ciliary epithelium, where they form the *blood-aqueous barrier*, and at the level of the retinal vascular endothelium and retinal pigment epithelium (RPE), where they form the *blood-retinal barrier*. While preventing pathogens from entering the eye, the blood-ocular barrier also restricts drugs from entering the eye (Hughes et al., 2005; Urtti, 2006)[1,2].

This barrier can be damaged by surgery, by conditions such as uveitis, diabetes, and ocular infection, and by certain treatments such as photocoagulation and cryopexy. When the blood-ocular barrier breaks down, drugs can enter and leave the eye more easily. A shift in Starling forces (forces controlling the fluid balance) can occur, resulting in macular edema. Serum can leak into the eye leading to cellular proliferation, and there can be aqueous hyposecretion.

Strategies for Delivering Drugs to the Posterior Segment

Conceptually, there are three approaches to delivering drugs to the eye:

(1) *Deliver large amounts of drugs systemically.* Traditionally drugs are administered *systemically* in amounts that are theoretically large enough to achieve therapeutic levels in the eye. In practice, however, the amounts of drugs actually reaching the posterior segment are limited by the blood-ocular barrier, which therefore requires very high doses to be administered systemically in order to achieve even borderline therapeutic retinal drug levels. The limiting factor to this approach is frequently the systemic toxicity associated with the

relatively high systemic drug levels needed to overcome the blood-ocular barrier.

(2) *Modify the blood-ocular barrier.* The second approach to drug delivery is to *modify the permeability* of the blood-ocular barrier to allow greater drug penetrance, and allow access to certain drugs and compounds [e.g. histamines, bradykinin agonists, and vascular endothelial growth factor (VEGF)] that can increase vascular permeability. This approach is rarely used.

(3) *Local delivery of drugs to the eye.* The third strategy involves delivering drugs *locally to the target tissues.* There is evidence to suggest that local delivery of drugs to the posterior segment is the most effective approach to the management of posterior segment diseases, and this approach has been the source of renewed enthusiasm.

Local Therapy

When considering local drug delivery to the posterior segment, several approaches need to be taken into account. They include transcorneal drug delivery, transscleral drug delivery, and intravitreal drug delivery.

Topical therapy is the most common mode of drug delivery into the eye, but it is mostly ineffective for posterior segment diseases. Transcorneal iontophoresis has been under extended development for years and has not yet been used for any indication. Periocular approaches and intravitreal injections have long been used and can be extremely effective. Intravitreal drug delivery systems are now beginning to be more widely used, with 3 systems (Vitrasert®, Retisert®, and Ozurdex™) currently approved by the Food and Drug Administration (FDA) and one other (Iluvien®) under current submission to the FDA.

Topical Drug Delivery
Penetration and distribution of a drug into the posterior tissues of the eye after topical administration can occur by diffusion into the iris root and

subsequently into the posterior chamber and segment, or through the pars plana without encountering the blood-retinal barrier (Hughes et al., 2005)[1] (fig. 1). The drugs can also enter the sclera by lateral diffusion followed by penetration of Bruch's membrane and the RPE. To a lesser extent, the drug can be absorbed into the systemic circulation either through the conjunctival vessels or via the nasolacrimal duct and gain systemic access to the retinal vessels.

Topically applied drugs reach the posterior segment via the transcorneal or transconjunctival pathways (Urtti, 2006; Chiou et al., 1982; Ahmed et al., 1985; Geroski et al., 2000)[2–5]. Transcorneal penetration involves crossing the corneal epithelial barrier, across into the anterior chamber, and then through the lens or the iris root.

Transscleral/conjunctival access is either across the sclera, choroid, choriocapillaris, and the RPE to the retina, or indirectly into the retrobulbar space and the optic nerve head (Ahmed et al., 1985)[4].

Transcorneal Route
The cornea is a unique tissue, which has an aqueous phase (stroma) sandwiched by 2 lipid layers (epithelium and endothelium). As a result, a drug that is both hydrophobic and hydrophilic can penetrate corneal tissue freely. If a drug is a pure polar or a pure nonpolar compound, it does not penetrate the cornea effectively. The corneal barrier is formed upon maturation of the epithelial cells. The apical corneal epithelial cells form tight junctions that limit paracellular drug permeation.

Therefore, lipophilic drugs typically have at least an order of magnitude higher permeability in the cornea than hydrophilic drugs. Despite the tightness of the corneal epithelial layer, transcorneal permeation is the main route of drug entrance from the lacrimal fluid to the aqueous humor. The amount of drug that penetrates does not depend on the volume of the drop once it is above 10 µl (Maurice, 2002)[6].

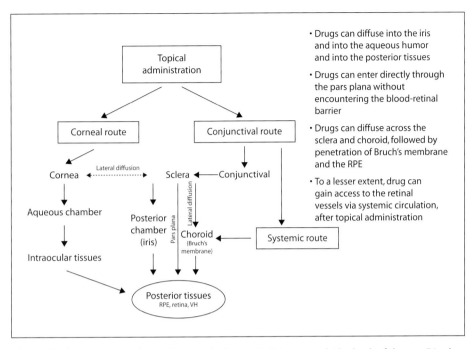

Fig. 1. Ocular transport scheme. How topically applied drugs reach the back of the eye (Hughes et al., 2005)[1].

The maximum concentration in the aqueous humor occurs between 0.5 and 3 h after instillation and there is a ×150,000 dilution of the drop for a hydrophilic drug and a ×1,500 dilution for a lipophilic drug (Maurice, 2002)[6].

Transscleral/Conjunctival Route
The sclera has a large and accessible surface area and a high degree of hydration that renders it conducive to water-soluble substances. It is relatively devoid of cells. Moreover, the sclera has few proteolytic enzymes or protein-binding sites that can degrade or sequester drugs. Scleral permeability does not appreciably decline with age (Olsen et al., 1995)[7].

Mechanically blocking off the corneal surface has little effect on drug penetration into the posterior tissues, suggesting that the transscleral/conjunctival route is the more important for posterior segment drug delivery.

Subconjunctival injection of a lipophobic tracer results in a ×1/100,000 decrease in retinal/vitreous levels. For a very lipophilic tracer, these quantities are about 10 times greater (Maurice, 2002)[6].

New Topical Therapies for Retinal and Choroidal Diseases
Several new topical therapies for retinal and choroidal diseases are under current development.

TargeGen 801 VEGF Receptor/src Kinase Inhibitor
TargeGen 801 VEGF receptor/src kinase inhibitor acts against VEGF receptor/PDGF receptor/ Src family kinases resulting in antipermeability, antiangiogenic, and anti-inflammatory effects. Pharmacokinetic data across multiple species have shown that the drug moves from the front to the back of the eye via a transscleral

route. The drug is delivered as a prodrug, with a molecular weight of 580, which is then converted to an active agent with a molecular weight of 476.

A phase I trial has been completed in 42 healthy volunteers who were given high- and low-dose TG100801, twice daily for 14 days. The drug was well tolerated at both doses. The phase II trial was initiated in patients with choroidal neovascularization due to age-related macular degeneration (AMD). While some clinical benefit was seen, the study was halted due to the formation of corneal deposits. Though the status of the drug is doubtful, next-generation compounds are being developed [unpublished data].

ATG3 (CoMentis) Nonselective nAChR Antagonist

Acetylcholine induces endothelial cell proliferation and migration and mediates angiogenesis in vivo. It is upregulated by hypoxia and is interdependent with the VEGF/fibroblast growth factor pathway. Mecamylamine is a potent small-molecule nonselective antagonist of nAChR with a molecular weight of 167.29. It penetrates to the retina-choroid following topical administration apparently by the transscleral/conjunctival route [unpublished data].

A phase II, randomized, double-masked, placebo-controlled clinical trial for 330 patients with choroidal neovascularization/AMD is currently ongoing.

Ocucure OC-10X

Ocucure OC-10X is a nontoxic vascular targeting agent with selective tubulin inhibition and a molecular weight of 300. The mechanism of action is selective tubulin inhibition with antiangiogenic and antiangiolytic activity. OC-10X is lipid soluble and hence crosses the human cornea. It achieves therapeutic concentrations in the retina and choroid. The downstream mechanism of action may be useful for combination therapy [unpublished data].

Othera OT-551

Othera OT-551 is a small prodrug molecule, which gets converted to TEMPOL (4-hydroxy-2,2,6,6-tetramethylpiperidine-n-oxyl) hydroxylamine. The multiple modes of action include antioxidant, antiangiogenic, and anti-inflammatory properties. It suppresses photooxidative damage in the RPE and photoreceptors and also downregulates disease-induced overexpression of NF-κB. It also inhibits angiogenesis stimulated by VEGF and other factors and is synergistic/additive with ranibizumab.

Othera OT-551 penetrates the cornea, sclera, and distributes to the retina. Phase II clinical trials are ongoing for geographic atrophy, neovascular AMD, and cataract. The phase II trial for geographic atrophy, however, did not show enough benefit to warrant continuation of the trial (Ni et al., 2009)[8].

Pazopanib

Pazopanib (GW786034) is a potent multitargeted receptor tyrosine kinase inhibitor against VEGF receptors 1, 2, and 3; platelet-derived growth factor receptors α and β, and the stem cell factor receptor (c-kit) (Kumar et al., 2007)[9]. It is under clinical development by GlaxoSmithKline for the treatment of AMD using topical administration. Pazopanib has shown significant activity in preclinical models of ocular neovascularization and tumor angiogenesis. A phase I study in healthy volunteers has been completed, as has a 28-day phase II trial in 70 patients with choroidal neovascularization associated with AMD. In the phase II study, patients were treated with Pazopanib eye drops 5 mg/ml once daily, 5 mg/ml 3 times daily, or 2 mg/ml 3 times daily for 28 days. Results have not yet been published but appear to be favorable. A phase III trial for wet AMD is anticipated for 2010.

Iontophoresis for Drug Delivery

A number of chemical and physical enhancement techniques have been developed in an attempt to compromise epithelial barrier function in a reversible manner. Ocular iontophoresis was first investigated in 1908 by the German investigator Wirtz. Iontophoresis involves the application of a small electric potential to maintain a constant current, which allows controlled drug delivery (Wirtz, 1908)[10].

The amount of compound delivered is directly proportional to the quantity of charge passed. The basic electrical principle that oppositely charged ions attract and same charged ions repel is the central tenet of iontophoresis. The ionized substances are driven into the tissue by electrorepulsion at either the anode (for positive drugs) or the cathode (for negatively charged drugs) (Guy, 2000)[11]. This ionic-electric field interaction, also called the Nernst-Planck effect, is the largest contributor to flux enhancement for small ions.

Other advantages include an improved onset time as well as a more rapid offset time, such that once the current is switched off, there is no further transport. Moreover, the current profile can be customized to achieve the desired drug input kinetics depending on whether continuous or pulsatile delivery is required. The electromigration of a molecule depends on the concentration of the drug, the magnitude of current, and the pH value.

Several investigators conducted clinical studies using transscleral iontophoresis of the anti-inflammatory corticosteroid, methylprednisolone hemisuccinate SoluMedrol®. Halhal et al. presented results in a study of patients with acute corneal graft rejection (Halhal et al., 2003)[12]. Iontophoretic treatment of methylprednisolone using 1.5 mA (3 mA/cm^2) for 4 min was performed once daily for 3 consecutive days, with no need for analgesia. Of the eyes treated, 88% demonstrated complete reversal of the rejection processes with no significant side effects.

Periocular/Sub-Tenon/Juxtascleral Drug Delivery
The posterior juxtascleral depot method delivers drugs into the sub-Tenon space onto bare sclera in a depot in the region of the macula.

This method of drug delivery avoids the risk of intraocular damage and endophthalmitis posed by an intravitreal injection. Much like subconjunctival injections, there is an increased risk of systemic drug exposure due to drug contact with orbital tissue when compared with intravitreal injections, though there is much less systemic exposure than occurs with either topical or systemic therapy.

Sub-Tenon Triamcinolone Acetonide
The sub-Tenon administration of triamcinolone acetonide is commonly practiced in clinical ophthalmology. This method provides two important goals. First it specifically delivers the drug to the site of desired activity while avoiding most systemic side effects secondary to systemic drug absorption. Second, the drug is slowly released while contained in a closed sub-Tenon compartment, thus local tissue levels of the drug are constant for a relatively long duration of time. The drug can be delivered in various methods, such as by cannula to the posterior sub-Tenon space or to the orbital floor.

This method of administration may cause a rise in intraocular pressure (IOP) and cataract progression; however, this risk appears to be relatively low (Byun et al., 2009)[13].

Sub-Tenon triamcinolone has been reported to be effective in the treatment of selected cases of refractory diabetic macular edema nonresponsive to laser photocoagulation (Bakri et al., 2005)[14]. It has also been utilized in the treatment of intermediate uveitis (Venkatesh et al., 2007)[15] and other etiologies of refractory macular edema.

Juxtascleral (Modified Sub-Tenon) Anecortave Acetate
Anecortave acetate (Retaane, Alcon) was formulated after removal of the 11β-hydroxyl group and the addition of the 21-acetate group in a typical steroid. Conceptually, the goal was to maintain the therapeutic benefit of the steroid but eliminate the likelihood of steroid-related ocular side effects,

primarily glaucoma and cataract. Anecortave inhibits vascular proliferation by decreasing extracellular protease expression and inhibiting endothelial cell migration. It is administered as a posterior juxtascleral depot of 15 mg/0.5 ml every 6 months using the 19-gauge, 56° posterior juxtascleral cannula. The clinical trials of anecortave acetate in wet AMD and primary open-angle glaucoma have been discontinued since they failed to show efficacy in phase III trials after initially showing benefit in phase II trials (Russell et al., 2007)[16].

Intravitreal Injections

Intravitreal injections have a long history of use in clinical practice. This method provides maximum drug concentrations within the vitreal cavity with minimal systemic absorption. Once used primarily to deliver antibiotic agents to treat endophthalmitis and retinitis and later used to deliver steroids to treat macular edema of various causes, this method is now widespread in the treatment of neovascular AMD, as well as macular edema secondary to vascular occlusive disease and diabetes.

The introduction of a needle through the sclera may be the port of entry of bacteria into the eye. The feared complication of bacterial endophthalmitis does not seem to be as common as once believed. Large-scale clinical trials have yielded low rates of endophthalmitis after intravitreal injections done utilizing topical povidone-iodine, sterile speculum, and topical anesthesia (0.09% for intravitreal ranibizumab) (Bhavsar et al., 2009)[17]. Other authors have reported similar low rates of post-injection endophthalmitis (up to about 2% in the MARINA study, up to 1.4% in the ANCHOR study) (Rosenfeld et al., 2006; Brown et al., 2006)[18,19].

Other main adverse effects reported in large-scale trials are retinal tears (0.4% in the MARINA study), rhegmatogenous retinal detachment (0.4% in the MARINA study, 0.7% in the ANCHOR study), vitreous hemorrhage (up to about 0.8% in both studies) and lens damage (0.4% in the MARINA study) during drug administration. Another known transient complication is an inflammatory reaction. A transient rise in IOP after injection seems to be common.

Intravitreal Drug Delivery Implants
Another way of delivering drugs to the posterior segment is through implants that allow the release of controlled amounts of drugs over time (sustained release). Of these, the ganciclovir implant (Vitrasert®) was the first to be approved by the FDA in 1996, for the treatment of cytomegalovirus retinitis. Subsequently, by using a similar technology containing fluocinolone acetonide, the Retisert® implant was approved in 2005 by the FDA for the treatment of uveitis (fig. 2). *The Ozurdex^{TM} implant,* which is biodegradable and contains dexamethasone, was approved by the FDA in 2009 for the treatment of macular edema caused by retinal vein occlusion. *The Iluvien® implant* containing fluocinolone has completed pivotal trials for diabetic macular edema and is currently under review by the FDA. Other implants are either under development or being tested in clinical trials, including the I-vation implant containing triamcinolone acetonide, the Neurotech encapsulated cell technology implant, which contains ciliary neurotrophic factor, and the brimonidine biodegradable implant.

Vitrasert® Ganciclovir Implant (Bausch and Lomb)
The ganciclovir implant has a drug core surrounded by two membranes, one of which is permeable (polyvinyl alcohol) and the other impermeable (ethylene vinyl acetate). The impermeable ethylene vinyl acetate membrane is discontinuous at the posterior aspect of the implant and releases the drug in a circular ring-like fashion. This structure is similar to that of the Retisert® fluocinolone acetonide implant. Insertion of the ganciclovir and fluocinolone implants requires a surgical incision of 5.5 and 3.5 mm, respectively, of the pars

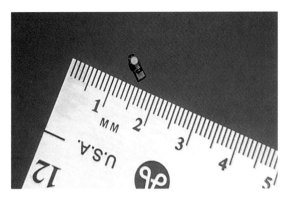

Fig. 2. Retisert® implant.

plana, and both implants are sutured to the eye wall. Neither one is biodegradable.

Local delivery of ganciclovir with the reservoir implant has been shown to be a much more effective way of delivering the drug to the vitreous than intravenous administration (the most efficient systemic drug delivery route). Clinical trials showed that the mean time to reactivation of cytomegalovirus retinitis was 210 days for eyes treated with a ganciclovir implant compared to 70 days for eyes treated with intravenous ganciclovir. The difference in drug quantities is remarkable and demonstrates the power of local therapy for chorioretinal disease. For example, when treating a 70-kg male patient, the ganciclovir implant containing 5 mg ganciclovir typically lasts for 8 months and achieves an intravitreal drug level of 4 μg/ml (Hughes et al., 2005)[1]. For the same treatment duration of 8 months, approximately 100,000 mg of drug would have been administered intravenously to control the disease (assuming induction doses of 5 mg/kg twice daily for 4 weeks to achieve quiescence followed by 6 weeks of maintenance therapy of 5 mg/kg once daily, with recurrence requiring resumption of induction therapy and a repeat of the cycle of 4 weeks induction/6 weeks maintenance throughout an 8-month period). Importantly, the intravenous therapy achieves an intravitreal drug level of only 1 μg/ml (Urtti, 2006)[2]. Thus, with

20,000 times more drug, the level of intravitreal ganciclovir achieved with intravenous injections is 4 times less than that achieved with the reservoir implant. These differences in drug levels may also be critical to ensure the efficacy of other therapeutic agents (Kuppermann et al., 1993; Martin et al., 1994)[20,21].

Retisert® Fluocinolone Acetonide Implant (Bausch and Lomb)

In 2005, the FDA approved an intraocular implant containing fluocinolone acetonide (Retisert®, Bausch and Lomb, Rochester, N.Y., USA) for the treatment of chronic noninfectious uveitis affecting the posterior segment of the eye. Retisert® is implanted into the eye via a surgical procedure entailing a 3.5-mm circumferential incision through the pars plana, and the implant is sutured to the eye wall. The implant is nonbiodegradable (fig. 3).

The fluocinolone implant investigated in the uveitis study has also been studied in a multicenter, randomized, controlled clinical trial for the treatment of diabetic macular edema. Patients in the study were randomized 2:1 to receive either a 0.59-mg fluocinolone implant or standard of care, defined as repeat laser treatment or observation.

Pearson et al. reported that at 36 months the implant resolved edema at the center of the macula and produced a 3-line or more improvement in visual acuity in a significant proportion of eyes studied (n = 197). At 36 months, no evidence of edema was present in 58% of implanted eyes compared with 30% of eyes that received the standard of care (p < 0.001). Visual acuity improvements of 3 lines or more occurred more frequently in implanted eyes (28 vs. 15%, p < 0.05) (Pearson et al., 2006)[22].

The most common serious adverse events in the implanted eyes were cataract development requiring extraction and an increase in IOP. Of the phakic implanted eyes, 95% required cataract surgery, and 35% experienced increased IOP. A filtering procedure was necessary in 28% of implanted

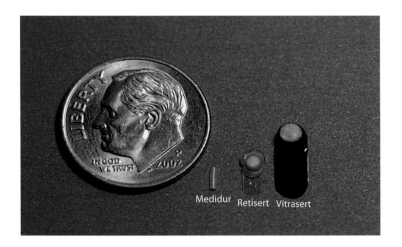

Fig. 3. Comparative sizes of Iluvien®, Retisert®, and Vitrasert®.

eyes, and explantation was performed in 5% of eyes to manage IOP.

Iluvien® Fluocinolone Acetonide Implant (Alimera)
A second fluocinolone acetonide sustained-delivery device has been developed. The injectable Medidur/Iluvien® fluocinolone acetonide implant (Alimera Sciences Inc., Alpharetta, Ga./pSivida, Watertown, Mass., USA) does not require sutures and can be inserted in an ophthalmologist's office. This drug delivery pellet is injected through a 25-gauge needle and floats freely in the vitreous cavity, typically embedding itself in the inferior vitreous base (fig. 4). The Iluvien® implant is not biodegradable and contains roughly half the amount of fluocinolone acetonide of the Retisert® implant.

Two pivotal phase III studies evaluating the Iluvien® implant in patients with diabetic macular edema were recently completed. The Fluocinolone Acetonide in Diabetic Macular Edema (FAME) studies enrolled 956 patients in the USA, Canada, Europe, and India, and evaluated 2 doses of fluocinolone (0.2 and 0.5 µg per day) compared to standard of care (essentially a laser control group). The top-line 2-year primary efficacy and safety data from this study were released in December 2009 and showed the following results: (1) efficacy

trial A: 26.8% of subjects in the low-dose group and 26.0% of those receiving a high dose had a 3-line improvement in best corrected visual acuity (BCVA) at 2 years; (2) efficacy trial B: 30.6 and 31.2% of subjects in the low- and high-dose group, respectively, had an increase in BCVA; (3) safety: the percentage of eyes with IOP greater than 30 mm Hg at any time point was 16.3% in the low-dose and 21.6% in the high-dose group. Surgical trabeculectomy was performed in 2.1% of low-dose patients and 5.1% of high-dose patients by 24 months. The company states that it will submit an application to the FDA for approval for its use (low dose) in patients with diabetic macular edema by the second quarter (pSivida Corporation, 2009)[23].

Ozurdex™ Dexamethasone Biodegradable Implant (Allergan)
The Ozurdex™ dexamethasone implant contains dexamethasone (350 or 700 µg) and poly(lactic-co-glycolic acid), which is a biodegradable copolymer. It hydrolyzes to lactic and glycolic acids, and the lactic acid produced is further metabolized to H_2O and CO_2. Glycolic acid is either excreted or enzymatically converted to other metabolized species. It is inserted in an office setting with a 22-gauge biplanar injection (fig. 5). Like

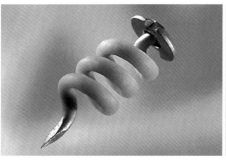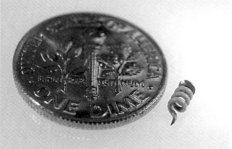

Fig. 4. I-vation sustained drug delivery system.

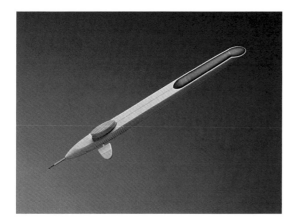

Fig. 5. Ozurdex™ dexamethasone implant.

the Iluvien® implant, the Ozurdex™ implant floats freely in the vitreous cavity and typically embeds itself in the inferior vitreous base. Unlike the Iluvien® implant, which even when emptied of drug leaves a husk permanently in the eye, the Ozurdex™ implant completely biodegrades in the eye once drug delivery is complete (fig. 6).

Two doses of dexamethasone in this biodegradable drug delivery system were evaluated in a 6-month, phase II, multicenter, randomized clinical trial. The phase II trial used a surgical cutdown to place a tableted version of the Ozurdex™ implant into the eye, whereas the phase III trials use a thinner, longer extruded version (rather than tableted

as in the phase II trial) of the Ozurdex™ implant, which is injected into the eye. The 315 patients in the phase II trial had persistent macular edema due to diabetic retinopathy (n = 172), retinal vein occlusion (n = 102), Irvine-Gass syndrome (n = 27), or uveitis (n = 14). In each patient, 1 eye was randomized either to treatment with a 350-µg dose of dexamethasone, a 700-µg dose of dexamethasone (both implants inserted into the vitreal cavity via a small pars plana incision), or observation.

Implantation with Ozurdex™ in this phase II trial resulted in a statistically significant increase in patients gaining 2 and 3 lines or more of visual acuity in a dose-dependent fashion at 90 and 180 days compared with observation (p < 0.025). The percentages of patients who gained 2 lines or more of visual acuity 180 days after implantation were 32.4% in the 700-µg group, 24.3% in the 350-µg group, and 21% in the observation group (p = 0.06). The percentages of patients who gained 3 lines or more of visual acuity 180 days after implantation were 18.1% in the 700-µg group, 14.6% in the 350-µg group, and 7.6% in the observation group (p = 0.02). The visual acuity improvements achieved with the 700-µg implant were consistent across all subgroups at day 90.

In addition, at the primary endpoint, 2% of the patients who were implanted with Ozurdex™ containing either 350 and 700 µg of dexamethasone had an increase in IOP of 10 mm Hg or more

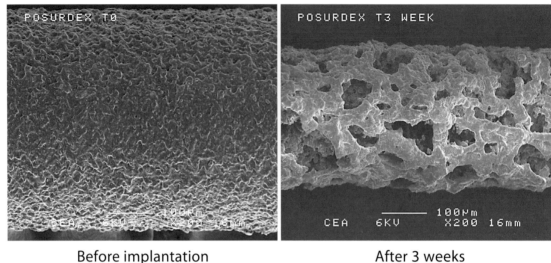

Before implantation   After 3 weeks

Fig. 6. Biodegradation of polymer matrix.

from baseline, compared with 1% of patients in the observation arm. All were successfully managed with either observation or topical IOP-lowering medication. Cataracts were present in 15% of the 350-μg group, 17.8% of the 700-μg group, and 12.4% of the observation group (p < 0.001 vs. observation) (Kuppermann et al., 2007)[24].

Based on the results of this successful phase II trial, several additional clinical trials evaluating the Ozurdex[TM] implant have been performed. Of greatest significance, 2 pivotal phase III trials, which enrolled over 1,209 patients, were completed evaluating Ozurdex[TM] for the treatment of macular edema caused by retinal vein occlusion. As a result of that trial, the FDA approved the Ozurdex[TM] implant for treatment of retinal vein occlusion-related macular edema in June 2009. In that study, in which about two thirds of the patients had branch retinal vein occlusion and one third had central retinal vein occlusion, patients were randomized to 1 of 3 groups: Ozurdex[TM] 700 μg dexamethasone; Ozurdex[TM] 350 μg dexamethasone; observation. They were then followed for 6 months. At the 6-month visit, patients received a second implant if visual acuity was worse

than 20/20 or central retinal thickness was above 250 μm. The primary efficacy endpoint of the trials was time to achieve a 15-letter gain in BCVA. Mean pretreatment visual acuity was 20/80. Mean central retinal thickness was over 500 μm in all 3 of the study groups. The results showed that the mean change in visual acuity peaked at 60 days and tapered off by 180 days in all 3 groups, at which time a cumulative 41% of treated patients had gained 3 or more lines of vision, compared with 23% of sham patients. About 20% of patients overall required only 1 treatment to achieve vision of 20/25 or better and central retinal thickness of 250 μm or better at the 1-year endpoint. Patients receiving a sham implant who went on to receive Ozurdex[TM] treatment at the 6-month time point in the open-label extension phase of the trial also showed a benefit but not as significant as those that received the Ozurdex[TM] at baseline. An IOP rise ≥25 mm Hg occurred in 1.2% of subjects in the 700-μg treatment group, 1.3% of subjects in the 350-μg group, and 0.8% of the sham group. In all groups, the increase in pressure peaked at day 60 and returned to baseline by day 180. All were managed medically or with observation, except

5 eyes that required filtering surgery (2 of which had neovascular glaucoma). Rates of cataract progression did not differ significantly between groups (7% in the 700-µg treatment group, 4% in the 350-µg group, and 5% in the sham group).

Additionally, a phase III trial evaluating the Ozurdex™ implant for the treatment of *diabetic macular edema* has completed enrollment and is in the follow-up phase. Moreover, a trial evaluating Ozurdex™ in combination with Lucentis for the treatment of choroidal neovascularization associated with AMD was completed and showed that adjunctive therapy with Ozurdex™ statistically significantly delays first as-needed ranibizumab injection based on the Kaplan-Meier product limit method (p = 0.016). The 75th percentile of injection-free interval was 12 weeks in the Ozurdex™ group versus 8 weeks in the control group over 6 months. Relative risk of not requiring additional as-needed ranibizumab injection was 3.28 (dexamethasone implant vs. sham, p = 0.048). There were no significant between-group differences in visual acuity or improvement in central retinal thickness. At every time point, fewer patients who were randomized to the Ozurdex™ group needed supplemental ranibizumab therapy compared to patients who had not received Ozurdex™. Treatment-related adverse events were similar between groups, except: increased IOP (9.9 vs. 3.4%) and conjunctival hemorrhage (6.6 vs. 0.8%) in the dexamethasone implant group versus control group (p ≤ 0.044). A trial evaluating the Ozurdex™ implant for the treatment of posterior uveitis has also been completed. That trial showed that the proportion of patients with *posterior uveitis* Ozurdex™ with resolution of vitreous haze at week 8 was significantly higher in patients receiving Ozurdex™ (46.8% in the 700-µg group and 35.5% in the 350-µg group) than in sham-treated patients (11.8%) (p < 0.001). This treatment benefit persisted through the final 26-week visit. The proportion of patients with at least a 15-letter improvement from baseline BCVA was also significantly greater in the Ozurdex™ groups compared

to the sham group at all study visits: 42.9% for Ozurdex™ 700 µg, 39.5% for Ozurdex™ 350 µg, and 6.6% for sham at the primary time point (p < 0.001). Overall the Ozurdex™ 700 µg implant demonstrated greater efficacy than the Ozurdex™ 350 µg implant. The percent of patients with an IOP ≥25 mm Hg peaked at 7.1% for Ozurdex™ 700 µg, 8.7% for Ozurdex™ 350 µg, and 4.2% for the sham group, with no statistically significant difference between groups at any study visit. Cataracts and subcapsular cataracts were reported as adverse events in 11/76 Ozurdex™ 700 µg patients, 10/74 Ozurdex™ 350 µg patients, and 8/75 sham patients (p = 0.769).

Triamcinolone Acetonide I-vation Sustained Drug Delivery System (SurModics)

This implant has a helical design and is implanted through a 25-gauge incision by surgical conjunctival cutdown. The surface area for drug delivery is increased by this novel helical design. This device is self-anchoring within the sclera and is removable (fig. 7). It is nonbiodegradable. The SurModics polymer coating technology has adjustable drug elution rates. The I-vation device contains triamcinolone acetonide as the therapeutic agent.

The prospective, randomized, double-masked Sustained Triamcinolone Release for Inhibition of Diabetic Macular Edema (STRIDE) trial assessed the safety and tolerability of the I-vation triamcinolone acetonide (SurModics, Irvine, Calif., USA) in 30 patients. In the study, patients were randomized to either a slow-release or fast-release implant, each containing 925 µg triamcinolone. They were also stratified by baseline visual acuity and by presence or absence of prior laser treatment.

From screening to 6 months, the proportion of patients with visual acuity of at least 70 ETDRS (Early Treatment Diabetic Retinopathy Study) letters (in the study eye) increased from 14 to 46% in the slow group and from 18 to 41% in the fast group. A gain of more than 15 letters occurred in 8% of patients in the slow group and in 18% of patients in the fast group. Both

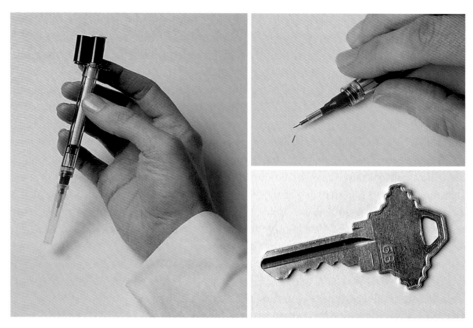

Fig. 7. Alimera Iluvien® FA implant.

implant formulations were associated with improvements in macular thickness. Every phakic eye in the study developed a visually significant cataract. Increases in IOP occurred in 50% of eyes, though none required surgery to treat the IOP increase. Further studies with I-vation triamcinolone acetonide have currently been suspended by the sponsor.

Brimonidine Biodegradable Implant (Allergan)
Brimonidine tartrate has been shown to have neuroprotectant effects on the optic nerve and retina in preclinical studies. A brimonidine implant containing 200 or 400 mg brimonidine tartrate was developed by Allergan using the same biodegradable platform as the Ozurdex™ dexamethasone implant. This implant is designed to release the drug for 6 months, then the poly(lactic-co-glycolic acid) polymer subsequently biodegrades to lactic acid and carbon dioxide over a period of a few additional months. Over 120 patients with

bilateral geographic atrophy were enrolled in a phase II trial (NCT00658619) and were injected with either implant or sham at baseline and again at 6 months. Results are anticipated in 2010.

Encapsulated Cell Technology (Neurotech)
This interesting drug delivery technology utilizes a unique cell-based approach. The surgically implanted pellet, which is sutured to the eye wall, contains modified RPE cells in an immune protected capsule. The RPE cells are programmed to produce therapeutic levels of ciliary neurotrophic factor, a neuroprotectant agent, for 3 years. The RPE cells, however, can be programmed to produce almost any complex molecule including bevacizumab and ranibizumab. This technology addresses a key problem of long-term drug delivery of complex molecules – how to manage long-term stability of proteins and other complex molecules at the physiologic intravitreal temperature of 37°C. In this case,

since the drug-eluting RPE cells are producing the molecules continuously, no long-term stability issues occur. A phase I trial for retinitis pigmentosa and a phase II trial for geographic atrophy have been completed.

Conclusion

In conclusion, many ocular diseases still need improved pharmacological solutions. First-generation drug delivery technology exists and is being further refined. Future devices will allow longer drug duration and increased target specificity. Longer-acting reservoir implants have good long-term control of disease but have the potential for drug or suppressive side effects. Shorter-acting biodegradable inserts have potentially less drug or suppressive side effects but may not control the disease as well in the long term. Different approaches may be used in different diseases to achieve maximum benefit with minimal risks.

Intraocular Self-Reporting Nanocrystals (Smart Dust) for Intraocular Drug Delivery

Nanoparticles are small porous particles made from drug-laden photonic crystals. Spectral properties of photonic crystals (empty vs. drug-laden) permit in vivo monitoring of residual drug in crystals. The nanostructure allows control of the temporal release profile. Dexamethasone has been shown to be stable for months in this nanostructure, and the release of drug results in a change of crystal color. Large molecules such as VEGF Fab can be loaded into crystals.

References

1 Hughes PM, Olejnik O, Chang-Lin JE, Wilson CG: Topical and systemic drug delivery to the posterior segments. Adv Drug Deliv Rev 2005;57:2010–2032.

2 Urtti A: Challenges and obstacles of ocular pharmacokinetics and drug delivery. Adv Drug Deliv Rev 2006;58:1131–1315.

3 Chiou GC, Watanabe K: Drug delivery to the eye. Pharmacol Ther 1982;17:269–278.

4 Ahmed I, Patton TF: Importance of the noncorneal absorption route in topical ophthalmic drug delivery. Invest Ophthalmol Vis Sci 1985;26:584–587.

5 Geroski DH, Edelhauser HF: Drug delivery for posterior segment eye disease. Invest Ophthalmol Vis Sci 2000;41:961–964.

6 Maurice DM: Drug delivery to the posterior segment from drops. Surv Ophthalmol 2002;47(suppl 1):S41–S52.

7 Olsen TW, Edelhauser HF, Lim JI, Geroski DH: Human scleral permeability. Effects of age, cryotherapy, transscleral diode laser, and surgical thinning. Invest Ophthalmol Vis Sci 1995;36:1893–903.

8 Ni Z, Hui P: Emerging pharmacologic therapies for wet age-related macular degeneration. Ophthalmologica 2009;223:401–410.

9 Kumar R, Knick VB, Rudolph SK, Johnson JH, Crosby RM, Crouthamel MC, et al: Pharmacokinetic-pharmacodynamic correlation from mouse to human with pazopanib, a multikinase angiogenesis inhibitor with potent antitumor and antiangiogenic activity. Mol Cancer Ther 2007;6:2012–2021.

10 Wirtz R: Die Ionentherapie in der Augenheilkunde. Klin Monbl Augenheilkd 1908;46:543–549.

11 Guy J: New therapies for optic neuropathies: development in experimental models. Curr Opin Ophthalmol 2000;11:421–429.

12 Halhal M, Renard G, Bejjani RA, Behar-Cohen F: Corneal graft rejection and corticoid iontophoresis: 3 case reports. J Fr Ophthalmol 2003;26:391–395.

13 Byun YS, Park YH: Complications and safety profile of posterior subtenon injection of triamcinolone acetonide. J Ocul Pharmacol Ther 2009;25:159–162.

14 Bakri SJ, Kaiser PK: Posterior subtenon triamcinolone acetonide for refractory diabetic macular edema. Am J Ophthalmol 2005;139:290–294.

15 Venkatesh P, Abhas Z, Garg S, Vohra R: Prospective optical coherence tomographic evaluation of the efficacy of oral and posterior subtenon corticosteroids in patients with intermediate uveitis. Graefes Arch Clin Exp Ophthalmol 2007;245:59–67.

16 Russell SR, Hudson HL, Jerdan JA, Anecortave Acetate Clinical Study Group: Anecortave acetate for the treatment of exudative age-related macular degeneration – A review of clinical outcomes. Surv Ophthalmol 2007;52(suppl 1):S79–S90.

17 Bhavsar AR, Googe JM Jr, Stockdale CR, Bressler NM, Brucker AJ, Elman MJ, Glassman AR, Diabetic Retinopathy Clinical Research Network: Risk of endophthalmitis after intravitreal drug injection when topical antibiotics are not required: the diabetic retinopathy clinical research network laser-ranibizumab-triamcinolone clinical trials. Arch Ophthalmic 2009;127:1581–1583.

18 Rosenfeld PJ, Brown DM, Heier JS, Boyer DS, Kaiser PK, Chung CY, Kim RY, MARINA Study Group: Ranibizumab for neovascular age-related macular degeneration. N Engl J Med 2006;355:1419–1431.

19 Brown DM, Kaiser PK, Michels M, Soubrane G, Heier JS, Kim RY, Sy JP, Schneider S, ANCHOR Study Group: Ranibizumab vs verteporfin for neovascular age-related macular degeneration. N Engl J Med 2006;355:1432–1444.

20 Kuppermann BD, Quiceno JI, Flores-Aguilar M, Connor JD, Capparelli EV, Sherwood CH, Freeman WR: Intravitreal ganciclovir concentration after intravenous administration in AIDS patients with cytomegalovirus retinitis: implications for therapy. J Infect Dis 1993;168:1506–1509.

21 Martin DF, Parks DJ, Mellow SD, Ferris FL, Walton RC, Remaley NA, Chew EY, Ashton P, Davis MD, Nussenblatt RB: Treatment of cytomegalovirus retinitis with an intraocular sustained-release ganciclovir implant. A randomized controlled clinical trial. Arch Ophthalmol 1994;112:1531–1539.

22 Pearson P, Levy B, Comstock T, Fluocinolone Acetonide Implant Study Group: Fluocinolone acetonide intravitreal implant to treat diabetic macular edema: 3-year results of a multi-center clinical trial. Invest Ophthalmol Vis Sci 2006;47: 5442.

23 pSivida Corporation: Form 8-K document submitted to the Securities and Exchange Commision (SEC). December 23, 2009.

24 Kuppermann BD, Blumenkranz MS, Haller JA, Williams GA, Weinberg DV, Chou C, Whitcup SM, Dexamethasone DDS Phase II Study Group: Randomized controlled study of an intravitreous dexamethasone drug delivery system in patients with persistent macular edema. Arch Ophthalmol 2007;125:309–317.

Prof. Anat Loewenstein
Department of Ophthalmology, Tel Aviv Medical Center
Sackler Faculty of Medicine, Tel Aviv University
6 Weizmann St.
Tel Aviv 64239 (Israel)
E-Mail anatl@tasmc.health.gov.il

Chapter 6

Coscas G (ed): Macular Edema.
Dev Ophthalmol. Basel, Karger, 2010, vol 47, pp 73–110

Diabetic Macular Edema

Francesco Bandello[a] · Maurizio Battaglia Parodi[a] · Paolo Lanzetta[b] ·
Anat Loewenstein[c] · Pascale Massin[d] · Francesca Menchini[b] ·
Daniele Veritti[b]

[a]Department of Ophthalmology, Scientific Institute San Raffaele, Milan, and [b]Department of Ophthalmology, University of Udine,
Udine, Italy; [c]Department of Ophthalmology, Tel Aviv Medical Center, Tel Aviv, Israel; [d]Department of Ophthalmology, Lariboisière
Hospital, Paris, France

Abstract

Diabetic macular edema (DME), defined as a retinal thickening involving or approaching the center of the macula, represents the most common cause of vision loss in patients affected by diabetes mellitus. In the last few years, many diagnostic tools have been proven useful in the detection and the monitoring of the features characterizing DME. On the other hand, several therapeutic approaches can now be proposed on the basis of the DME-specific characteristics. The aim of the present chapter is to thoroughly delineate the clinical and morphofunctional characteristics of DME and its current treatment perspectives. The pathogenesis and the course of DME require a complex approach with multidisciplinary intervention both at the systemic and local levels.

Copyright © 2010 S. Karger AG, Basel

Introduction and Definition

Despite continued improvement in diagnostic screening techniques and the proven efficacy of laser treatment in preventing visual loss, diabetic retinopathy (DR) remains the leading cause of legal blindness in working-age populations of industrialized countries.

Future perspectives are not encouraging: the World Health Organization estimates that more than 180 million people worldwide have diabetes and this number is expected to raise to epidemic proportions within the next 20 years, fuelled by increased life expectancy, sedentary lifestyle, and obesity (King et al., 1998)[1]. Although our understanding of biochemical and hemodynamic stimuli and mediators that ultimately lead to microvascular changes in diabetic patients has progressively improved, and despite a substantial body of scientific evidence that underlies current treatment recommendations for DR, this disease remains a *major public health problem* with significant socioeconomic implications, affecting approximately 50% of diabetic subjects.

Vision loss due to DR may result from several mechanisms. Macular edema or capillary nonperfusion may directly impair central vision. Retinal and/or disk neovascularization in the course of proliferative diabetic retinopathy (PDR) can cause severe and often irreversible visual loss due to vitreous/preretinal hemorrhage and tractional retinal detachment. While complications of PDR lead more frequently to severe visual loss, the *most common cause* of visual impairment among diabetic patients is diabetic macular edema (DME), accounting for about three fourths of cases of visual loss.

The development of macular edema is not limited to diabetic patients but represents a common response to a broad spectrum of potential problems caused by retinal disease. The predilection of the edema to the macular region is probably secondary to the higher susceptibility of the macula to both ischemic and oxidative stress and to its peculiar anatomical features, for example, loose intercellular adhesion and an absence of Müller cells in the fovea.

The pathogenesis of DME is complex and multifactorial and mainly results from the disruption of the blood-retinal barrier (BRB), leading to accumulation of fluid and serum macromolecules in the intercellular space (Antonetti et al., 1999)[2]. Accelerated apoptosis of pericytes and endothelial cells, acellular capillaries, basement membrane thickening, and capillary occlusion all contribute to endothelial damage and breakdown of the inner BRB.

Significant variations in the incidence and prevalence of DME have been reported in various epidemiologic studies, depending on the type of diabetes (type I or II), the treatment modality (insulin, oral hypoglycemic agents, or diet only), and the mean duration of diabetes. DME can develop at any stage of DR, but it occurs more frequently as the duration of diabetes and the severity of DR increase. In the Wisconsin Epidemiologic Study of Diabetic Retinopathy (WESDR), the 10-year rate of developing DME was 20.1% in patients with type I diabetes, 13.9% in patients with type II diabetes not using insulin, and 25.4% in type II diabetes patients using insulin. DME prevalence increases with the severity of DR: it effects 3% of eyes with mild nonproliferative diabetic retinopathy (NPDR), rises to 38% of eyes with moderate to severe NPDR, and reaches 71% of eyes with PDR.

The natural history of DME is characterized by a slow progression of *retinal thickening* until the center of the macula is involved, causing visual

acuity deterioration. Spontaneous resolution of DME is rare and usually secondary to improvement in systemic risk factors, such as glycemic control, hypertension, or hypercholesterolemia. If untreated, 29% of eyes with DME and foveal involvement experience moderate visual loss (doubling of the visual angle) after 3 years. Spontaneous visual recovery is also unusual, with improvement of at least 3 Early Treatment Diabetic Retinopathy Study (ETDRS) lines occurring in 5% of cases.

Definition and Classification

The diagnosis of macular edema is clinical. Traditionally, the gold standard for diagnosing DME is stereoscopic fundus photography. In clinical practice, noncontact fundus biomicroscopy is often employed, and it can be useful, especially when there is significant retinal thickening. In early or borderline cases, however, contact lens biomicroscopy is considered more sensitive.

Fluorescein angiography is not necessary for diagnosing DME, but it provides a qualitative assessment of vascular leakage, helps in identifying treatable lesions, and is essential for assessing the presence of an enlargement of the foveal avascular zone (FAZ), which may be associated with poor visual prognosis (Antonetti et al., 1999)[2].

Conventionally, DME is defined as retinal thickening or presence of hard exudates within 1 disk diameter of the center of the macula. The term 'clinically significant macular edema' (CSME) was coined to characterize the severity of the disease and to provide a threshold level to apply laser photocoagulation (table 1) (Early Treatment Diabetic Retinopathy Study Research Group, 1985)[3].

In addition to this ophthalmoscopic classification, DME can be classified into focal and diffuse. *Focal macular edema* is characterized by the presence of localized areas of retinal thickening, derived from focal leakage of individual microaneurysms or clusters of microaneurysms. Fluorescein

Bandello · Battaglia Parodi · Lanzetta · Loewenstein · Massin · Menchini · Veritti

Table 1. ETDRS definition of CSME

- Thickening of the retina at or within 500 µm of the center of the macula
- Hard exudates at or within 500 µm of the center of the macula, if associated with thickening of adjacent retina
- A zone or zones of retinal thickening at least 1 disk area in extent, any part of which is within 1 disk diameter of the center of the macula

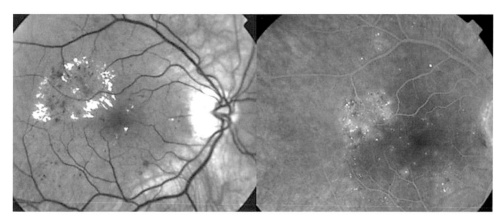

Fig. 1. Focal DME. Left: red-free photograph shows circinate ring of hard exudates surrounding microaneurysms. Right: fluorescein angiography reveals leakage from hyperfluorescent punctate lesions corresponding to microaneurysms.

angiography clearly demonstrates that microaneurysms are the major source of dye leakage (fig. 1). Areas of focal leakage are often demarcated by a partial or complete ring of hard exudates with a circinate appearance.

Diffuse macular edema is derived from extensively damaged capillaries, microaneurysms, and arterioles, and it is characterized by a more widespread thickening of the macula secondary to generalized abnormal permeability of the retinal capillary bed that appears to be diffusely dilated (fig. 2). Diffuse macular edema tends to be symmetric and without significant exudation. Ocular and systemic risk factors for the development and progression of diffuse DME are an increasing microaneurysm count, advanced retinopathy,

vitreomacular traction, adult-onset diabetes, renal disease, and severe hypertension.

Cystoid macular edema, often associated with diffuse macular edema, results from a generalized breakdown of the BRB with fluid accumulation in a petaloid pattern, primarily in the outer plexiform and inner nuclear layers. The presence or absence of cystoid appearance, however, does not directly influence the prognosis and management of DME.

In clinical practice, the distinction between focal and diffuse edema is not always clear, and a wide variety of *mixed forms* are observed. These two patterns of leakage can be clearly visualized by fluorescein angiography. It is important to note that leakage on fluorescein angiography is not

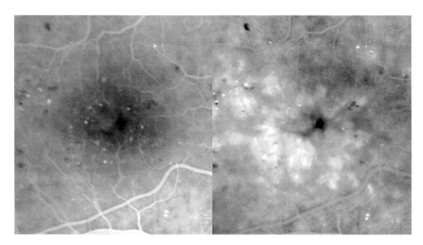

Fig. 2. Diffuse DME. Fluorescein angiography (left: early phase; right: late phase) shows leakage throughout the posterior pole with late dye pooling at the macula in a petaloid pattern.

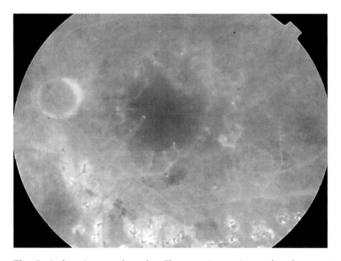

Fig. 3. Ischemic maculopathy. Fluorescein angiography shows extensive capillary nonperfusion at the macula, with enlargement and irregularity of the FAZ.

always synonymous with retinal edema, since it does not necessarily indicate retinal thickening.

Once the diagnosis of CSME and the decision to treat have been made, fluorescein angiography is extremely useful in helping to decide the treatment strategy and in determining the vascular perfusion. Ischemic or nonperfused macular edema is an important variant of DME, and it can be revealed only by fluorescein angiography.

Ischemic maculopathy is defined by the presence of rarefaction and occlusion of the perifoveal capillary network, with doubling of the extension of the FAZ (fig. 3). Normally the FAZ is approximately 350–750 µm in diameter. Even in

Bandello · Battaglia Parodi · Lanzetta · Loewenstein · Massin · Menchini · Veritti

the absence of macular edema in diabetic eyes, abnormalities of the FAZ are often seen, and include irregular margins and widening of the intercapillary spaces.

On a pathogenic basis, DME can be further classified into prevalently retinovascular or nonretinovascular, the latter definition including different clinical entities, such as diabetic retinal pigment epitheliopathy, tractional macular edema, and macular edema with taut, attached posterior hyaloid. In most cases, different pathogenic components are combined, making it difficult to decide which component is prevalent and what treatment is the most indicated.

The common pathway that results in DME is *disruption of the BRB*. The mechanism of the BRB breakdown is multifactorial: it is caused by changes in the tight junction, pericyte loss, endothelial cell loss, retinal vessel leukostasis, upregulation of vesicular transport, retinal vessel dilation, and vitreoretinal traction.

Prevalently retinovascular DME is characterized by abnormal permeability of retinal capillaries, and it includes previously described focal or diffuse DME caused by pathological changes primarily of retinal vascular origin, including pericyte dropout, microaneurysm formation, and generalized breakdown of the inner BRB. Fluorescein angiography is indispensable to distinguish between prevalently retinovascular and nonretinovascular macular edema. In prevalently retinovascular macular edema, early fluorescein angiograms clearly define microvascular abnormalities as the major source of late dye leakage.

In 1995, an unusual form of diabetic maculopathy was described for the first time, in which the retinal pigment epithelium (RPE) and the subretinal space played a main role (Weinberger et al., 1995)[4]. Fluorescein angiograms of 1,850 patients with NPDR were examined, and 1% of cases exhibited an area of diffuse RPE leakage spread around the macular region in the late phase; no cystic changes or cystoid macular edema were present in any of the eyes. This condition was named *diabetic retinal pigment epitheliopathy*.

DME may be caused or exacerbated by persistent *vitreomacular traction* by residual cortical vitreous on the macula following posterior vitreous detachment, macular traction due to tractional proliferative membrane, thickened and taut posterior hyaloid that may exert tangential macular traction and cause edema (Lewis et al., 1992; Harbour et al., 1996)[5,6]. On biomicroscopy, a thick, taut, glistening posterior hyaloid is visible, while fluorescein angiography exhibits a characteristic early hypofluorescence, and deep, diffuse round late leakage, often from vascular arcade to arcade (fig. 4). Unlike what occurs in prevalently retinovascular DME, in these cases there is no topographic correspondence between microvascular abnormalities visible in the early phase of the angiography and late leakage.

Optical coherence tomography (OCT) is a noninvasive, noncontact instrument, which provides cross-sectional, high-resolution images of the retina and a quantitative assessment of retinal thickness with a high degree of accuracy and reproducibility. The advantage of OCT in diagnosing CSME as compared to fundus biomicroscopy is its ability to provide an objective, quantitative, measure of retinal thickness as well as additional morphological details.

Correlation between OCT and fluorescein angiography findings in the course of CSME is fairly good: about 60% of patients with foveal thickening and homogeneous intraretinal optical reflectivity on OCT have focal leakage on fluorescein angiography, while more than 90% of patients with diffuse cystoid leakage exhibit foveal thickening with decreased optical reflectivity in the outer retinal layers or foveal thickening with subretinal fluid accumulation on OCT (Kang et al., 2004)[7]. Furthermore, OCT clearly visualizes the vitreoretinal interface and reveals the presence and extent of vitreomacular traction and epiretinal membrane (fig. 5).

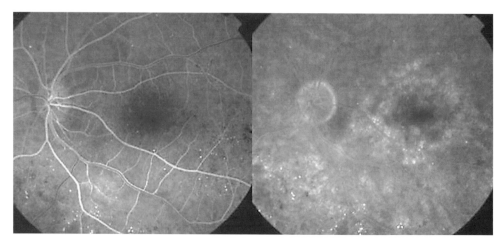

Fig. 4. Macular edema associated with taut, attached posterior hyaloid. In early (left) angiographic phases, hypofluorescence and minimal diabetic changes are evident. In the late (right) phase, fluorescein angiography shows diffuse leakage around the macular area.

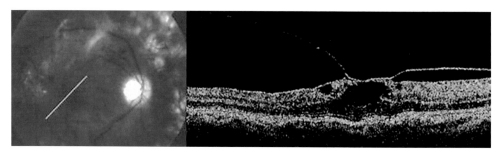

Fig. 5. Localized vitreous traction. Red-free photograph (left) shows the presence of vitreous strand adherent to the macula. The presence of a focal traction, causing loss of physiologic foveal depression, is clearly visualized by OCT (right).

An *international clinical disease severity scale* has been developed for DR and DME (table 2). This scale, based on the ETDRS classification of DR and on the data collected in clinical trials and epidemiologic studies of DR, was proposed with the aim to improve communication between ophthalmologists and primary care physicians involved in diabetic patient care. Validation studies of the international scales are under way. According to the International Clinical Diabetic Retinopathy and Diabetic Macular Edema Disease Severity Scales, eyes with apparent DME are separated from those with no apparent thickening or lipid in the macula (DME present and absent); an additional division is based on the distance of retinal thickening and/or lipid from the fovea (mild, moderate, and severe) (Wilkinson et al., 2003)[8].

Epidemiology

DME occurs in approximately 14% of diabetics and can be found in both type I and type II patients (Girach and Lund-Andersen, 2007)[9]. The

Bandello · Battaglia Parodi · Lanzetta · Loewenstein · Massin · Menchini · Veritti

Table 2. International clinical DME disease severity scale (Wilkinson et al., 2003)[8]

Proposed disease severity level	Findings on dilated ophthalmoscopy
Diabetic macular edema apparently absent	No apparent retinal thickening or hard exudates in posterior pole
Diabetic macular edema apparently present	Some apparent retinal thickening or hard exudates in posterior pole
If diabetic macular edema is present, it can be classified into:	
Diabetic macular edema present	• Mild diabetic macular edema: some retinal thickening or hard exudates in posterior pole but distant from the center of the macula
	• Moderate diabetic macular edema: retinal thickening or hard exudates approaching the center of the macula but not involving the center
	• Severe diabetic macular edema: retinal thickening or hard exudates involving the center of the macula

reported risk factors for occurrence and progression of DME, most of which are derived from large studies such as the WESDR and the UK Prospective Diabetes Study, are duration of diabetes, degree of metabolic control, elevated glycosylated hemoglobin A_{1c}, severity of DR, hypertension, low socioeconomic status, and older age (Girach and Lund-Andersen, 2007; Williams et al., 2004)[9,10].

Additional risk factors for progression of DME have been reported including dyslipidemia, microalbuminuria, and proteinuria. (Among the WESDR patients with gross proteinuria at baseline, 95% had an increased risk for progression to DME.) Pregnancy may cause progression of DME and PDR with postpartum regression in some patients and persistent edema in others. Elevated plasma levels of IL-6 were also strongly related to the severity of macular edema (Girach and Lund-Andersen, 2007)[9].

Prevalence

Prevalence studies on type II diabetes show that 2–8.2% of diabetic patients had macular edema 5 years after the diagnosis, while 28% had the condition 20 years after the diagnosis. For type I diabetic patients, 0.0% had macular edema 5 years after the diagnosis, while 29% had the condition 20 years after the diagnosis (Williams et al., 2004)[10].

A study of a mixed population in the United States found a slightly different prevalence of macular edema: 36.7% of diabetic African Americans had DR and 11.1% had macular edema; 37.4% of diabetic Hispanics had DR and 10.7% had macular edema; 24.8% of diabetic Caucasians had DR and 2.7% had macular edema, and 25.7% of diabetic Chinese had DR and 8.9% had macular edema (Varma et al., 2004)[11].

Patients treated with insulin were found to have a higher prevalence of macular edema. Fifteen years after the diagnosis, 18% of type I and 20% of type II diabetic patients treated with insulin had macular edema, while only 12% of type I and type II diabetic patients not treated with insulin had macular edema. The prevalence of CSME varies worldwide. Among American Caucasians, CSME was found in 6% of type I diabetic patients and in 2–4% of type II diabetic patients. The African American population shows a prevalence of 8.6% of CSME in type II and in the mixed cohort, and the Hispanic population shows a prevalence of 6.2% in the mixed cohort (Williams et al., 2004; Varma et al., 2004)[10,11].

The prevalence of CSME in the type II diabetic population in South America is 3.4–5.5%, while 5.4% of type II diabetics in Europe had CSME. In the UK specifically, 2.3–6.4% of type I diabetics and 6.4–6.8% of the mixed cohort had CSME. The prevalence of CSME in the type II diabetic population of South Asia was 6.4–13.3%, and 2.3% specifically in China. With regard to the duration of the disease, the prevalence of CSME was 5% in type I and 2% in type II during the first years after diagnosis and an increase to 20% in type I patients over 25 years was noted (Williams et al., 2004)[10].

Incidence

The incidence of CSME is reported to be correlated with the increase in the number of retinal microaneurysms (Girach and Lund-Andersen, 2007)[9] and the duration of the disease. In American Caucasians with a diabetes duration of over 10 years, the incidence of CSME has been reported to be 20.1% in type I patients and 13.9% in type II patients. When a mixed cohort of the Australian population was studied, an incidence as high as 7% per year was reported. In the Scandinavian population, the incidence of CSME in type I diabetic patients over a 4-year period was 3.4%. The 4-year incidence of CSME in type I and type II insulin-treated diabetic patients was found to be 4.3 and 5.1%, while type II noninsulin-treated patients had a 1.3% incidence (Williams et al., 2004)[10].

Diagnosis

Macular edema is clinically defined as retinal thickening of the macula as seen on biomicroscopy. When moderate, the thickening may be difficult to diagnose, and contact lenses with good stereoscopy, such as Centralis Direct® (Volk), or noncontact lenses of 60, 78, or 90 dpt could be used.

The biomicroscopic assessment of the retinal thickness is subjective, and the clinical examination can only quantify thicknesses at above 1.6 times the normal rate (Brown et al., 2004)[12]. Today, the OCT evaluation for retinal thickness is objective.

Ancillary Tests

Fluorescein Angiography
Fluorescein angiography visualizes leakage from incompetent vessels that have lost their ability to prevent the egress of dye into the retinal tissue. Additionally, in the early phase of the angiogram, capillary dilatation may be seen in the perifoveal region. Late pooling of the dye may be evident assuming a petaloid pattern when accumulation of dye involves the perifoveal region or it may show a honeycomb appearance when occurring outside the perifoveal area.

Fluorescein angiography shows the cause of leakage from microaneurysms or macular capillaries. It may also enable assessment as to the extent of macular nonperfusion, which has a significant prognostic value. Fluorescein leakage is not, however, sufficient to diagnose macular edema; a simple diffusion of fluorescein without retinal thickening is not included as part of the definition of macular edema.

Optical Coherence Tomography
OCT imaging helps in immediately estimating intraretinal modifications, pinpointing the eventual existence of infraclinical foveolar detachment, assessing the vitreoretinal juncture, and precisely

measuring the thickened retina (Massin et al., 2006)[13]. In the case of DME, OCT demonstrates increased retinal thickness with areas of low intraretinal reflectivity prevailing in the outer retinal layers and the loss of foveal depression.

Spectral domain OCT (SD-OCT) can show small cysts, sometimes in the inner retina, even when retinal thickening is moderate (fig. 6, 7). Hard exudates are detected as spots of high reflectivity with low reflective areas behind them and are found primarily in the outer retinal layers. Two distinct features (Otani et al., 1999)[14] can be observed: cystoid spaces, which appear as small round hyporeflective lacunae with high-signal elements bridging the retinal layers, and outer retinal swelling, characterized by an ill-defined, widespread hyporeflective area of thickening. It is distinguished from serous retinal detachment by the absence of the highly anterior reflective boundary. Small spots with high reflectivity may be seen with SD-OCT, which may be due to protein or lipid deposits secondary to an early breakdown of the BRB (fig. 7) (Bolz et al., 2009)[15].

OCT is particularly useful in detecting a feature combined with macular edema not easily seen on biomicroscopy, i.e. *serous retinal detachment* (fig. 7) (Ozdemir et al., 2005, Catier et al., 2005)[16,17]. Serous retinal detachment, seen in 15% of eyes with DME, appears as a shallow elevation of the retina, with an optically clear space between the retina and the RPE, and a distinct outer border of the detached retina. The pathogenesis and the functional consequences of serous retinal detachment associated with cystoid macular edema are still unknown. However, in a series of 78 eyes with macular edema examined on OCT, the presence of serous retinal detachment was not correlated with poorer visual acuity (Catier et al., 2005)[17]. It has been shown that a serous retinal detachment could be present combined with moderate retinal thickening and disappear when DME worsens (Gaucher et al., 2008)[18]. It may be a sign of early dysfunction of the outer BRB.

OCT seems particularly relevant to analyze the *vitreomacular relationship*. Indeed OCT is much more accurate than biomicroscopy in determining the status of a posterior hyaloid when it is only slightly detached from the macular surface (Gaucher et al., 2005)[19]. In some cases of DME, the posterior hyaloid on OCT is thick and hyperreflective. It is partially detached from the posterior pole and taut over it but remains attached to the disk and to the top of the raised macular surface, on which it exerts an obvious vitreomacular traction (fig. 8). In these cases, vitrectomy is beneficial (Lewis et al., 1992; Massin et al., 2003; Thomas et al., 2005; Pendergast et al., 2000)[5,20–22]. In other cases, the posterior hyaloid appears slightly reflective, detached from the retinal surface in the perifoveolar area, and attached at the foveolar center. This aspect is quite common and corresponds to early posterior vitreous detachment (fig. 7) (Gaucher et al., 2005; Uchino et al., 2001)[19,23].

One major advantage of OCT is that it allows *measurement of retinal thickness* from the tomograms by means of computer image-processing techniques (Hee et al., 1995, 1998)[24,25]. OCT allows retinal thickness to be calculated as the distance between the anterior and posterior highly reflective boundaries of the retina, which are located by a thresholding algorithm. The anterior boundary corresponds to the internal limiting membrane (ILM) and is well defined because of the contrast between the nonreflective vitreous and the backscattering of the retina. In SD-OCT, the posterior boundary is located as the hyperreflective band visible just above the RPE band, which is thought to correspond to the signal of the photoreceptor and especially to the junction between the inner and outer photoreceptor segments. Finally, on SD-OCT, the posterior boundary is located differently according to the various devices. Since the commercialization of OCT systems, several types of software have become available to quantify macular thickening. Hee and associates have developed a standardized mapping

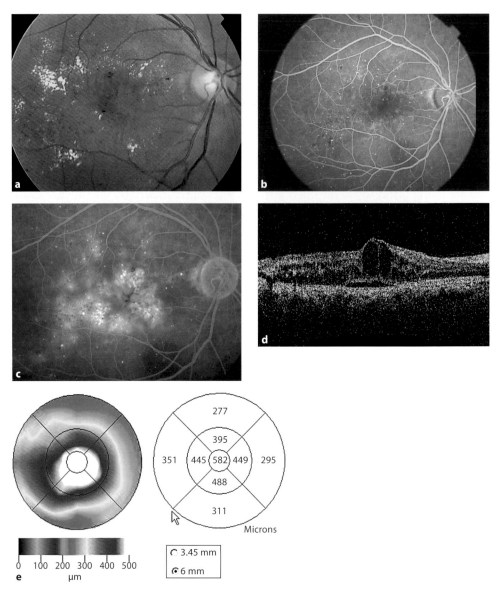

Fig. 6. Severe DME. **a** Color fundus photography: severe macular edema with numerous microaneurysms and retinal hemorrhages at the posterior pole, associated with retinal exudates and two large central cysts. **b** Early frame of the angiography: numerous microaneurysms associated with intraretinal microvascular abnormalities, and capillary closure. **c** Late frame of the angiography: cystoid macular edema. **d** OCT scan (Cirrhus OCT, Zeiss) showing severe retinal thickening with loss of the foveal depression, accumulation of fluid predominantly in the outer retinal layers and in a subfoveal serous retinal detachment, and two large central cysts occupying the entire thickness of the retina. **e** Corresponding OCT mapping.

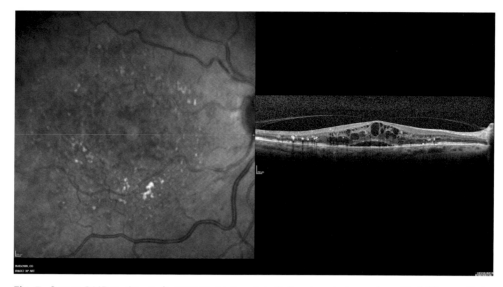

Fig. 7. Severe DME on Spectralis OCT (Heidelberg). Left: Fundus photography with OCT scan. Right: Severe retinal thickening with serous retinal detachment. Several intraretinal cysts are visible, prevailing in the outer retinal layers, but small cysts are located in the inner layers as well. Retinal exudates appear as spots of high reflectivity with low reflective areas behind them, and small spots with high reflectivity are also seen with SD-OCT which may be due to protein or lipid deposits. In addition, a perifoveolar detachment of the posterior hyaloid is well visible. The line of the photoreceptors is relatively well preserved.

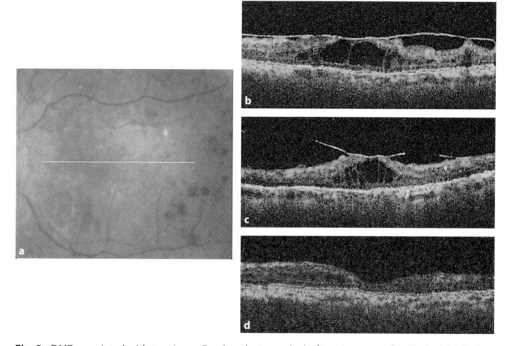

Fig. 8. DME associated with traction. **a** Fundus photography before vitrectomy. **b**, **c** Retinal thickening is combined with a thickened epiretinal membrane. **d** After vitrectomy, retinal thickness had decreased, with a normal foveal depression.

OCT protocol, which consists of 6 radial tomograms 6 mm long in a spoke pattern centered on the fovea, and it has the advantage of concentrating measurements in the central fovea (Hee et al., 1998)[25]. The retinal thickness is computed for a total of 600 macular locations along these 6 intersecting lines.

Retinal thickness is displayed in two different manners: first as a 2-dimensional color-coded map of retinal thickness in the posterior pole, with brighter colors indicating areas of increased retinal thickness and, for quantitative evaluation, retinal thickness is reported as a numeric average of the 9 ETDRS-type areas. With the Humphrey Stratus OCT, new macular mapping algorithms have become available. The fast macular mapping protocol allows the 6 radial scans, each containing 128 A-scans, to be performed in a single session of 1.92 s. The high-density scan protocol consists of 6 separate 6-mm radial lines, each containing 512 points, obtained in 1.28 s, taking a total time of 7.32 s to acquire the entire set.

Regarding SD-OCT, a new type of macular mapping is proposed: macular mapping in a 3-dimensional cube, a system for scanning multiple parallel lines, which provides a more homogenous distribution of measured points within the macular region and is also a real source of 3-dimensional image reconstruction. A number of studies have demonstrated good reproducibility of OCT measurements of single scans and retinal mapping in normal eyes and in eyes with DME (Massin et al., 2001; Polito et al., 2005)[26,27]. Excellent reproducibility of retinal thickness measurements with the SD-OCT has been reported as well, especially with Spectralis OCT (Wolf-Schnurrbusch et al., 2009; Menke et al., 2009)[28,29]. The Diabetic Retinopathy Clinical Research Network (DRCR. net) has calculated that for the Stratus OCT, an 11% change or more of macular thickness can be considered as clinically significant (Diabetic Retinopathy Clinical Research Network, 2007)[30]. Finally, OCT may allow detection of early thickening of the macular area, which may be calculated

as follows: when the mean retinal thickness of an area is greater than the mean thickness +2 SD in the corresponding area in healthy subjects (Strom et al., 2002)[31].

Medical Care

Systemic Control

Solid evidence has been provided regarding the principle that the control of systemic risk factors is strictly related to the course of macular edema secondary to DR. The attention of researchers has been especially focused on the effect of hyperglycemia, and many single studies, together with several multicenter clinical trials, have clearly demonstrated that persistent hyperglycemia is strongly associated with the incidence and progression of macular edema (Klein et al., 1989; Klein et al., 1995; Klein et al., 1998; Vitale et al., 1995; Diabetes Control and Complications Trial Research Group, 1997; Diabetes Control and Complications Trial Research Group, 2000; Aroca et al., 2004; Roy and Affouf, 2006; White et al., 2008; UK Prospective Diabetes Study Group, 1998; UK Prospective Diabetes Study Group, 1998; Matthews et al., 2004; Kohner et al., 2001; Kohner, 2008; Adler et al., 2000)[32–46].

Lower levels of glycosylated hemoglobin, in particular, have turned out to be associated with a lower incidence of macular edema, independent of the duration of diabetes mellitus. An increase of 1% in the glycosylated hemoglobin value between baseline and subsequent follow-up was associated with a 22% increase in the 21-year cumulative incidence of macular edema (Klein et al., 2009)[47]. These data are similar to those obtained by the Diabetes Control and Complications Trial, which found that intensive glycemic control was associated with a 46% reduction in the incidence of macular edema at the end of the trial, and with a 58% reduction 4 years later in the patients undergoing intensive treatment (3 or more daily insulin injections or a continuous subcutaneous insulin infusion), in comparison to those in the conventional group (with 1 or 2 daily injections of insulin) (Diabetes Control and Complications Trial Research Group, 2000)[37].

A possible consequence of strict metabolic control is represented by the potential development of severe hypoglycemic episodes (Diabetes Control and Complications Trial Research Group, 1997; Davis et al., 2007)[36,48]. A rapid worsening of the macular edema can occur following a too fast improvement of glycemic control and a gradual metabolic balance is generally advisable.

Systolic blood pressure was found to be associated with the incidence of macular edema by several studies (Klein et al., 1989; Klein et al., 1995; Klein et al.,1998; Vitale et al., 1995; Aroca et al., 2004; Roy and Affouf, 2006; Klein et al., 2009; Jaross et al., 2005)[32–35,38,39,47,49]. Rigid control of hypertension is also mandatory in an effort to reduce the progression of microvascular damage typical of DR, including macular edema (Matthews et al., 2004; Funatsu and Yamashita, 2003)[43,50]. In particular, the level of blood pressure, rather than the type of drug used, is critical in an attempt to limit the course of macular edema, as shown by the UK Prospective Diabetes Study (Matthews et al., 2004)[43]. Moreover, some investigators have indicated that, among the blood pressure-controlling drugs, special consideration should be given to angiotensin II-converting enzyme inhibitors (Sjolie, 2007)[51].

A number of investigations have also described an association between the prevalence of diabetic nephropathy, as manifest by microalbuminuria or gross proteinuria, and the incidence and progression of macular edema (West et al., 1980; Knuiman et al., 1986; Jerneld, 1988; Kostraba et al., 1991; Cruickshanks et al., 1993; Klein et al., 1993; Romero et al., 2007)[52–58].

Smoking has inconsistently been found to be associated with the prevalence and incidence of macular edema (Klein et al., 1983; Moss et al., 1996)[59,60]. Smoking might influence the course of macular edema due to its effect on coagulation and the inflammatory response to the disease. Regardless of its association, smoking should be avoided because of its relation to increased risk of death and other systemic complications.

Lastly, hyperlipidemia has been linked to the occurrence of retinal hard exudates and macular edema in patients with DR (Sjolie, 2007; Chew et al., 1996)[51,61]. The control of serum lipid level through pharmacologic therapies, including simvastatin, can retard the progression of macular edema and can lead to the reduction of hard deposition and microaneurysm formation (Sen et al., 2002; Rechtman et al., 2007)[62,63]. In essence, a number of investigations have clearly pointed out that good systemic control can effectively slow the natural evolution of macular edema secondary to DR.

Objectives of systemic therapy must address several aspects, including the attainment of good glycemic control, both by achieving the target glycosylated hemoglobin and minimizing the variability in the serum glucose levels and by obtaining blood pressure stabilization.

Special attention must be paid to make the risk of severe hypoglycemia occurrence as minimal as possible. On the basis of these data, the ophthalmologist must recommend that the patients comply with the suggested therapy, have their glycemia, glycosylated hemoglobin, and blood pressure frequently checked, and have regular physical examinations with their general practitioner and retina specialist, in any attempt to steer clear of the ocular complications of diabetes mellitus.

Ocular Pharmacotherapy

Corticosteroids
Photocoagulation is the standard of care for DME. However, a substantial group of patients are unresponsive to laser therapy and fail to improve after photocoagulation. It has been reported that 3 years after initial grid treatment, visual acuity

improved in 14.5% of patients with DME, did not change in 60.9%, and decreased in 24.6% (Lee and Olk, 1991)[64]. Thus, other treatment modalities for DME are being investigated.

In recent years, the *intravitreal administration of steroids* has provided promising results for the treatment of DME. The anti-inflammatory, angiostatic, and antipermeability properties of these compounds have gained interest in chronic retinal conditions such as DME. A complete understanding of the mechanism of action of corticosteroids has not been fully clarified. However, corticosteroids have been shown to interfere with many regulatory components of gene expression inhibiting the expression of vascular endothelial growth factor (VEGF) and key proinflammatory genes (tumor necrosis factor α and other inflammatory chemokines), while inducing gene functioning as anti-inflammatory factors [pigment epithelium-derived growth factor (PEDF)] (Tsaprouni et al., 2002; Juergens et al., 2004; Tong et al., 2006; Kim et al., 2007; Zhang et al., 2006)[65–69]. The anti-inflammatory activity of steroids is also related to the inhibition of the phospholipase A_2 pathway, to the lower release of inflammatory cell mediators, and to the reduced leukocyte chemotaxis (Abelson and Butrus, 1994)[70]. Additionally, triamcinolone acetonide (TA) seems to reduce the expression of matrix metalloproteinases (MMPs) and downregulates intercellular adhesion molecule 1 on choroidal endothelial cells (Mizuno et al., 2007)[71].

Intravitreal Triamcinolone Acetonide Injection
Intravitreal TA has been used for treatment of DME in a number of randomized clinical trials and has demonstrated significant improvements in morphological and functional outcomes (Audren et al., 2006; Jonas et al., 2006; Gillies et al., 2006)[72–74]. A carefully designed prospective, randomized trial conducted by the DRCR.net investigated the efficacy and safety of 1- and 4-mg doses of preservative-free intravitreal TA in comparison with focal or grid laser photocoagulation (Diabetic Retinopathy Clinical Research Network, 2008)[75]. In this study, photocoagulation was shown to be more effective over time and had fewer side effects than TA.

Several published reports disclose that a significant proportion of patients with diffuse DME, resulting from a generalized breakdown of the inner BRB, have poor prognosis despite grid laser photocoagulation (Lee and Olk, 1991)[64]. Intravitreal TA has also been tested with favorable results in cases of diffuse DME refractory to laser treatment. Even if the mentioned reports differ in drug dosage and follow-up length, a positive trend in visual acuity can be found in the TA groups (3.1–8.1 ETDRS letters improvement) as compared with control groups (0.1–3.6 ETDRS letters loss) at least in the short term (Audren et al., 2006; Jonas et al., 2006; Gillies et al., 2006; Hauser et al., 2008; Kim et al., 2008)[72–74,76,77]. It has been observed that adequate concentrations of TA could provide therapeutic effects for approximately 3 months after 4-mg intravitreal TA injection (Beer et al., 2003)[78]. A maximum effect duration of 140 days has been suggested (Audren et al., 2004)[79].

Intravitreal TA injections carry considerable risks, including acute infectious endophthalmitis, pseudoendophthalmitis, and iatrogenic retinal breaks. A recent review reported an estimated incidence rate of endophthalmitis after intravitreal administration of TA of 1.4% per injection (24/1,739) (Jager et al., 2004)[80]. In the DRCR.net study, no cases of endophthalmitis or inflammatory pseudo-endophthalmitis were reported after any of the 1,649 intravitreal injections.

A significant increase in intraocular pressure was seen in 10% of eyes included in the laser group, 20% of those treated with 1 mg TA and 40% of those injected with 4 mg TA. Among phakic eyes at baseline, cataract surgery was performed before the 2-year outcome visit in 13% of eyes in the laser group, and in 23 and 51% of cases treated with 1 and 4 mg intravitreal TA, respectively (Diabetic Retinopathy Clinical Research Network, 2008)[75]. It must be pointed out that different commercially available TA formulations have been used in the different trials.

Peribulbar Triamcinolone Acetonide Injection
Evidence has shown the efficacy of the transscleral pathway in delivering drug to the macular retina (Geroski et al., 2001; Olsen et al., 1995; Kato et al., 2004)[81–83]. Transscleral delivery of TA is routinely used for the treatment of various inflammatory eye diseases and has been proposed for the treatment of DME. Some studies report that intravitreal injection of TA may be more effective than posterior juxtascleral infusion for the treatment of refractory DME (Bonini-Filho et al., 2005; Cardillo et al., 2005; Ozdek et al., 2006)[84–86]. Recently, a modified formulation of TA injected via juxtascleral infusion was proposed (Veritti et al., 2009)[87], which proved a sustained effect of 6 months.

Corticosteroid Implants
Several intravitreal steroid-releasing implants have been designed in an attempt to provide long-term drug delivery to the macular region. These include nonbiodegradable and biodegradable dexamethasone, fluocinolone acetonide, and TA implants.

Dexamethasone is synthetic glucocorticoid, which is relatively small, water-soluble and has a pharmacokinetic half-life of about 3 h and a biological half-life of 36–45 h (Graham and Peyman, 1974; Hardman et al., 2001)[88,89]. Consequently, a sustained-release formulation is attractive to prolong its efficacy in the target tissue.

Posurdex-Ozurdex[TM] (Allergan Inc., Irvine, Calif., USA) is a biodegradable extended-release form of dexamethasone. The polymer matrix composed of poly-lactide-co-glycolide copolymer releases dexamethasone over approximately 1 month with a potential therapeutic effect for about 4–6 months (Fialho et al., 2008)[90]. It is injected via the pars plana with a 22-gauge device. Recently, Ozurdex[TM] has been approved by the Food and Drug Administration (FDA) for the treatment of macular edema secondary to retinal vein occlusion.

The Ozurdex[TM] implant has been evaluated in 315 eyes with persistent (≥90 days despite treatment) macular edema associated with diabetes, retinal vein occlusion, uveitis, and postcataract surgery. A group of 172 diabetic patients were randomized to 3 groups: 350-μg implant, 700-μg implant, or observation. At 3 months, a gain in visual acuity of 2 lines or more was achieved in 33% of eyes in the 700-μg implant group and in 12% of eyes in the observation group. Among all cases of macular edema, at 6 months a visual acuity gain of at least 2 lines was obtained in 32.4% (p < 0.06), 24.3 and 21% of eyes in the 350-μg implant group, the 700-μg implant group, and observation group, respectively (Kuppermann et al., 2007)[91]. A dose-response effect favoring the higher dose was also seen on fluorescein angiography with a reduction of central macular thickness and leakage.

An intraocular pressure increase of 10 mm Hg or more from baseline was found in 12% of the dexamethasone 350-μg group, in 17% of the dexamethasone 700-μg group, and in 3% of the observation group. No significant difference was found in the number of reports of cataract among the different study groups.

Phase II studies are evaluating the safety and efficacy of the intravitreal implant of dexamethasone with laser treatment versus laser treatment alone in patients with DME (NCT00464685) and the effect of the implant in vitrectomized eyes with DME (NCT00799227). Phase III trials are investigating the efficacy of the Posurdex[TM] implant for the treatment of DME (NCT00168389).

Fluocinolone acetonide is a synthetic steroid with a solubility of 1/24 in aqueous solution of dexamethasone and a short systemic half-life. Fluocinolone acetonide can be released in a linear manner in vivo over an extended period of time by nonerodible drug delivery devices (Ashton et al., 1994; Jaffe et al., 2000)[92,93].

Retisert® (Bausch and Lomb, Rochester, N.Y., USA) is a nonbiodegradable polymer intravitreal implant designed to release 0.59 mg of fluocinolone acetonide to the posterior segment at an initial rate of 0.6 μg/day decreasing over the first month to a steady state of 0.3–0.4 μg/day. Drug release can last for a period of 30 months (Hsu, 2007)[94]. Retisert® has been approved for clinical use in patients with uveitis and has shown a proper safety profile with good toleration and no detectable systemic drug absorption in preclinical studies.

A multicenter, randomized, controlled clinical trial was conducted to determine the safety and efficacy of a sustained-release fluocinolone acetonide intravitreal implant in patients with DME. The 3-year study results compared the implantation of the 0.59 mg fluocinolone acetonide with the standard of care (repeat laser or observation). A group of 197 patients were involved in the study with 128 receiving the implant. After 3 years, there was no evidence of edema in 58% of eyes receiving the implant versus 30% of control eyes (p < 0.001). A visual acuity improvement of 3 lines or more was seen in 28% of the patients with the implant and in 15% of the control group (p < 0.05).

During the follow-up, 95% of phakic implanted eyes required cataract surgery. Intraocular pressure elevation was found in 35% of treated eyes (Pearson et al., 2006)[95].

Iluvien® (Alimera Sciences, Alpharetta, Ga., USA) is a nonerodable injectable fluocinolone intravitreal implant, which delivers a low dose of drug for up to either 18 or 36 months and either 0.2 or 0.5 μg of drug per day. This product is currently in phase III clinical trials comparing 0.2 and 0.5 mg fluocinolone acetonide intravitreal insert and standard of care in DME (NCT00490815-NCT00344968).

I-vation (SurModics, Eden Prairie, Minn., USA) is a nonbiodegradable, helical, metal alloy implant coated with polybutyl methacrylate, polyethylene vinyl acetate polymers, and TA.

Drug delivery and duration rates can be tuned varying the ratios of the constituent polymers. This system is implanted through a 25-gauge device. In a phase I safety study, 31 patients with DME were randomized to receive the TA implant in either the slow-release or fast-release formulation. Interim data at 18 months are available for 24 patients. No surgical complications and uncontrollable intraocular pressure elevation above 22 mm Hg were reported. Endophthalmitis occurred in 1 case. Mean visual acuity improvement was 18 letters and mean retinal thickness reduction was 237 μm at 18 months (Eliott et al., 2008)[96]. A phase IIb trial for I-vation TA was suspended following the publication of the DRCR.net study.

Verisome® (Icon Bioscience Inc., Sunnyvale, Calif., USA) is a biodegradable implant designed to be injected intravitreously and release TA for up to 1 year. Preclinical studies have demonstrated sustained levels of the drug in the vitreous for up to 6 months (6.9 mg formulation) and 12 months (13.8 mg formulation). This implant appears to be well tolerated in rabbit eyes (Hu et al., 2008)[97]. A phase I clinical trial is currently been conducted to investigate safety of this drug release device in cystoid macular edema patients.

Vascular Endothelial Growth Factor Inhibitors
In the pathophysiologic sequence of events leading to DME, chronic hyperglycemia induces oxidative damage to endothelial cells and an inflammatory response (Gardner et al., 2002)[98]. The subsequent overexpression of a number of growth factors, including VEGF, insulin-like growth factor 1, angiopoietin 1 and 2, stromal-derived factor 1, fibroblast growth factor 2, and tumor necrosis factor α, leads to BRB breakdown in the ischemic retina (Grant et al., 2004)[99]. Thus, anti-VEGF agents, interfering with a critical stimulus for the development of BRB breakdown, have been investigated in the treatment of DME.

Pegaptanib
Pegaptanib sodium (Macugen, Eyetech Pfizer) is an anti-VEGF aptamer, a small piece of RNA that self-folds into a shape that binds to and blocks the effects of $VEGF_{165}$ isoform. The drug is approved by the FDA and European Medicines Evaluation

Agency for the treatment of neovascular age-related macular degeneration (AMD), and it has recently been studied in a phase II trial for DME. The Macugen Diabetic Retinopathy Study was a phase II study comparing the use of 3 different doses of pegaptanib (0.3, 1, or 3 mg) with a sham injection. It evaluated 3 injections 6 weeks apart followed by subsequent injections at 6-week intervals at the discretion of the investigators.

Patients assigned to the pegaptanib group had better outcomes in terms of visual acuity (34 vs. 10% ≥10-letter gain; p = 0.003) and retinal thickness (68 vs. 4 μm decrease; p = 0.02), and had a reduced need for focal or scatter laser photocoagulation as compared to the sham group (Cunningham et al., 2005)[100]. This trend continued but was not statistically significant after 36 weeks. A multicenter phase III trial is currently recruiting patients to evaluate the safety and efficacy of pegaptanib sodium in eyes with DME (NCT00605280).

Ranibizumab

Ranibizumab (Lucentis, Genentech) is a humanized antigen-binding fragment directed against VEGF. It is currently labeled for the treatment of wet AMD and is approved by the FDA and the European Medicines Evaluation Agency. Ranibizumab has shown short-term efficacy against DME in a series of nonrandomized and randomized clinical trials.

In a pilot study, 10 DME eyes were treated with 5 ranibizumab injections of 0.5 mg at baseline and at months 1, 2, 4, and 6 and a mean improvement in vision of 12.3 letters at month 7 was found (p = 0.005) (Nguyen et al., 2006)[101]. Mean decrease in central OCT thickness was 246 μm at the end of follow-up (p = 0.005) (Nguyen et al., 2006)[101].

The Ranibizumab for Edema of the Macula in Diabetes (READ) study was a phase I/II open-label evaluation of 20 eyes injected with ranibizumab 0.5 mg at baseline, and at months 1, 2, 4, and 6. One year following initial injection, treated eyes demonstrated a mean gain of 7 letters from baseline and resolution of 77% of excess thickening over normal by OCT measurements (Shah et al., 2006)[102].

The Ranibizumab for Edema of the Macula in Diabetes 2 (READ-2) was a phase II randomized clinical trial, which studied 126 patients. Patients were randomized to receive ranibizumab for 6 months, photocoagulation alone, or ranibizumab for 6 months plus photocoagulation. At 6 months, the mean change in visual acuity score was +7 letters in eyes treated with ranibizumab, –1 letter in eyes treated with photocoagulation, and +4 letters in eyes treated with photocoagulation and ranibizumab (Nguyen et al., 2008)[103].

The phase II Safety and Efficacy of Ranibizumab in Diabetic Macular Edema With Center Involvement (RESOLVE) trial demonstrated the effects of ranibizumab when administered using a retreatment regime guided by visual acuity and tomographic response to treatment. It included 151 patients with a central macular thickness of 300 μm or more and a best corrected visual acuity letter score of between 39 and 73. Eyes were randomized to receive 3 monthly injections with either 0.3 or 0.5 mg ranibizumab or placebo (sham group). After the initial 3 injections, treatment was administered on a pro re nata basis. If edema resolution was incomplete, then the dose of ranibizumab was doubled after 1 month. Photocoagulation after 3 injections was given if needed. At 12 months, the pooled ranibizumab group (n = 102) gained +10.2 letters compared to the sham group that lost a mean of 1 letter (p < 0.001). Mean central retinal thickness decreased by 200 μm in the ranibizumab group compared to 40 μm in the sham group (Massin et al., 2008)[104].

A phase III study on Efficacy and Safety of Ranibizumab in Patients With Visual Impairment Due to Diabetic Macular Edema (RESTORE) is under way to assess the effects of ranibizumab (0.5 mg) as adjunctive or monotherapy to laser treatment after 12 months of treatment in subjects with visual impairment due to DME (NCT00687804). Two additional phase III randomized controlled studies, the Ranibizumab Injection in Subjects With Clinically Significant Macular Edema With Center Involvement Secondary to Diabetes Mellitus (RISE) (NCT00473330) and Ranibizumab Injection in Subjects With Clinically Significant Macular Edema With Center Involvement Secondary to Diabetes Mellitus (RIDE) (NCT00473382), are currently recruiting patients. As has been the case with treatment approaches for AMD-related choroidal neovascularization, combination therapy is also being studied for the treatment of DME. A DRCR.net phase III study is evaluating intravitreal ranibizumab or TA in combination with laser photocoagulation for DME (NCT00444600).

Bevacizumab
Bevacizumab (Avastin; Genentech) is a full-length humanized antibody against VEGF. It is widely used off-label in the treatment of wet AMD. It is approved for the treatment of metastatic cancer and a randomized, phase II DRCR.net trial evaluated short-term effect of intravitreal bevacizumab demonstrating a beneficial action in DME (Scott et al., 2007)[105].

A randomized, placebo-controlled clinical trial compared the efficacy of 3 intravitreal injections of bevacizumab alone or combined with intravitreal triamcinolone in the first injection versus sham injection. A total of 115 eyes were randomly assigned to 1 of 3 groups (bevacizumab alone, bevacizumab combined with intravitreal triamcinolone, or sham injection). Central macular thickness was reduced significantly in both treatment groups. At week 24, retinal thickness reduction was 95.7 μm in the bevacizumab group, 92.1 μm in the combination group, compared with a mean increase of 34.9 μm in the control group. Significant gains in visual acuity were noted compared with the sham group (monotherapy: p = 0.01; combination therapy: p = 0.006). The addition of a steroidal drug in this study had no significant effect on retinal thickness but did result in a trend toward earlier visual improvements

(Ahmadieh et al., 2008)[106]. Similar overall results were also found in another randomized study (Soheilian et al., 2009)[107].

The Intravitreal Triamcinolone Acetonide Versus Intravitreal Bevacizumab for Refractory Diabetic Macular Edema (IBEME) study was a trial comparing morphological and functional outcomes in 28 patients treated with a single injection of either bevacizumab or TA in DME. Central macular thickness was significantly reduced in the triamcinolone group compared with the bevacizumab group at weeks 4, 8, 12, and 24. Visual acuity was significantly higher in the triamcinolone group at weeks 8 and 12. A significant increase in intraocular pressure was seen only in the triamcinolone group at week 4 (Paccola et al., 2008)[108]. Phase III randomized, controlled studies of intravitreal bevacizumab, alone or in combination with TA and laser photocoagulation, are currently recruiting participants (NCT00737971, NCT00682539, NCT00545870, NCT00370669).

Pharmacologic Vitreolysis
The vitreoretinal interface plays an important role in the pathogenesis of many retinal disorders including DME. In the absence of posterior vitreous detachment, the vitreous cortex is adherent to the internal limiting lamina of the inner retina. This junction is thought to participate in the pathophysiology of DME. Surgical management of DME often aims at separating the posterior hyaloid from the ILM (Gandorfer et al., 2002)[109].

Several authors have proposed enzymatic and nonenzymatic methods to cleave the vitreoretinal adhesion and liquefy the central vitreous as an adjunct to vitreoretinal surgery, as a method to resolve vitreous traction or to clear vitreous opacities (Trese, 2000; Hermel and Schrage, 2007)[110,111]. Enzymatic manipulation of the vitreous (chemical vitrectomy) can potentially relieve vitreoretinal traction and change oxygen and cytokine levels in the vitreous cavity (Stefansson and Loftsson, 2006; Quiram et al., 2007)[112,113].

Vitreolysis has been proposed using hyaluronidase (Vitrase®, ISTA Pharmaceuticals). It shows no toxicity and appears to be effective, promising the clearance of vitreous hemorrhage and treatment of DR (Kuppermann et al., 2005; Kuppermann et al., 2005)[114,115]. Other potential enzymes that may allow for nonsurgical treatment of DME include plasmin and microplasmin (ThomboGenics NV, Leuven, Belgium), a truncated form of human plasmin (Trese, 2000; Sakuma et al., 2005)[110,116].

Other Drugs

Novel prophylactic and therapeutic interventions in DR are being investigated in either systemic or ocular delivery. Ocular pharmacologic therapies include MMP inhibitors and PEDF inducers as an alternative to growth factor modulators and steroids.

Infliximab is an engineered antibody directed against tumor necrosis factor α. It is used intravenously in the treatment of systemic inflammatory diseases and has been evaluated for the treatment of uveitis in a number of clinical studies (Lindstedt et al., 2005; Theodossiadis et al., 2007)[117,118]. Direct intravitreal administration has been investigated in a rabbit model and has been proven safe at a dose of up to 1.7 mg (Giansanti et al., 2008)[119]. A trial is currently recruiting participants to evaluate safety and tolerability of intravitreal infliximab in human subjects with refractory DME or choroidal neovascularization (NCT00695682). PF-04523655 is a short interfering RNA that interferes with the expression of the RTP-801 gene by means of the RNA interference pathway. In preclinical models, inhibition of the RTP-801 gene produced increased vascular permeability and inhibition of new vessels. A phase II trial has been planned to investigate safety and efficacy of PF-04523655 in DME (NCT00701181).

Bevasiranib is a short interfering RNA designed to silence the VEGF gene. The RNAi Assessment of Bevasiranib in DME, or RACE trial, was a pilot phase II investigation of the safety and preliminary efficacy of bevasiranib in patients with DME. This randomized trial studied 3 dose levels of bevasiranib and showed a decrease in macular thickness between weeks 8 and 12 (New and Indevelopment Treatments For Diabetic Macular Edema, 2009)[120].

VEGF-Trap is a fusion protein of portions of VEGF receptors 1 and 2 and the Fc region of a human IgG. It binds all VEGF isoforms and has been studied in a phase I study, which showed a good safety profile and encouraging efficacy results (Do et al., 2009)[121]. Four of 5 patients had improvements in visual acuity of 6–10 letters at 4 weeks after injection, with a mean decrease in central retinal thickness of 115 μm. A phase II trial is currently recruiting participants (NCT00789477).

Sirolimus is an immunosuppressant drug approved for systemic use in renal transplantation. It inhibits the mammalian target of rapamycin. It can be injected either subconjunctivally or intravitreally and has shown positive interim data from a phase I study in patients with DME. Results from this prospective study of 50 patients demonstrated that sirolimus was safe and well tolerated at all doses tested with 2 different routes of administration (Macusight announces positive results, 2009)[122]. A phase II, randomized dose-ranging clinical study to assess the safety and efficacy of subconjunctival injections of sirolimus in patients with DME is currently recruiting participants (NCT00656643).

MMPs are endogenous peptidases that degrade extracellular matrix elements allowing for endothelial migration. Intraocular MMP inhibition has been investigated in animal studies. Intravitreal injection of prinomastat has been demonstrated to be both safe and effective in animal models of uveal melanoma and post-traumatic proliferative vitreoretinopathy (Ozerdem et al., 2000)[123].

PEDF is an endogenous inhibitor of angiogenesis and its levels correlate directly with oxygen concentrations in animal models (Gao et al., 2001)[124]. In a murine model of angiogenic retinopathy, administration of PEDF showed complete inhibition of retinal vascular abnormalities (Stellmach et al., 2001; Duh et al., 2002)[125,126]. These results suggest that PEDF may be used as a pharmacologic intervention in DR. However, significantly elevated concentration levels of PEDF have been found in patients with active PDR (Duh et al., 2004)[127]. The relationship between VEGF and PEDF vitreous concentrations, and the importance of their ratio in the development of DME have yet to be fully clarified. Encapsulated cell technology is a treatment modality developed by Neurotech (Lincoln, R.I., USA), which involves the implantation in the vitreous cavity of a semipermeable polymer capsule. The small capsule contains cells that have been genetically modified to produce desired proteins or peptides. The structure of the hollow fiber membrane is designed to allow influx of oxygen and nutrients while guaranteeing immune privilege. Encapsulated cell technology can also be engineered to secrete anti-angiogenic and anti-inflammatory factors. Encapsulated cell technology is being investigated in phase II clinical trials including subjects with geographic atrophy and retinitis pigmentosa.

Surgical Care

Photocoagulation

Many studies have demonstrated a beneficial effect of laser photocoagulation on DME, and it remains the standard of care. The ETDRS, which identified macular edema as a study objective, provided the most comprehensive directives for the management of affected patients and the strongest support for the therapeutic benefit of photocoagulation. In the ETDRS, focal/grid laser photocoagulation of eyes with edema involving or threatening the fovea reduced the 3-year risk of moderate visual loss (defined as a loss of ≥15 letters) by approximately 50%, from 24% in the control group, to 12% in the laser group (Early Treatment Diabetic Retinopathy Study Research Group, 1985)[3].

As a result, the clinical and therapeutic approach to DME is largely based on the findings and conclusions of the ETDRS. Laser photocoagulation leads to visual improvement in a minority of patients. For the majority of cases, the goal of laser treatment is to stabilize visual acuity, and patients should be informed of this when laser photocoagulation is planned. Furthermore, the visual and functional prognosis in the subgroup of patients with diffuse DME is poor, and in those cases, macular edema is often refractory to multiple treatments.

With the advent of new imaging modalities, it has come into question if the presence of CSME on fundus biomicroscopy is still to be considered as the best indicator to apply laser. In the ETDRS, the diagnosis of macular edema was based on clinical examination, regardless of visual acuity, and fluorescein angiography was used to help direct laser treatment. In recent years, the use of OCT has gained increasing popularity as an objective tool to measure retinal thickness and other aspects associated with DME. Standard OCT assessment of macular edema has been adopted in multicenter trials in patients with DME and has been demonstrated to correlate well with fundus biomicroscopy (Strom, 2002)[31].

Recent studies have demonstrated a good correlation between OCT and fluorescein angiography in patients with CSME, with a greater sensitivity of OCT to detect earlier stages of macular edema (Kang, 2004; Jittpoonkuson et al., 2009)[7,128]. Combined fluorescein angiography and OCT data could be helpful to disclose the pathogenesis of the edema, to diagnose and optimize early treatment, when necessary, thereby reducing visual loss. It remains to be evaluated with longitudinal studies if earlier treatment decisions based on fluorescein angiographic and tomographic features reflect a more favorable visual prognosis.

Mechanism of Action of Laser Photocoagulation

The specific mechanisms of action of laser photocoagulation in DME are still unclear. Pigments involved in the process of light absorption during laser photocoagulation are xanthophylls (outer and inner plexiform layers), melanin (RPE cells, choroidal melanocytes), and hemoglobin (retinal and choroidal vessels).

The primary effect of laser treatment is thermal damage, mainly induced at the level of the RPE. However, concurrent damage to the adjacent choriocapillary and outer retinal layers, such as the photoreceptors, usually occurs as a consequence of heat transmission. Two different mechanisms of action can be hypothesized: direct and indirect.

The effectiveness of focal laser photocoagulation could be due, at least partially, to direct thrombosis caused by absorption of light by hemoglobin with consequent closure of leaky microaneurysms. Several hypotheses suggesting an indirect effect of laser photocoagulation have been proposed, and these seem to be supported by the efficacy of grid treatment alone (without focal, direct treatment of microaneurysms), light photocoagulation, and micropulse techniques (Bandello et al., 2005)[129]. One possible explanation is that the laser-induced destruction and consequent reduction of retinal, RPE, and choriocapillaris tissue following treatment could lead to direct oxygen diffusion from the choriocapillaris to the inner retina, through the laser scars, ultimately relieving retinal hypoxia (Stefansson, 2001)[130].

Furthermore, laser photocoagulation could reduce the oxygen demand by destroying the outer retinal layers, allowing an increased oxygen supply to the inner retina. Contrasting evidence exists on this point: some authors demonstrate an increased preretinal oxygen partial pressure in photocoagulated areas, while others revealed choriocapillaris loss and reduction of retinal capillaries in areas of laser photocoagulation (Wolbarsht and Landers, 1980; Molnar et al., 1985)[131,132].

Recently, both conventional continuous-wave laser and micropulse laser demonstrated to induce reduction of outer retinal oxygen consumption and increased oxygen level within the retina in animal models (Stefansson et al., 1981)[133]. The latter finding supports the hypothesis that loss of retinal capillary after laser photocoagulation would result in the reduction of abnormal leaking vessels and consequent improvement of macular edema (Yu et al., 2005)[134].

Another theory proposes that laser treatment may stimulate improvement of retinal oxygenation and induce autoregulatory vasoconstriction of macular arterioles and venules, thus reducing retinal blood flow and consequently macular edema (Wilson et al., 1988)[135]. Some investigators have hypothesized that laser injury to the RPE induces both anatomic remodeling and functional restoration. Laser photocoagulation may restore the RPE barrier, leading to cell proliferation, resurfacing, and inducing the production of cytokines that antagonize the permeabilizing effect of VEGF (Guyer et al., 1992; Han et al., 1992; Gottfredsdottir et al., 1993; Xiao et al., 1999; Ogata et al., 2001)[136–140].

Despite theoretical advantages of some wavelengths over others, several studies have shown a similar efficacy for all the wavelengths (yellow, green, red, infrared) commonly used for the treatment of DME.

Timing of Laser Photocoagulation

An indispensable requirement for successful laser treatment is the presence of prevalently retinovascular DME. There is no proven indication for laser treatment when the cause of macular edema is tractional (epiretinal membrane, taut, attached posterior hyaloid), and often in such cases laser photocoagulation is even contraindicated, since treatment could worsen the tractional component.

Analysis of early- and late-frame fluorescein angiography provides information about the nature of the edema and its possible causal mechanisms. Prevalently retinovascular DME is typically characterized by an exact correspondence between microvascular abnormalities, well defined in the early phases, and dye leakage evident in the late frames. On the contrary, biomicroscopic examination, however carefully performed, allows an evaluation of the presence of retinal thickening, but only occasionally (especially for focal edema where there are circinate lipid exudates in which leaking lesions are often obvious within the lipid ring) consents to disclose the exact cause of macular edema.

Fluorescein angiography is currently the most reliable diagnostic technique to identify retinovascular DME and should be mandatory for early and adequate laser treatment. Furthermore, fluorescein angiography identifies the presence and severity of macular ischemia that, if extensive, contraindicates laser photocoagulation.

Laser treatment is most effective when initiated before visual acuity declines, therefore treatment should be initiated as soon as CSME is detected (Early Treatment Diabetic Retinopathy Study Research Group, 1985; Early Treatment Diabetic Retinopathy Study Research Group, 1995)[3,141]. When treatment is planned, risks and benefits of laser photocoagulation should be discussed with the patient. Patients should be informed that the treatment aim is to stabilize vision and prevent further visual loss, and that visual improvement, although possible, is uncommon. In asymptomatic patients with excellent visual acuity (20/20), it is possible to consider deferring focal laser treatment and scheduling close follow-up appointments (every 2–4 months). In such cases, assessment of the proximity of exudates to the fovea, status of the fellow eye, scheduled cataract surgery, and presence of retinopathy approaching high-risk characteristics should guide treatment decision. In patients with optimal visual acuity, treatment can be deferred in the presence of macular edema without central involvement.

If careful, serial examinations and documentation (fundus stereophotography is a valuable tool to document clinical findings and to allow comparison) reveal progression of the edema toward the center. Patients should be considered for laser treatment especially if treatable lesions are located 500 μm outside of the macular center. When panretinal photocoagulation is needed for severe NPDR or nonhigh-risk PDR in eyes with macular edema, it is preferable to perform focal photocoagulation before panretinal photocoagulation, starting treatment in the nasal and inferior sectors, since there is evidence that panretinal photocoagulation as used in the ETDRS may exacerbate macular edema. However, panretinal and focal laser photocoagulation should be concomitantly performed in the presence of CSME and high-risk PDR (if retinal or disk neovascularization is extensive or vitreous/preretinal hemorrhage has occurred recently).

A follow-up examination for individuals with CSME should be scheduled within 3–4 months of laser treatment. Retreatment of up to 300 μm (unless there is perifoveal capillary dropout) or including the FAZ should be considered if macular edema persists or recurs. Close monitoring, at least every 3–4 months, should be planned and retreatment deferred if visual acuity has improved and an objective reduction of retinal thickness is observed.

Treatment Procedures

Even though the principles of macular laser therapy were established about 20 years ago, the ETDRS recommendations still constitute the basis of the current treatment guidelines.

Laser photocoagulation techniques for DME can traditionally be classified as focal or grid (fig. 9). The ETDRS treatment strategy involves treating discrete areas of leaking microaneurysms considered to produce retinal thickening or hard exudates with focal photocoagulation.

The grid technique was applied to treat areas of diffuse leakage, including microaneurysms, intraretinal microvascular abnormalities, leaking capillary segments, and areas of nonperfusion. Both techniques are usually performed after pupil dilation and under topical anesthesia, with the application of a contact lens.

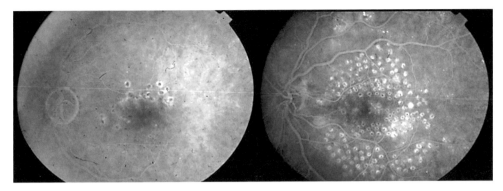

Fig. 9. Examples of laser treatment techniques. Left: focal. Right: grid.

Focal Treatment

The ETDRS protocol requires the direct treatment of all focal points of leakage located between 500 and 3,000 μm from the center of the macula. At the initial session, lesions located between 300 and 500 μm from the macular center could be optionally treated if visual acuity is 20/40 or worse, and if treatment would not destroy the remaining perifoveal capillary network.

Initial treatment requires a whitening of microaneurysms with 50- to 100-μm spots for a duration of 0.1 s. Repeat focal burns are applied, if needed, to obtain the desired effect, especially for microaneurysms larger than 40 μm. Retreatment is required if macular edema persists and the above-mentioned criteria are not met. Clusters of microaneurysms could be treated with larger and confluent spots (200–500 μm), if lesions are not located within 750 μm from the center of the macula. Additional treatment is recommended if 4 months following initial treatment, residual CSME with treatable lesions is seen on examination. Intervals between laser sessions need to be at least 4 months.

Focal Treatment: Practical Guidelines

Laser strategy for macular edema has changed and evolved over the years in order to maintain the same results and reduce potential complications.

There is a trend toward larger spot sizes, longer exposure times, and lower energy levels. Most retinal specialists do not directly treat microaneurysms, as performed in the ETDRS, since 'whitening' or 'darkening' of the aneurysms is not necessary and requires higher energy. Light, small-sized (100–200 μm in diameter) burns to leaking microaneurysms in the macula (500–3,000 μm from the center of the macula but not within 500 μm of the disk), with a relatively long exposure time of 0.1–0.3 s, are preferable if patients provide adequate compliance and immobility (table 3).

Initial power setting varies according to media opacities, degree of fundus pigmentation, and type of wavelength employed. Laser wavelengths with great affinity for hemoglobin are preferred (yellow, green). Red and infrared laser wavelengths can be useful in the presence of cataract; blue and blue-green wavelengths should not be employed due to their potential to damage the ILM and their absorption by macular xanthophyll. When using krypton red or diode infrared lasers, it is recommended to employ low energy and longer exposure time. If an infrared diode laser is chosen, retinal whitening should be barely visible, otherwise there is a high risk of provoking tears of the Bruch's membrane. Independent of the wavelength selected, power should be gradually increased, by 10–20 mW, until the desired effect is

Table 3. Parameters for focal photocoagulation

Spot size	100–200 μm
Exposure time	0.1–0.3 s
Change in microaneurysm color	Whitening/darkening of microaneurysms is not required, but at least a mild gray-white burn beneath all microaneurysms
Power increase	10–20 mW

Table 4. Parameters for grid photocoagulation

Spot size	100–200 μm
Exposure time	0.1–0.3 s
Burn intensity	Light whitening (barely visible burns)
Power increase	10–20 mW
Spot spacing	At least 1 spot width apart

reached. Whitening of microaneurysms is not required, but at least a mild gray-white burn should be evident beneath all microaneurysms. Exposure time should be as long as possible to obtain the desired effect, unless the target area is paracentral: in such cases, shorter exposure times are preferred. It is advisable to avoid overtreating, which causes almost inevitably large chorioretinal atrophy and scotomata.

As established by the ETDRS, initial focal treatment should not be applied to focal lesions located within 300–500 μm from the center of the FAZ: treatment can be applied within 500 μm if at 4-month follow-up retinal thickening persists, if such treatment does not destroy the perifoveal capillary network and visual acuity is worse than 20/40. In the presence of numerous microaneurysms that would require the destruction of extensive retinal areas and the risk of progressive confluence of the laser scars, it is advisable to perform a grid treatment.

Grid Treatment
In the ETDRS, the grid strategy for diffuse macular edema consisted of burns of 50–200 μm in size, a duration of 0.1 s, and of lighter intensity than that required for panretinal photocoagulation, placed one burn width apart. Laser spots could be placed in the papillomacular bundle but not within 500 μm from the margin of the optic disk and the center of the macula. Retreatment criteria were the same as for focal laser: further treatment was advisable if residual CSME was present on examination at 4-month intervals.

Grid Photocoagulation: Practical Guidelines
In the grid technique, a grid or pattern of nonconfluent spots (100–200 μm spot size, with 1 burn width spacing) is placed to the entire leaking area and/or segments of capillary nonperfusion, producing a light-gray burn (table 4). Three to 4 concentric rows of spots with a ring-like pattern are usually applied. The grid is centered on the FAZ

and extended up to 2 papillary diameters or to the margin of a pre-existing panphotocoagulative treatment, including the interpapillomacular bundle (but not within 500 µm from the disk).

Laser power is lower compared to that used for focal treatment, since the target of grid photocoagulation should be to obtain a barely visible whitening at the level of the retina and RPE. Since the severity of retinal thickening and the degree of fundus pigmentation may vary in the course of diffuse edema, photocoagulative parameters must be modified many times during each session, requiring higher power in more edematous areas. Therefore, it is sensible to start laser treatment in areas scarcely thickened and then proceed to treat more thickened zones, gradually increasing the power by 10 mW. Special care should be taken in treating large intraretinal hemorrhages, particularly if green and yellow wavelengths are used, since their absorption by innermost retinal layers can damage the ILM and the nerve fiber layer. In such cases, red or infrared wavelengths must be used.

In some patients, due to extensive retinal thickness, it can be difficult to ascertain the exact localization of the edge of the FAZ. In these cases, it is rational to begin with a conservative treatment. Following initial laser photocoagulation, the leakage and edema are likely to decrease, permitting an easier recognition of the FAZ and consenting to bring the treatment up to the edge of the FAZ. In case of bilateral grid treatment, it is advisable to spare the median raphe in order to avoid paracentral scotomata.

Modified Grid Photocoagulation

In clinical practice, it is common to encounter mixed forms of DME, where focal and diffuse leakage are combined and clearly visible on fluorescein angiography. In such cases, the use of a modified grid technique that has been shown to have comparable efficacy to the ETDRS grid is advisable. Modified grid photocoagulation was introduced more than 15 years ago (Lee and

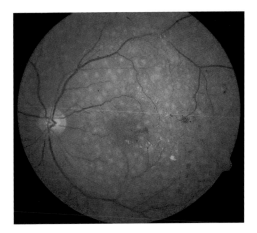

Fig. 10. Mild macular grid.

Olk, 1991; Early Treatment Diabetic Retinopathy Study Research Group, 1987; Ferris and Davis, 1999)[64,142,143].

This technique primarily consists in a grid treatment to areas of diffuse leakage, with occasional focal treatment of localized leakage situated either within or outside areas of diffuse edema. Grid treatment leads to visual improvement in 14.5% of treated eyes, stabilization in 60.9%, and worsening in 24.6% of eyes. Modified grid photocoagulation is applied to edematous perifoveal retina, including the edge of the FAZ, using 2–3 rows of 100-µm spots, placed 100 µm apart. The remaining areas of retinal thickening and/or capillary nonperfusion are then treated with 150- to 200-µm spots, placed 200 µm apart. The end point of laser treatment is to obtain a barely visible light intensity burn at the level of the retina and RPE. Associated focal leakage is treated with 100- to 150-µm spots to achieve a slightly darker burn. Additional treatment is usually applied after 3–4 months, if residual retinal thickening involving the center of the FAZ is noted.

An alternative approach is the mild macular grid (fig. 10). With this technique, mild, widely spaced, 50-µm burns are applied to the entire area considered for grid treatment, including unthickened retina and avoiding the foveal region. A total of 200–300 evenly distributed, light burns are usually performed. However, the mild macular grid technique appears to be less effective than the modified ETDRS laser, leading to a slightly worse visual acuity outcome and slightly smaller reduction in retinal thickening compared to the latter one (Olk, 1986)[144].

Complications of Photocoagulation
Although effective, the ETDRS technique involves placing burns close to the center of the macula, with potential complications. Complications of laser treatment can occur, although most side effects are transient and resolve spontaneously, and therefore the possible adverse effects should be discussed with the patient. Iris stromal burns caused by inappropriate focusing of the laser beam on the retina are much more common following panretinal photocoagulation and rarely observed after macular treatment.

Perception of symptomatic paracentral scotomata is often the result of confluence of adjacent spots placed close to the fovea. This complication is more common when the blue-green wavelength is used in macular treatment, due to the absorption of this particular wavelength by the nerve fiber layer. One of the most serious complications of focal and grid techniques associated with permanent visual loss is inadvertent foveolar burn. This can be avoided by careful observation of the macular topography, possibly with the aid of a recent fluorescein angiography, which helps in finding foveal landmarks. If the edema is massive and the exact localization of the macula is difficult, selecting the cobalt blue filter of the slit lamp can be useful: the fovea can be located through the selective absorption of the blue light by the macular xanthophylls. Alternatively, the operator may ask the patient to fixate on the laser beam; however, in the course of edema, the fixation point may not correspond to the anatomical fovea. A nonexperienced operator can be misled by the use of inverting fundus lenses, therefore it is always useful to locate the macula before and during treatment. If the patient is uncooperative, moves, or is unable to understand the operator's instruction during treatment, short exposure times or peribulbar anesthesia may be indicated. It is important to avoid excessively intense and/or short-duration burns, especially for focal laser photocoagulation, since there is the risk of rupture of the Bruch's membrane and consequent iatrogenic choroidal neovascularization (fig. 11). In this case, an immediate hemorrhage may herald the Bruch's membrane tear, but a clinically visible break is not always observable.

Choroidal neovascularization arising from areas where Bruch's membrane was ruptured can develop 2 weeks to 5 months after treatment (Olk, 1990)[146]. Iatrogenic choroidal neovascularization, usually type II and subretinal, can be successfully treated with photodynamic therapy, and usually a single treatment is sufficient to obtain the formation of a fibrovascular scar (author's personal experience). To reduce the risk of this complication, it is recommended to use the lowest intensity needed to obtain a light-gray burn, a spot size greater than 50 μm, and avoid repeated burns over a single microaneurysm.

Epiretinal fibrosis is an uncommon complication of macular laser treatment, usually secondary to intense treatment and direct treatment of intraretinal hemorrhage. Another serious complication, usually associated with poor visual prognosis, is the development of subretinal fibrosis (Guyer et al., 1992; Han et al., 1992; Writing Committee for the Diabetic Retinopathy Clinical Research Network, 2007)[136,137,146]. Only 8% of cases of subretinal fibrosis are directly related to focal laser photocoagulation. In these cases, strands of subretinal fibrosis originating from laser scars are noted, suggesting that a rupture of the Bruch's membrane secondary to high-intensity burns is the causal mechanism. Most of the cases are correlated with the presence of extensive hard exudates, especially following the reabsorption of macular edema. In

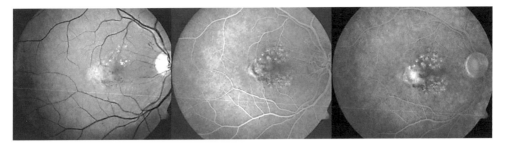

Fig. 11. Iatrogenic choroidal neovascularization. Red-free photograph (left) and early (center) and late (right) fluorescein angiography reveal the presence of a classic choroidal neovascularization which arose from a laser burn following grid photocoagulation for DME.

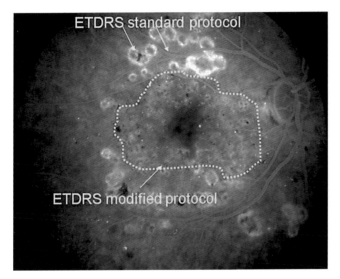

Fig. 12. ETDRS-modified protocol versus standard ETDRS photocoagulation: difference in laser burns. Laser burns applied superiorly to the macula and performed using the standard ETDRS parameters are larger and confluent compared to the spots placed in a grid pattern using a smaller spot diameter and lower intensity.

these cases, subretinal fibrosis results from fibrous metaplasia of the RPE stimulated by the presence of the exudates. The most important predictive factors for the development of subretinal fibrosis include the presence of severe exudation in the macula, usually seen as plaque of hard exudates, and elevated serum lipids prior to laser photocoagulation (Writing Committee for the Diabetic Retinopathy Clinical Research Network, 2007)[146]. The ETDRS reported the presence of subretinal fibrosis in 31% of patients with intense exudation versus 0.05% of eyes without hard exudates.

Scar enlargement over time is a complication described following grid treatment for diffuse DME in about 5% of treated eyes (Lewis et al., 1990)[147]. Causal mechanism is usually intense treatment, which may lead to RPE hyperplastic changes and atrophy. If small-sized, intense burns are applied close to the fovea, scar enlargement may lead to significant visual loss. The occurrence of this complication following macular treatment for DME is much less than that seen in eyes treated with photocoagulation for choroidal neovascularization, and the progressive trend toward lower energy and larger spot sizes has reduced its frequency (fig. 12) (Schatz et al., 1991; Fong et al., 1997)[148,149].

Advancements in Laser Photocoagulation

Light and Subthreshold Laser Photocoagulation
Laser photocoagulation is a photothermal process in which heat is produced by the absorption of laser energy in targeted tissues. This treatment modality is the standard of care for a number of retinal and choroidal diseases. The current end point of laser photocoagulation is an ophthalmoscopically visible retinal whitening, the sign that the retina itself has been thermally damaged. This thermal tissue injury is the origin of many potential complications of laser photocoagulation including preretinal and subretinal fibrosis, choroidal neovascularization, and progressive expansion of laser scans. Light, minimally invasive laser treatment for clinically significant DME has been compared to conventional photocoagulation in a prospective, randomized clinical trial (Bandello et al., 2005)[129]. Low levels of energy were employed to produce barely visible burns at the level of the RPE. This 29-eye study suggested that light photocoagulation is as effective as conventional laser treatment in the reduction of foveal retinal thickness and improvement of visual acuity. Recently, subthreshold nonvisible retinal laser irradiation has been proposed as a less invasive treatment modality, associated with less side effects and maintained efficacy (Lanzetta et al., 2001)[150].

Micropulse Retinal Photocoagulation
Subthreshold nonvisible photocoagulation with repetitively pulsed (micropulse) photocoagulators has been proposed to avoid or minimize unnecessary retinal damage. In micropulse irradiation, laser pulses (pulse envelopes) contain a series (pulse train) of very brief micropulses. The pulse train of micropulses has a characteristic frequency (repetition rate in hertz) and duty cycle (percentage of time that the laser is on during the pulse envelope).

Typically, a train of repetitive, short- and low-energy laser pulses is used to confine laser damage to the minimum level that is sufficient to evoke a biological response, leaving unaffected the surrounding tissue. Each pulse induces a temperature rise that decays quickly in the interpulse time, so the thermal gradient in adjacent structures stays below the threshold to obtain visible damage. Such laser treatment does not leave a visible sign of laser exposure on the retina tissue and is therefore not ophthalmoscopically detectable (Dorin, 2003)[151]. However, OCT may be used to detect early changes in retinal reflectivity during subclinical and retinal sparing photocoagulation (Lanzetta et al., 2008)[152]. The Oculight SLx laser system (Iridex Corporation, Mountain View, Calif., USA) is an infrared (810 nm) diode laser, which can be used either for continuous-wave conventional photocoagulation or for subthreshold micropulse photocoagulation.

A typical micropulse treatment modality employs a 200-ms exposure enveloping 100 micropulses of 0.3 ms (500 Hz, 15% duty cycle). Repetitively pulsed laser irradiation seems to localize the thermal effect to the RPE layer. The very short micropulses offer little time for heat conduction from the RPE cells to the surrounding tissue. The efficacy of subthreshold diode laser photocoagulation in clinically significant DME was evaluated in 18 eyes with a minimum foveal thickness of 223 μm treated with micropulse laser irradiation (Luttrull and Spink, 2006)[153]. Three months after treatment, 67% of cases were improved with a mean foveal thickness reduction of 298 μm (Luttrull and Spink, 2006)[153]. Micropulse and continuous-wave 810-nm diode laser photocoagulation was used to treat 59 patients with DME (Friberg and Karatza, 1997)[154]. Among the study population, 40 cases had no previous treatment. Six months after laser irradiation, 76% of newly treated eyes with DME and 67% of previously treated eyes had clinical resolution of their edema. Vision improved or stabilized in 91 and 73% of newly treated and retreated patients, respectively. Micropulse laser treatment has also been investigated in 39 eyes with macular edema secondary to branch retinal vein occlusion or diabetic maculopathy (Moorman and Hamilton, 1999)[155]. Reduction in macular edema was seen in 56.5% of eyes and 97% of cases maintained or improved vision at the 6-month follow-up visit.

Long-term visual outcome of subthreshold micropulse diode laser photocoagulation for clinically significant diffuse DME has been reported for 25 eyes included in a noncomparative case series (Sivaprasad et al., 2007)[156]. Visual acuity stabilized or improved in 84% of treated eyes by the end of the first year. By the third year of follow-up, 92% of cases maintained vision. Clinically significant DME decreased in 92% of the eyes and resolved in 88% during the first year. By the second year, 92% showed complete resolution of DME. Recurrent clinically significant DME was noted in 28% of patients during the third year of follow-up.

Recently, the results of a prospective, randomized controlled trial comparing subthreshold micropulse diode laser photocoagulation and conventional green laser for clinically significant DME have been reported (Figueira et al., 2009)[157]. Eighty-four eyes (53 patients) were randomly assigned to micropulse or conventional laser photocoagulation. No statistical difference in change of visual acuity, contrast sensitivity, and retinal thickness was found between the 2 groups at 0, 4, and 12 months. Fundus photos were obtained from 82 eyes at 12 months and laser scars were detected in 14% of cases treated with micropulse laser irradiation and in 59% of eyes from the conventional laser group.

Selective Retina Treatment

Selective retina treatment is a laser modality regime that can be used for retinal diseases associated with a degeneration of the RPE. The goal of treatment is to selectively harm RPE cells without damaging the photoreceptors (and thus avoiding scotomata), the neural retina, and the choroid (Brinkmann et al., 2006)[158]. Typically, heat diffuses from the absorbing RPE at a speed of approximately 1 μm/s. Thus, traditional laser expositions of 100 ms and more leads to significant heat conduction. Selective retina treatment involves the delivery of 30 light pulses of 1.7 μs at a repetition rate of 100 Hz using a 527-nm frequency doubled Q-switched Nd:YLF laser. Repeated irradiation with those very-short-duration pulses seems to confine energy to the RPE while sparing the photoreceptors.

Whereas after standard argon laser photocoagulation a grayish-white spot is ophthalmoscopically perceivable, lesions produced with selective retina treatment are not visible but are detectable by fluorescein angiography. This differs from micropulse retinal photocoagulation in which laser spots are not visible with ophthalmoscopy and fluorescein angiography. Possibly, submillisecond and submicrosecond repetitive pulse laser treatment are dissimilar in the localization of laser irradiance effects to RPE cells or their melanin granules.

The effects of selective retina treatment Q-switched laser pulses of only 8 ns have recently been investigated in a rabbit model with a double-frequency Nd:YAG laser (532 nm) (Framme et al., 2008)[159]. Ophthalmoscopic and angiographic damage thresholds were determined to be 266 and 72 mJ/cm^2, respectively, for a repetition of 10 pulses. Histologic examination of lesions revealed damaged RPE with an intact Bruch's membrane. However, selective damage of the RPE without affecting the photoreceptors can only rarely be achieved due to the small safety range.

Recently, selective retina treatment has been evaluated in 19 patients with various macular disorders (including DME) with 200-ns and 1.7-µs laser pulses. Ophthalmic and angiographic threshold irradiances were recorded. Among the 200-ns treatments, nearly all could be individuated angiographically (angiographic threshold: 115 µJ) but could not be visualized ophthalmoscopically. ED_{50} cell damage threshold energies were 99.6 µJ for 200-ns laser pulses and 196.3 µJ for 1.7-µs pulses (Framme et al., 2008)[160].

Retinal Regeneration Therapy
Retinal regeneration therapy (Ellex Medical, Adelaide, Australia) has been proposed as a laser treatment modality that uses extremely short pulses to stimulate the RPE to produce a renewal process, with a reduction in retinal disease progression. The goal of retinal regeneration therapy is to cause RPE cell migration in a sort of biostimulation, releasing MMPs. The Ellex retinal regeneration therapy laser system uses a Q-switched double-frequency Nd:YAG laser to produce a single 3-ns pulse at 532 nm.

A preliminary report on 29 eyes with DME treated with retinal regeneration therapy has been presented (Hamilton, 2007)[161]. Central macular thickness at 3 months decreased by more than 5% in 55% of eyes, remained stable in 24% of cases, and increased in 20% of eyes. A majority of patients manifested an improvement in visual acuity, while no evidence of laser damage to the photoreceptor cells was demonstrated by microperimetry (Hamilton, 2007)[161].

Semiautomated Patterned Scanning Laser Photocoagulation
The Pattern Scan Laser (Pascal, Optimedica Corporation, Santa Clara, Calif., USA) is a double-frequency Nd:YAG diode-pumped solid-state laser, which produces laser beams with a wavelength of 532 nm and can deliver multiple spots

in predetermined patterns. It is based on a galvanometric scanner system (Blumenkranz et al., 2006)[162]. Two output channels send x-axis and y-axis coordinates to an x-y galvanometer, which changes the mirror angle for the laser pulse delivery. The Pascal photocoagulator can deliver a series of different pattern arrays.

The operator can select the pattern, the number of spots, and spacing between them. Predetermined patterns include single-spot, square arrays, octants, quadrants, full and modified macular grid, triple arcs, and single-line arcs. To allow the system to apply multiple spots, pulse durations are reduced to 10–20 ms. Shorter pulse durations are also associated with reduced pulse energy requirements and with decreased heat conduction to the surrounding tissues. Theoretically, the decreased anterior diffusion would lead to less damage to the inner retina and nerve fiber layer and the lower posterior diffusion would be associated with less discomfort to the patient. This leaves space for less invasive treatment modalities and less time-consuming procedures.

Typically, the Pascal photocoagulator allows a uniform whitening with less scar expansion. The feasibility of a rapid application of a precise array of spots allows the physician to deliver adequate-spaced treatment in the absence of an ophthalmoscopically visible end point. This can be particularly suitable for subthreshold laser irradiation, permitting a more accurate placement of subthreshold lesions in a predetermined pattern.

Conclusion
In recent years, advances in laser therapy for retinal disease have been directed toward reducing the unnecessary disruptive effect that laser photocoagulation causes to retinal tissues. To obtain such treatment, pulse duration should be lowered to reduce thermal conduction and spare the neural retina. However, short exposure times may reduce the safety power range between a threshold photocoagulation burn and photo-disruptive

Table 5. Vitrectomy results on eyes with diffuse macular edema combined with taut and thickened posterior hyaloid

Studies	Eyes	Improvement in VA of ≥2 lines	Anatomical improvement	Follow-up months
(Lewis et al., 1992)[5]	10	6 (60%)	10 (100%)	16
(Van Effenterre et al., 1993)[163]	22	22 (100%)	19 (86%)	14
(Harbour et al., 1996)[6]	7	4 (57%)	6 (86%)	12
(Pendergast et al., 2000)[22]	55	27 (49%)	52 (95%)	23
(Gandorfer et al., 2000)[109]	10	10 (100%)	10 (100%)	16
(Massin et al., 2003)[20]	7	5 (70%)	7 (100%)	18

VA = Visual acuity.

phenomena. Therefore, an appropriate treatment window should be prudently individuated. Furthermore, there is the need for the physician to know when an appropriate laser dose has been delivered in the absence of a visible end point with a dedicated on-line detection system.

Vitrectomy

Lewis and Van Effentere were the first to provide results on surgery for tractional DME (Lewis et al., 1992; Van Effentere et al., 1993)[5,163]. This intervention consists of a vitrectomy with a posterior vitreous cortex peeling. Pendergast and colleagues (Pendergast et al., 2000)[22] later confirmed the beneficial results observed in the first studies. It covers a retrospective study of 55 eyes with an average of 23 months of follow-up. Following the vitrectomy, 27 eyes (49%) regained at least 2 lines of visual acuity, 23 eyes (42%) had stable visual acuity, and 5 eyes (9%) had a loss of at least 2 lines. The authors describe a decrease in clinical features of cystoid macular edema for 52 patients (95%), and the complete disappearance for 45 patients (92%).

Other studies have confirmed a beneficial result of vitrectomy for tractional DME (table 5) (Harbour et al., 1996; Massin et al., 2003; Gandorfer et al., 2000)[6,20,164]. The functional prognosis is even better when vitrectomy is performed at an early stage.

Authors have also reported their experience of vitrectomy for macular edema, without any vitreomacular traction syndrome. The results are more controversial, as they are retrospective and have not yet been confirmed (Ikeda et al., 1999; Ikeda et al., 2000; Otani and Kishi, 2000; Yamamoto et al., 2001)[165–168].

The results of 5 randomized studies have recently been published (table 6) (Kumar et al., 2007; Patel et al., 2006; Stolba et al., 2005; Thomas et al., 2005; Yanyali et al., 2005)[169–173]. These studies compare the outcome of vitrectomy, including the peeling of the ILM in 3 studies, to laser treatment in 4 studies, and to the spontaneous evolution of macular edema in 1 study (Stolba et al., 2005)[171]. The studies, however, have a small patient base and the results are contradictory. Only Yanyali and colleagues have shown beneficial results of vitrectomy in a study comprising 24 eyes, both in terms of visual acuity and in reduction of the macular

Table 6. Results of randomized studies on vitrectomy for eyes with diffuse macular edema syndrome without vitreomacular traction

Studies	Eyes	Type of intervention	Improvement in VA of ≥2 lines	Mean decrease of retinal thickening on OCT
(Stolba et al., 2005)[171]	56	PPV + ILM vs. spontaneous evolution	52% 13%	63 μm null
(Thomas et al., 2005)[21]	40	PPV + ILM vs. laser	NS	73 μm 29 μm
(Yanyali et al., 2005)[173]	24	PPV + ILM vs. laser	50% 25%	219 μm 29 μm
(Patel et al., 2006)[170]	15	PPV vs. laser	NS	27 μm (NS) 107 μm
(Kumar et al., 2007)[169]	12	PPV + ILM vs. laser	6 (50%), NS 3 (25%)	300 μm 106 μm

NS = Not significant; PPV = pars plana vitrectomy.

thickening, but the follow-up is short. In addition, the patients from the 'laser' group have only received one photocoagulation session. Stolba and colleagues demonstrated significant improvement of visual acuity but had a less successful result related to macular thickening. Thomas and colleagues as well as Patel and colleagues did not demonstrate any significant difference between the 2 treatments, although Patel and colleagues showed a slight preference for laser treatment. Kumar and colleagues did not obtain a significant difference in improved visual acuity between groups.

Thus, the randomized studies have currently not demonstrated any advantage for recommending a vitrectomy for DME without associated traction.

Follow-Up and Prognosis

The evolution of DME is slow. It may wax and wane, probably under the effect of systemic factors, such as high blood pressure and glycemia

(Massin-Korobelnik et al., 1994; Polito et al., 2006)[174,175]. In the control group of the ETDRS trial, only 15% of patients with CSME had significant visual loss after a 3-year follow-up (Early Treatment Diabetic Retinopathy Study Research Group, 1985)[3]. The long-term prognosis of DME, however, is poor in eyes with persistent macular edema.

Factors of poor visual prognosis include long duration of edema, severe macular nonperfusion, subfoveal plaque exudates, or subfoveal fibrosis.

Conclusion

DME remains among the first causes of visual loss in the working-age population, and its frequency will increase due to significant development of diabetes mellitus incidence throughout the world.

Laser treatment is the gold standard of therapy for reducing visual loss from DME. Attempts have been made over recent years to make laser treatment less invasive and with fewer associated complications. In some clinical trials, light and subthreshold laser approaches have appeared as effective as the classic technique. Although there is still a lack of strong supporting evidence, a less destructive technique using a reduced amount of energy is currently favored by many ophthalmologists in their daily practice.

Significant improvement in diagnostic tools has greatly changed the management of DME. The advent of OCT and its pervasive clinical use has been particularly important in determining a correct interpretation of pathogenic mechanisms involved in the appearance of macular edema, particularly when an anomalous adherence of posterior hyaloid makes pars plana vitrectomy a more rational approach than laser photocoagulation.

OCT is also needed when quantification of edema is the basis for determining efficacy of different treatment modalities, both in multicenter clinical trials and in daily practice.

The advent of the intravitreal approach for treatment of posterior segment disease by using different compounds is one of the most important innovations in the field of macular edema of the last few years.

Steroids and anti-VEGF drugs can now be injected inside the eye, reaching high concentrations with few or no systemic side effects. Multicenter clinical trials have already been completed or are under way, and in the next few years, new compounds will become available making treatment of DME more effective.

Considering the complexity of DME pathogenesis, it is also possible that a combination of different therapeutic approaches will soon become the standard of care for this disease.

References

1 King H, Aubert RE, Herman WH: Global burden of diabetes, 1995–2025: prevalence, numerical estimates, and projections. Diabetes Care 1998;21:1414–1431.

2 Antonetti DA, Lieth E, Barber AJ, Gardner TW: Molecular mechanisms of vascular permeability in diabetic retinopathy. Semin Ophthalmol 1999;14:240–248.

3 Early Treatment Diabetic Retinopathy Study Research Group: Photocoagulation for diabetic macular edema. Early Treatment Diabetic Retinopathy Study report number 1. Arch Ophthalmol 1985;103:1796–1806.

4 Weinberger D, Fink-Cohen S, Gaton D, Priel E, Yassur Y: Non-retinovascular leakage in diabetic maculopathy. Br J Ophthalmol 1995;79:728–731.

5 Lewis H, Abrams GW, Blumenkranz MS, Campo RV: Vitrectomy for diabetic macular traction and edema associated with posterior hyaloidal traction. Ophthalmology 1992;99:753–759.

6 Harbour JW, Smiddy WE, Flynn HWJ, Rubsamen PE: Vitrectomy for diabetic macular edema associated with a thickened and taut posterior hyaloid membrane. Am J Ophthalmol 1996;121:405–413.

7 Kang SW, Park CY, Ham DI: The correlation between fluorescein angiographic and optical coherence tomographic features in clinically significant diabetic macular edema. Am J Ophthalmol 2004;137:313–322.

8 Wilkinson CP, Ferris FL, Klein RE, Lee PP, Agardh CD, Davis M, Dills D, Kampik A, Pararajasegaran R, Verdaguer JT, Global Diabetic Retinopathy Project Group: Proposed international clinical diabetic retinopathy and diabetic macular edema disease severity scales. Ophthalmology 2003;110:1677–1682.

9 Girach A, Lund-Andersen H: Diabetic macular oedema: a clinical overview. Int J Clin Pract 2007;61:88–97.

10 Williams R, Airey M, Baxter H, Forrester J, Kennedy-Martin T, Girach A: Epidemiology of diabetic retinopathy and macular oedema: a systemic review. Eye 2004;18:963–983.

11 Varma R, Torres M, Peña F, Klein R, Azen S, Los Angeles Latino Eye Study Group: Prevalence of diabetic retinopathy in adult Latinos. Ophthalmology 2004;111:1298–1306.

12 Brown JC, Solomon SD, Bressler SB, et al: Detection of diabetic foveal edema. Contact lens biomicroscopy compared with optical coherence tomography. Arch Opthalmol 2004;122:330–335.

13 Massin P, Girach A, Erginay A, Gaudric A: Optical coherence tomography: a key to the future management of patients with diabetic macular oedema. Acta Ophthalmol Scand 2006;84:466–474.

14 Otani T, Kishi S, Maruyama Y: Patterns of diabetic macular edema with optical coherence tomography. Am J Ophthalmol 1999;127:688–693.

15 Bolz M, Schmidt-Erfurth U, Deak G, Mylonas G, Kriechbaum K, Scholda C: Optical coherence tomographic hyperreflective foci: a morphologic sign of lipid extravasation in diabetic macular edema. Ophthalmology 2009;116:914–920.

16 Ozdemir H, Karacorlu M, Karacorlu S: Serous macular detachment in diabetic cystoid macular oedema. Acta Ophthalmol Scand 2005;83:63–66.

17 Catier A, Tadayoni R, Paques M, et al: Optical coherence tomography characterization of macular edema according to various etiology. Am J Ophthalmol 2005;140:200–206.

18 Gaucher D, Sebah C, Erginay A, et al: Optical coherence tomography features during the evolution of serous retinal detachment in patients with diabetic macular edema. Am J Ophthalmol 2008;145:289–296.

19 Gaucher D, Tadayoni R, Erginay A, et al: Optical coherence tomography assessment of the vitreorelationship in diabetic macular edema. Am J Ophthalmol 2005;139:807–813.

20 Massin P, Duguid G, Erginay A, et al: Optical coherence tomography for evaluating diabetic macular edema before and after vitrectomy. Am J Ophthalmol 2003;135:169–177.

21 Thomas D, Bunce C, Moorman C, Laidlaw AH: Frequency and associations of a taut thickened posterior hyaloid, partial vitreomacular separation, and subretinal fluid in patients with diabetic macular edema. Retina 2005;25:883–888.

22 Pendergast SD, Hassan TS, Williams GA, et al: Vitrectomy for diffuse diabetic macular edema associated with a taut premacular posterior hyaloid. Am J Ophthalmol 2000;130:178–186.

23 Uchino E, Uemura A, Ohba N: Initial stages of posterior vitreous detachment in healthy eyes of older persons evaluated by optical coherence tomography. Arch Ophthalmol 2001;119:1475–1479.

24 Hee MR, Puliafito CA, Wong C, Duker JS, Reichel E, Rutledge B, et al: Quantitative assessment of macular edema with optical coherence tomography. Arch Ophthalmol 1995;113:1019–1029.

25 Hee MR, Puliafito CA, Duker JS, Reichel E, Coker JG, Wilkins JR, et al: Topography of diabetic macular edema with optical coherence tomography. Ophthalmology 1998;105:360–370.

26 Massin P, Haouchine B, Gaudric A: Macular traction detachment and diabetic edema associated with posterior hyaloidal traction. Am J Ophthalmol 2001;132:599–600.

27 Polito A, Del Borrello M, Isola M, et al: Repeatability and reproducibility of fast macular thickness mapping using stratus optical coherence tomography. Arch Ophthalmol 2005;123:1330–1337.

28 Wolf-Schnurrbusch UE, Ceklic L, Brinkmann CK, et al: Macular thickness measurements in healthy eyes using six different optical coherence tomography instruments. Invest Ophthalmol Vis Sci 2009;50:3432–3437.

29 Menke MN, Dabov S, Knecht P, Sturm V: Reproducibility of retinal thickness measurements in healthy subjects using spectralis optical coherence tomography. Am J Ophthalmol 2009;147:467–472.

30 Krzystolik MG, Strauber SF, Aiello LP, et al, Diabetic Retinopathy Clinical Research Network: Reproducibility of macular thickness and volume using Zeiss optical coherence tomography in patients with diabetic macular edema. Ophthalmology 2007;114:1520–1525.

31 Strom C, Sander B, Larsen N, et al: Diabetic macular edema assessed with optical coherence tomography and stereo fundus photography. Invest Ophthalmol Vis Sci 2002;43:241–245.

32 Klein R, Moss SE, Klein BE, et al: The Wisconsin Epidemiologic Study of Diabetic Retinopathy. 11. The incidence of macular edema. Ophthalmology 1989;96:1501–1510.

33 Klein R, Klein BE, Moss SE, Cruickshanks KJ: The Wisconsin Epidemiologic Study of Diabetic Retinopathy. 15. The long-term incidence of macular edema. Ophthalmology 1995;102:7–16.

34 Klein R, Klein BE, Moss SE, Cruickshanks KJ: The Wisconsin Epidemiologic Study of Diabetic Retinopathy. 17. The 14-year incidence and progression of diabetic retinopathy and associated risk factors in type 1 diabetes. Ophthalmology 1998;105:1801–1815.

35 Vitale S, Maguire MG, Murphy RP, et al: Clinically significant macular edema in type I diabetes: incidence and risk factors. Ophthalmology 1995;102:1170–1176.

36 Diabetes Control and Complications Trial Research Group: Hypoglycemia in the Diabetes Control and Complications Trial. Diabetes 1997;46:271–286.

37 Diabetes Control and Complications Trial/Epidemiology of Diabetes Interventions and Complications Research Group: Retinopathy and nephropathy in patients with type 1 diabetes four years after a trial of intensive therapy. N Engl J Med 2000;342:381–389.

38 Aroca PR, Salvat M, Fernandez J, Mendez I: Risk factors for diffuse and focal macular edema. J Diabetes Complications 2004;18:211–215.

39 Roy MS, Affouf M: Six-year progression of retinopathy and associated risk factors in African American patients with type 1 diabetes mellitus: the New Jersey 725. Arch Ophthalmol 2006;124:1297–1306.

40 White NH, Sun W, Cleary PA, Danis RP, Davis MD, Hainsworth DP, Hubbard LD, Lachin JM, Nathan DM: Prolonged effect of intensive therapy on the risk of retinopathy complications in patients with type 1 diabetes mellitus: 10 years after the Diabetes Control and Complications Trial. Arch Ophthalmol 2008;126:1707–1715.

41 UK Prospective Diabetes Study (UKPDS) Group: Intensive blood glucose control with sulphonylureas or insulin compared with conventional treatment and risk of complications in patients with type 2 diabetes (UKPDS 33). Lancet 1998;352:837–853.

42 UK Prospective Diabetes Study Group: Tight blood pressure control and risk of macrovascular and microvascular complications in type 2 diabetes: UKPDS 38. BMJ 1998;317:708–713.

43 Matthews DR, Stratton IM, Aldington SJ, et al: Risk of progression of retinopathy and visual loss related to tight control of blood pressure in type 2 diabetes mellitus (UKPDS 69). Arch Ophthalmol 2004;122:1631–1640.

44 Kohner EM, Stratton IM, Aldington SJ, Holman RR, Matthews DR, UK Prospective Diabetes Study (UKPDS) Group: Relationship between the severity of retinopathy and progression to photocoagulation in patients with type 2 diabetes mellitus in the UKPDS (UKPDS 52). Diabet Med 2001;18:178–184.

45 Kohner EM: Microvascular disease: what does the UKPDS tell us about diabetic retinopathy? Diabet Med 2008;25:20–24.

46 Adler AI, Stratton IM, Neil HA, et al: Association of systolic blood pressure with macrovascular and microvascular complications of type 2 diabetes (UKPDS 36): prospective observational study. BMJ 2000;321:412–419.

47 Klein R, Knudtson MD, Lee KE, et al: The Wisconsin Epidemiologic Study of Diabetic Retinopathy. 23. The twenty-five-year incidence of macular edema in persons with type 1 diabetes. Ophthalmology 2009;116:497–503.

48 Davis MD, Beck RW, Home PD, Sandow J, Ferris FL: Early retinopathy progression in four randomized trials comparing insulin glargine and NPH (corrected) insulin. Exp Clin Endocrinol Diabetes 2007;115:240–243.

49 Jaross N, Ryan P, Newland H: Incidence and progression of diabetic retinopathy in an Aboriginal Australian population: results from the Katherine Region Diabetic Retinopathy Study (KRDRS). Report No 2. Clin Experiment Ophthalmol 2005;33:26–33.

50 Funatsu H, Yamashita H: Pathogenesis of diabetic retinopathy and the renin-angiotensin system. Ophthalmic Physiol Opt 2003;23;495–501.

51 Sjolie AK: Prospects for angiotensin receptor blockers in diabetic retinopathy. Diabetes Res Clin Pract 2007;76: S31–S39.

52 West KM, Erdreich LJ, Stober JA: A detailed study of risk factors for retinopathy and nephropathy in diabetes. Diabetes 1980;29:501–508.

53 Knuiman MW, Welborn TA, McCann VJ, et al: Prevalence of diabetic complications in relation to risk factors. Diabetes 1986;35:1332–1339.

54 Jerneld B: Prevalence of diabetic retinopathy: a population study from the Swedish island of Gotland. Acta Ophthalmol 1988;188:3–32.

55 Kostraba JN, Klein R, Dorman JS, et al: The Epidemiology of Diabetes Complications Study. 4. Correlates of diabetic background and proliferative retinopathy. Am J Epidemiol 1991;133:381–391.

56 Cruickshanks KJ, Ritter LL, Klein R, Moss SE: The association of microalbuminuria with diabetic retinopathy: the Wisconsin Epidemiologic Study of Diabetic Retinopathy. Ophthalmology 1993;100:862–867.

57 Klein R, Moss SE, Klein BE: Is gross proteinuria a risk factor for the incidence of proliferative diabetic retinopathy? Ophthalmology 1993;100:1140–1146.

58 Romero P, Baget M, Mendez I, et al: Diabetic macular edema and its relationship to renal microangiopathy: a sample of type I diabetes mellitus patients in a 15-year follow-up study. J Diabetes Complications 2007;21:172–180.

59 Klein R, Klein BE, Davis MD: Is cigarette smoking associated with diabetic retinopathy? Am J Epidemiol 1983;118:228–238.

60 Moss SE, Klein R, Klein BE: Cigarette smoking and ten-year progression of diabetic retinopathy. Ophthalmology 1996;103:1438–1442.

61 Chew EY, Klein ML, Ferris FL III, et al: Association of elevated serum lipid levels with retinal hard exudate in diabetic retinopathy. Early treatment diabetic retinopathy study (ETDRS) Report 22. Arch Ophthalmol 1996;114:1079–1084.

62 Sen K, Misra A, Kumar A, Pandey RM: Simvastatin retards progression of retinopathy in diabetic patients with hypercholesterolemia. Diabetes Res Clin Pract 2002;56:1–11.

63 Rechtman E, Harris A, Garzozi HJ, Ciulla TA: Pharmacologic therapies for diabetic retinopathy and diabetic macular edema. Clin Ophthalmol 2007;1:383–391.

64 Lee CM, Olk RJ: Modified grid laser photocoagulation for diffuse diabetic macular edema. Long-term visual results. Ophthalmology 1991;98:1594–1602.

65 Tsaprouni LG, Ito K, Punchard N, Adcock IM: Triamcinolone acetonide and dexamethasome suppress TNF-alpha-induced histone H4 acetylation on lysine residues 8 and 12 in mononuclear cells. Ann NY Acad Sci 2002;973:481–483.

66 Juergens UR, Jager F, Darlath W, Stober M, Vetter H, Gillissen A: Comparison of in vitro activity of commonly used topical glucocorticoids on cytokine- and phospholipase inhibition. Eur J Med Res 2004;9:383–390.

67 Tong JP, Lam DS, Chan WM, Choy KW, Chan KP, Pang CP: Effects of triamcinolone on the expression of VEGF and PEDF in human retinal pigment epithelial and human umbilical vein endothelial cells. Mol Vis 2006;12:1490–1495.

68 Kim YH, Choi MY, Kim YS, et al: Triamcinolone acetonide protects the rat retina from STZ-induced acute inflammation and early vascular leakage. Life Sci 2007;81:1167–1173.

69 Zhang SX, Wang JJ, Gao G, Shao C, Mott R, Ma JX: Pigment epithelium-derived factor (PEDF) is an endogenous antiinflammatory factor. FASEB J 2006;20:323–325.

70 Abelson MB, Butrus S: Corticosteroids in ophthalmic practice; in Abelson MB, Neufeld AH, Topping TM (eds): Principles and Practice of Ophthalmology. Philadelphia, WB Saunders, 1994, p 1014.

71 Mizuno S, Nishiwaki A, Morita H, Miyake T, Ogura Y: Effects of periocular administration of triamcinolone acetonide on leukocyte-endothelium interactions in the ischemic retina. Invest Ophthalmol Vis Sci 2007;48:2831–2836.

72 Audren F, Erginay A, Haouchine B, et al: Intravitreal triamcinolone acetonide for diffuse macular oedema: 6-month results of a prospective controlled trial. Acta Ophthalmol Scand 2006;84:624–630.

73 Jonas JB, Kamppeter BA, Harder B, Vossmerbaeumer U, Sauder G, Spandau UH: Intravitreal triamcinolone acetonide for diabetic macular edema: a prospective, randomized study. J Ocul Pharmacol Ther 2006;22:200–207.

74 Gillies MC, Sutter FK, Simpson JM, Larsson J, Ali H, Zhu M: Intravitreal triamcinolone for refractory diabetic macular edema: two-year results of a double-masked, placebo-controlled, randomized clinical trial. Ophthalmology 2006;113:1533–1538.

75 Diabetic Retinopathy Clinical Research Network: A randomized trial comparing intravitreal triamcinolone acetonide and focal/grid photocoagulation for diabetic macular edema. Ophthalmology 2008;115:1447–1449, 1449.e1–10.

76 Hauser D, Bukelman A, Pokroy R, et al: Intravitreal triamcinolone for diabetic macular edema: comparison of 1, 2, and 4 mg. Retina 2008;28:825–830.

77 Kim JE, Pollack JS, Miller DG, Mittra RA, Spaide RF: ISIS-DME: a prospective, randomized, dose-escalation intravitreal steroid injection study for refractory diabetic macular edema. Retina 2008;28:735–740.

78 Beer PM, Bakri SJ, Singh RJ, Liu W, Peters GB 3rd, Miller M: Intraocular concentration and pharmacokinetics of triamcinolone acetonide after a single intravitreal injection. Ophthalmology 2003;110:681–686.

79 Audren F, Tod M, Massin P, et al: Pharmacokinetic-pharmacodynamic modeling of the effect of triamcinolone acetonide on central macular thickness in patients with diabetic macular edema. Invest Ophthalmol Vis Sci 2004;45:3435–3441.

80 Jager RD, Aiello LP, Patel SC, Cunningham ET Jr: Risks of intravitreous injection: a comprehensive review. Retina 2004;24:676–698.

81 Geroski DH, Edelhauser HF: Transscleral drug delivery for posterior segment disease. Adv Drug Deliv Rev 2001;52:37–48.

82 Olsen TW, Edelhauser HF, Lim JI, Geroski DH: Human scleral permeability. Effects of age, cryotherapy, transscleral diode laser, and surgical thinning. Invest Ophthalmol Vis Sci 1995;36:1893–1903.

83 Kato A, Kimura H, Okabe K, Okabe J, Kunou N, Ogura Y: Feasibility of drug delivery to the posterior pole of the rabbit eye with an episcleral implant. Invest Ophthalmol Vis Sci 2004;45:238–244.

84 Bonini-Filho MA, Jorge R, Barbosa JC, Calucci D, Cardillo JA, Costa RA: Intravitreal injection versus sub-Tenon's infusion of triamcinolone acetonide for refractory diabetic macular edema: a randomized clinical trial. Invest Ophthalmol Vis Sci 2005;46:3845–3849.

85 Cardillo JA, Melo LA Jr, Costa RA, et al: Comparison of intravitreal versus posterior sub-Tenon's capsule injection of triamcinolone acetonide for diffuse diabetic macular edema. Ophthalmology 2005;112:1557–1563.

86 Ozdek S, Bahceci UA, Gurelik G, Hasanreisoglu B: Posterior subtenon and intravitreal triamcinolone acetonide for diabetic macular edema. J Diabetes Complications 2006;20:246–251.

87 Veritti D, Lanzetta P, Perissin L, Bandello F: Posterior juxtascleral infusion of modified triamcinolone acetonide formulation for refractory diabetic macular edema: one-year follow-up. Invest Ophthalmol Vis Sci 2009;50:2391–2397.

88 Graham RO, Peyman GA: Intravitreal injection of dexamethasone. Treatment of experimentally induced endophthalmitis. Arch Ophthalmol 1974;92:149–154.

89 Hardman JG, Limbird LE, Molinoff PB: Goodman & Gilman's The Pharmacological Basis of Therapeutics, ed 9. New York, McGraw Hill, 2001.

90 Fialho SL, Behar-Cohen F, Silva-Cunha A: Dexamethasone-loaded poly(epsilon-caprolactone) intravitreal implants: a pilot study. Eur J Pharm Biopharm 2008;68:637–646.

91 Kuppermann BD, Blumenkranz MS, Haller JA, et al: Randomized controlled study of an intravitreous dexamethasone drug delivery system in patients with persistent macular edema. Arch Ophthalmol 2007;125:309–317.

92 Ashton P, Blandford DL, Pearson PA, Jaffe GJ, Martin DF, Nussenblatt RB: Review: implants. J Ocul Pharmacol 1994;10:691–701.

93 Jaffe GJ, Yang CH, Guo H, Denny JP, Lima C, Ashton P: Safety and pharmacokinetics of an intraocular fluocinolone acetonide sustained delivery device. Invest Ophthalmol Vis Sci 2000;41:3569–3575.

94 Hsu J: Drug delivery methods for posterior segment disease. Curr Opin Ophthalmol 2007;18:235–239.

95 Pearson P, Levy B, Comstock T, Fluocinolone Acetonide Implant Study Group: Fluocinolone acetonide intravitreal implant to treat diabetic macular edema: 3-year results of a multicenter clinical trial. Annu Meet Assoc Res Vis Ophthalmol, Ft Lauderdale, May 4, 2006.

96 Eliott D, Dugel PU, Cantrill HL, et al: I-vation TA: 18 month results from phase I safety and preliminary efficacy study. Annu Meet Assoc Res Vis Ophthalmol, Ft Lauderdale, 2008.

97 Hu M, Huang G, Karasina F, Wong VG: Verisome, a novel injectable, sustained-release, biodegradable, intraocular drug delivery system and triamcinolone acetonide. Annu Meet Assoc Res Vis Ophthalmol, Ft Lauderdale, 2008.

98 Gardner TW, Antonetti DA, Barber AJ, LaNoue KF, Levison SW: Diabetic retinopathy: more than meets the eye. Surv Ophthalmol 2002;47(Suppl 2):S253–S262.

99 Grant MB, Afzal A, Spoerri P, Pan H, Shaw LC, Mames RN: The role of growth factors in the pathogenesis of diabetic retinopathy. Expert Opin Investig Drugs 2004;13:1275–1293.

100 Cunningham ET Jr, Adamis AP, Altaweel M, et al: A phase II randomized double-masked trial of pegaptanib, an anti-vascular endothelial growth factor aptamer, for diabetic macular edema. Ophthalmology 2005;112:1747–1757.

101 Nguyen QD, Tatlipinar S, Shah SM, et al: Vascular endothelial growth factor is a critical stimulus for diabetic macular edema. Am J Ophthalmol 2006;142:961–969.

102 Shah SM, Nguyen QD, Tatlipinar S, et al: One-year results of the READ study: ranibizumab for edema of the macula in diabetes. Retina Soc Annu Meet, Cape Town, 2006.

103 Nguyen QD, Heier JS, Shah SM, et al, The READ 2 Investigators: Six-month results of the READ 2 study: ranibizumab for edema of the macula in diabetes, a phase 2 clinical trial. Am Acad Ophthalmol 2008 Annu Meet, Atlanta, 2008.

104 Massin PG: Ranibizumab in diabetic macular edema. Joint Meet Am Acad Ophthalmol Eur Soc Ophthalmol, Atlanta, 2008.

105 Scott IU, Edwards AR, Beck RW, et al: A phase II randomized clinical trial of intravitreal bevacizumab for diabetic macular edema. Ophthalmology 2007;114:1860–1867.

106 Ahmadieh H, Ramezani A, Shoeibi N, et al: Intravitreal bevacizumab with or without triamcinolone for refractory macular edema: a placebo-controlled, randomized clinical trial. Graefes Arch Clin Exp Ophthalmol 2008;246:483–489.

107 Soheilian M, Ramezani A, Obudi A, et al: Randomized trial of intravitreal bevacizumab alone or combined with triamcinolone versus macular photocoagulation in diabetic macular edema. Ophthalmology 2009;116:1142–1150.

108 Paccola L, Costa RA, Folgosa MS, Barbosa JC, Scott IU, Jorge R: Intravitreal triamcinolone versus bevacizumab for treatment of refractory diabetic macular oedema (IBEME study). Br J Ophthalmol 2008;92:76–80.

109 Gandorfer A, Rohleder M, Kampik A: Epiretinal pathology of vitreomacular traction syndrome. Br J Ophthalmol 2002;86:902–909.

110 Trese MT: Enzymatic vitreous surgery. Semin Ophthalmol 2000;15:116–121.

111 Hermel M, Schrage NF: Efficacy of plasmin enzymes and chondroitinase ABC in creating posterior vitreous separation in the pig: a masked, placebo-controlled in vivo study. Graefes Arch Clin Exp Ophthalmol 2007;245:399–406.

112 Stefansson E, Loftsson T: The Stokes-Einstein equation and the physiological effects of vitreous surgery. Acta Ophthalmol Scand 2006;84:718–719.

113 Quiram PA, Leverenz VR, Baker RM, Dang L, Giblin FJ, Trese MT: Microplasmin-induced posterior vitreous detachment affects vitreous oxygen levels. Retina 2007;27:1090–1096.

114 Kuppermann BD, Thomas EL, de Smet MD, Grillone LR: Pooled efficacy results from two multinational randomized controlled clinical trials of a single intra-vitreous injection of highly purified ovine hyaluronidase (Vitrase) for the management of vitreous hemorrhage. Am J Ophthalmol 2005;140:573–584.

115 Kuppermann BD, Thomas EL, de Smet MD, Grillone LR: Safety results of two phase III trials of an intravitreous injection of highly purified ovine hyaluronidase (Vitrase) for the management of vitreous hemorrhage. Am J Ophthalmol 2005;140:585–597.

116 Sakuma T, Tanaka M, Mizota A, Inoue J, Pakola S: Safety of in vivo pharmacologic vitreolysis with recombinant microplasmin in rabbit eyes. Invest Ophthalmol Vis Sci 2005;46:3295–3299.

117 Lindstedt EW, Baarsma GS, Kuijpers RW, van Hagen PM: Anti-TNF-alpha therapy for sight threatening uveitis. Br J Ophthalmol 2005;89:533–536.

118 Theodossiadis PG, Markomichelakis NN, Sfikakis PP: Tumor necrosis factor antagonists: preliminary evidence for an emerging approach in the treatment of ocular inflammation. Retina 2007;27:399–413.

119 Giansanti F, Ramazzotti M, Vannozzi L, et al: A pilot study on ocular safety of intravitreal infliximab in a rabbit model. Invest Ophthalmol Vis Sci 2008;49:1151–1156.

120 New and in-development treatments for diabetic macular edema. http://www.retinalphysician.com/article.aspx?article=101898 (accessed April 4, 2009).

121 Do DV, Nguyen QD, Shah SM, et al: An exploratory study of the safety, tolerability and bioactivity of a single intravitreal injection of vascular endothelial growth factor Trap-Eye in patients with diabetic macular oedema. Br J Ophthalmol 2009;93:144–149.

122 Macusight announces positive initial results from phase 1 study of sirolimus in diabetic macular edema. http://www.frazierhealthcare.com/pdf/Macusight_100107.pdf (accessed April 4, 2009).

123 Ozerdem U, Mach-Hofacre B, Cheng L, et al: The effect of prinomastat (AG3340), a potent inhibitor of matrix metalloproteinases, on a subacute model of proliferative vitreoretinopathy. Curr Eye Res 2000;20:447–453.

124 Gao G, Li Y, Zhang D, Gee S, Crosson C, Ma J: Unbalanced expression of VEGF and PEDF in ischemia-induced retinal neovascularization. FEBS Lett 2001;489:270–276.

125 Stellmach V, Crawford SE, Zhou W, Bouck N: Prevention of ischemia-induced retinopathy by the natural ocular antiangiogenic agent pigment epithelium-derived factor. Proc Natl Acad Sci USA 2001;98:2593–2597.

126 Duh EJ, Yang HS, Suzuma I, et al: Pigment epithelium-derived factor suppresses ischemia-induced retinal neovascularization and VEGF-induced migration and growth. Invest Ophthalmol Vis Sci 2002;43:821–829.

127 Duh EJ, Yang HS, Haller JA, et al: Vitreous levels of pigment epithelium-derived factor and vascular endothelial growth factor: implications for ocular angiogenesis. Am J Ophthalmol 2004;137:668–674.

128 Jittpoonkuson T, Garcia P, Rosen RB: Correlation between fluorescein angiography and spectral domain optical coherence tomography in the diagnosis of cystoid macular edema. Br J Ophthalmol, E-pub ahead of print.

129 Bandello F, Polito A, Del Borrello M, Zemella N, Isola M: 'Light' versus 'classic' laser treatment for clinically significant diabetic macular oedema. Br J Ophthalmol 2005;89:864–870.

130 Stefansson E: The therapeutic effects of retinal laser treatment and vitrectomy. A theory based on oxygen and vascular physiology. Acta Ophthalmol Scan 2001;79:435–440.

131 Wolbarsht ML, Landers MBI: The rationale of photocoagulation therapy for proliferative diabetic retinopathy: a review and a model. Ophthalmic Surg Lasers 1980;11:235–245.

132 Molnar I, Poitry S, Tsacopoulos M, et al: Effect of laser photocoagulation on oxygenation of the retina in miniature pigs. Invest Ophthalmol Vis Sci 1985;26:1410–1414.

133 Stefansson E, Landers MBI, Wolbarsht ML: Increased retinal oxygen supply following panretinal photocoagulation and vitrectomy and lensectomy. Trans Am Acad Ophthalmol Soc 1981;79:307–334.

134 Yu D, Cringle S, Su E, Yu PK, Humayun MS, Dorin G: Laser-induced changes in intraretinal oxygen distribution in pigmented rabbits. Invest Ophthalmol Vis Sci 2005;46:988–999.

135 Wilson DJ, Finkelstein D, Quigley HA, Green RW: Macular grid photocoagulation. An experimental study on the primate retina. Arch Ophthalmol 1988;106:100–105.

136 Guyer DR, D'Amico DJ, Smith CW: Subretinal fibrosis after laser photocoagulation for diabetic macular edema. Am J Ophthalmol 1992;113:652–656.

137 Han DP, Mieler WF, Burton TC: Submacular fibrosis after photocoagulation for diabetic macular edema. Am J Ophthalmol 1992;113:513–521.

138 Gottfredsdottir MS, Stefansson E, Jonasson F, Gislason I: Retinal vasoconstriction after laser treatment for diabetic macular edema. Am J Ophthalmol 1993;115:64–67.

139 Xiao M, McLeod D, Cranley J, Williams G, Boulton M: Growth factor staining patterns in the pig retina following retinal laser photocoagulation. Br J Ophthalmol 1999;83:728–736.

140 Ogata N, Ando A, Uyama M, Matsumura M: Expression of cytokines and transcription factors in photocoagulated human retinal pigment epithelial cells. Graefes Arch Clin Exp Ophthalmol 2001;239:87–95.

141 Early Treatment Diabetic Retinopathy Study Research Group: Focal photocoagulation treatment of diabetic macular edema. Relationship of treatment effect to fluorescein angiographic and other retinal characteristics at baseline. ETDRS report number 19. Arch Ophthalmol 1995;113:1144–1155.

142 Early Treatment Diabetic Retinopathy Study Research Group: Treatment techniques and clinical guidelines for photocoagulation of diabetic macular edema. Early Treatment Diabetic Retinopathy Study report number 2. Ophthalmology 1987;94:761–774.

143 Ferris FL III, Davis MD: Treating 20/20 eyes with diabetic macular edema. Arch Ophthalmol 1999;117:675–676.

144 Olk RJ: Modified grid argon (blue-green) laser photocoagulation for diffuse diabetic macular edema. Ophthalmology 1986;93:938–950.

145 Olk RJ: Argon green (514 nm) versus krypton red (647 nm) modified grid laser photocoagulation for diffuse diabetic macular edema. Ophthalmology 1990;97:1101–1113.

146 Writing Committee for the Diabetic Retinopathy Clinical Research Network: Comparison of modified early treatment diabetic retinopathy study and mild macular grid laser photocoagulation strategies for diabetic macular edema. Arch Ophthalmol 2007;125:469–480.

147 Lewis H, Schachat AP, Haimann MH, et al: Choroidal neovascularization after laser photocoagulation for diabetic macular edema. Ophthalmology 1990;97: 503–511.

148 Schatz H, Madeira D, McDonald R: Progressive enlargement of laser scars following grid laser photocoagulation for diffuse diabetic macular edema. Arch Ophthalmol 1991;109:1549–1551.

149 Fong DS, Segal PP, Myers F, et al: Subretinal fibrosis in diabetic macular edema. ETDRS report number 23. Early Treatment Diabetic Retinopathy Study Research Group. Arch Ophthalmol 1997;115:873–877.

150 Lanzetta P, Dorin G, Pirracchio A, Bandello F: Theoretical bases of non-ophthalmoscopically visible endpoint photocoagulation. Semin Ophthalmol 2001;16: 8–11.

151 Dorin G: Subthreshold and micropulse diode laser photocoagulation. Semin Ophthalmol 2003;18:147–153.

152 Lanzetta P, Polito A, Veritti D: Subthreshold laser. Ophthalmology 2008;115:216–216.e1.

153 Luttrull JK, Spink CJ: Serial optical coherence tomography of subthreshold diode laser micropulse photocoagulation for diabetic macular edema. Ophthalmic Surg Lasers Imaging 2006;37:370–377.

154 Friberg TR, Karatza EC: The treatment of macular disease using a micropulsed and continuous wave 810-nm diode laser. Ophthalmology 1997;104:2030–2038.

155 Moorman CM, Hamilton AM: Clinical applications of the MicroPulse diode laser. Eye 1999;13(Pt 2):145–150.

156 Sivaprasad S, Sandhu R, Tandon A, Sayed-Ahmed K, McHugh DA: Subthreshold micropulse diode laser photocoagulation for clinically significant diabetic macular oedema: a three-year follow-up. Clin Experiment Ophthalmol 2007;35:640–644.

157 Figueira J, Khan J, Nunes S, et al: Prospective randomized controlled trial comparing subthreshold micropulse diode laser photocoagulation and conventional green laser for clinically significant diabetic macular oedema. Br J Ophthalmol 2009;93:1341–1344.

158 Brinkmann R, Roider J, Birngruber R: Selective retina therapy (SRT): a review on methods, techniques, preclinical and first clinical results. Bull Soc Belge Ophtalmol 2006;302:51–69.

159 Framme C, Schuele G, Kobuch K, Flucke B, Birngruber R, Brinkmann R: Investigation of selective retina treatment (SRT) by means of 8 ns laser pulses in a rabbit model. Lasers Surg Med 2008;40:20–27.

160 Framme C, Walter A, Prahs P, Theisen-Kunde D, Brinkmann R: Comparison of threshold irradiances and online dosimetry for selective retina treatment (SRT) in patients treated with 200 nanoseconds and 1.7 microseconds laser pulses. Lasers Surg Med 2008;40:616–624.

161 Hamilton P: Selective laser retinal pigment epithelium treatment for diabetic macular edema. Retina Subspecialty Day AAO Annu Meet, New Orleans, 2007.

162 Blumenkranz MS, Yellachich D, Andersen DE, et al: Semiautomated patterned scanning laser for retinal photocoagulation. Retina 2006;26:370–376.

163 Van Effenterre G, et al: Macular edema caused by contraction of the posterior hyaloids in diabetic retinopathy. Surgical treatment of a series of 22 cases. J Fr Ophthalmol 1993;16:602–610.

164 Gandorfer A, Messmer EM, Ulbig MW, Kampik A: Resolution of diabetic macular edema after surgical removal of the posterior hyaloid and the inner limiting membrane. Retina 2000;20:126–133.

165 Ikeda T, Sato K, Katano T, Hayashi Y: Vitrectomy for cystoid macular oedema with attached posterior hyaloid membrane in patients with diabetes. Br J Ophthalmol 1999;83:12–14.

166 Ikeda T, Sato K, Katano T, Hayashi Y: Improved visual acuity following pars plana vitrectomy for diabetic cystoid macular edema and detached posterior hyaloid. Retina 2000;20:220–222.

167 Otani T, Kishi S: Tomographic assessment of vitreous surgery for diabetic macular edema. Am J Ophthalmol 2000;129:487–494.

168 Yamamoto T, Akabane N, Takeuchi S: Vitrectomy for diabetic macular edema: the role of posterior vitreous detachment and epimacular membrane. Am J Ophthalmol 2001;132:369–377.

169 Kumar A, Sinha S, Azad R, Sharma YR, Vohra R: Comparative evaluation of vitrectomy and dye-enhanced ILM peel with grid laser in diffuse diabetic macular edema. Graefes Arch Clin Exp Ophthalmol 2007;245:360–368.

170 Patel JI, Hykin PG, Schadt M, et al: Diabetic macular oedema: pilot randomised trial of pars plana vitrectomy vs macular argon photocoagulation. Eye (Lond) 2006;20:873–881.

171 Stolba U, Binder S, Gruber D, Krebs I, Aggermann T, Neumaier B: Vitrectomy for persistent diffuse diabetic macular edema. Am J Ophthalmol 2005;140:295–301.

172 Thomas D, Bunce C, Moorman C, Laidlaw DA: A randomized controlled feasibility trial of vitrectomy versus laser for diabetic macular oedema. Br J Ophthalmol 2005;89:81–86.

173 Yanyali A, Nohutcu AF, Horozoglu F, Celik E: Modified grid laser photocoagulation versus pars plana vitrectomy with internal limiting membrane removal in diabetic macular edema. Am J Ophthalmol 2005;139:795–801.

174 Massin-Korobelnik P, Gaudric A, Coscas G: Spontaneous evolution and treatment of diabetic cystoid macular edema. Graefes Arch Ophthalmol 1994;232:279–289.

175 Polito A, Borello M, Polini G, et al: Diurnal variation in clinically significant diabetic macular edema measured by the Stratus OCT. Retina 2006;26:14–20.

Prof. Francesco Bandello
Department of Ophthalmology, University Vita-Salute
Scientific Institute San Raffaele
Via Olgettina, 60, IT–20132 Milano (Italy)
E-Mail bandello.francesco@hsr.it

Chapter 7

Coscas G (ed): Macular Edema.
Dev Ophthalmol. Basel, Karger, 2010, vol 47, pp 111–135

Retinal Vein Occlusions

Jost Jonas[a] · Michel Paques[b] · Jordi Monés[d] · Agnès Glacet-Bernard[c]

[a]Department of Ophthalmology, Faculty of Clinical Medicine Mannheim, University of Heidelberg, Mannheim, Germany; [b]Quinze-Vingts Hospital and Vision Institute, Paris, and [c]Ophthalmologic Department, Hôpital Intercommunal de Créteil, University Paris XII, Créteil, Paris, France; [d]Institut de la Màcula i de la Retina, Barcelona, Spain

Abstract

Retinal vein occlusions (RVOs) have been defined as retinal vascular disorders characterized by dilatation of the retinal veins with retinal and subretinal hemorrhages and macular edema, and/or retinal ischemia. Fluorescein angiography (FA) remains essential for the diagnosis and prognosis of RVO, allowing recognition of the diverse types of RVO, such as perfused or nonperfused, as well as detection of the different modalities in natural history. FA is the most effective method to determine the presence (or absence) of macular cystoid edema, its extension, persistence, regression, or the degree of ischemia. Spectral domain optical coherence tomography (SD-OCT) helps to quantify the changes in retinal thickness, the amount of cystoid macular edema, and supplies additional information, such as whether the accumulated fluid is located mostly within the retinal layers or additionally in the subretinal space. SD-OCT can display the presence and integrity of the outer limiting membrane and of the inner and outer segments of the photoreceptors, useful information for prognosis and a guide for treatment in the management of RVO. Laser photocoagulation in a 'grid' pattern over the area, demonstrated as leaking by FA, remains the 'reference treatment for macular edema due to branch retinal vein occlusion', according to the recent results of the SCORE Trial. Recent case series studies and prospective randomized trials strongly suggest an antiedematous effect of intravitreal steroids and an associated improvement in vision. These studies have suggested that intravitreal steroids (triamcinolone, fluocinolone, dexamethasone in a slow-release device) and intravitreal anti-VEGF drugs (bevacizumab, ranibizumab, pegabtanib) may at least temporarily reduce foveal edema and correspond-ingly improve visual function. Surgical treatment modalities have been reported for RVOs. The positive action of vitrectomy seems durable; the combination of surgery and intravitreal injection of steroids and/or an injection of tissue plasminogen activator could permit a more rapid and lasting action. However, strong data from randomized trials are warranted.

Copyright © 2010 S. Karger AG, Basel

Retinal vein occlusions (RVOs) have been defined as retinal vascular disorders characterized by engorgement and dilatation of the retinal veins with secondary, mostly intraretinal hemorrhages and mostly intraretinal (and partially subretinal) edema, retinal ischemia including cotton wool spots, retinal exudates, and macular edema (Hayreh, 1964; Hayreh, 1965; Coscas et al., 1978; Hayreh, 1983; The Central Vein Occlusion Study, 1993; The Central Vein Occlusion Study Group M report, 1995; The Central Vein Occlusion Study Group N report, 1995; Hayreh et al., 1990; Coscas et al., 1984)[1–9].

As soon as the foveal region is involved in macular edema, central visual acuity drops, leading to a progressive or sometimes acute painless loss in vision.

RVOs are differentiated into:
- *central retinal vein occlusion* (CRVO), if the whole venous retinal system is involved and

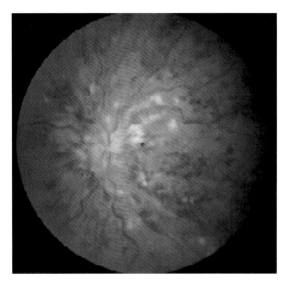

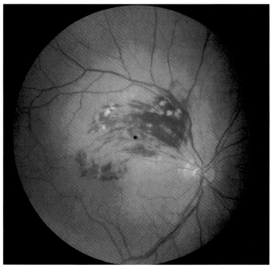

Fig. 1. Fundus photograph showing a CRVO.

Fig. 2. Fundus photograph showing a superior temporal BRVO.

if the presumed site of an increased venous outflow resistance is located in the lamina cribrosa and/or posterior to it[a] (fig. 1);
- *branch retinal vein occlusion* (BRVO), if the venous engorgement involves only branches of the whole retinal venous system. Depending on the site where the engorgement starts, one can further subdivide the group into BRVOs which originate in the optic disk, and BRVOs which originate at an arteriovenous crossing (fig. 2).

Based on the seminal works by Hayreh, the degree of ischemia has been used to further classify the RVOs into the ischemic type and into the nonischemic type (Hayreh, 1964; Hayreh, 1965; Coscas et al., 1978)[1–3]. In the ischemic RVO, there are well-established stigmata of inner retinal ischemia, including marked retinal capillary nonperfusion, marked amount of cotton wool spots, visual acuity of counting fingers or less, perimetric defects so that only the Goldmann target V4e could be seen, a relative afferent papillary defect of more than 1.2 logarithmic units, and later, intraocular neovascularization. In the nonischemic (or perfused) RVO, there is essentially a stasis of retinal venous circulation and macular edema associated with leakage from the altered retinal capillary bed.

Epidemiology

RVO is one of the most common causes of retinal vascular abnormality and a frequent cause of visual loss. Being recognized at least as early as 1855 (Liebreich, 1855)[10], it has been the subject of more than 3,000 publications. Current estimates

---

[a] If the superior or the inferior hemisphere of the fundus is involved, the presumed site of the occlusion is one of the two trunks of the intraneural central retinal vein where this congenital abnormality exists. This entity (hemicentral retinal vein occlusion) is considered a variant of CRVO.

of the prevalence of RVO are derived from major population-based studies, such as the Blue Mountains Eye Study, the Beaver Dam Eye Study, and a combined analysis of the Atherosclerosis Risk in Communities and Cardiovascular Health Studies (Klein et al., 2000; Mitchell et al., 1996; Wong et al., 2005)[11–13].

More recent data have been published from other *racial/ethnic groups*: the Beijing Eye Study (Liu et al., 2007)[14], the Multiethnic Study of Atherosclerosis (Cheung et al., 2008)[15] and the Singapore Malay Eye Study (Lim et al., 2008)[16]. The reported *prevalence of RVO* varied widely across these studies, ranging from 0.3% (Mitchell et al., 1996)[12] to 1.6%. The variability in prevalence rates is likely related to the small number of RVO cases in any single study, differing study methodologies (e.g. retinal photography), and possible racial/ethnic differences in distributions of RVO risk factors. As a result of these limitations, estimations of RVO prevalence are relatively imprecise.

Furthermore, most single studies rarely report on the *prevalence of different RVO subtypes,* namely CRVO and BRVO, which are important to distinguish as they have different risk factors (Hayreh et al., 2001; O'Mahoney et al., 2008)[17,18], prognosis, and treatment (Hayreh, 2005; McIntosh et al., 2006; Mohamed et al., 2006)[19–21].

A recent multicenter study pooled individual level data of more than 70,000 adults in 15 studies around the world (Rogers et al., 2009)[22]. The prevalence rates per 1,000 persons were 4.42 for BRVO and 0.80 for CRVO, with these prevalence rates being age- and gender-standardized to the 2008 world population aged 30 years and older. The prevalence of RVO was similar between men and women, and increased with age.

Overall, the prevalence of BRVO was highest in Asians and Hispanics and the lowest in whites, although the overlapping confidence intervals suggested racial/ethnic differences were not statistically significant. In the Multiethnic Study of Atherosclerosis (Cheung et al., 2008)[15], the only

study with 4 racial/ethnic groups examined in 1 study, the crude prevalence of any RVO was similar across whites, blacks, Chinese, and Hispanics.

It is worth noting that in the Multiethnic Study of Atherosclerosis, sample sizes of each ethnic group were relatively small, particularly the Chinese subgroup (n = 724), and that all participants were United States residents who were free from clinical cardiovascular disease (i.e., generally healthier study samples). Therefore, the Multiethnic Study of Atherosclerosis might not be sufficiently powered to detect meaningful ethnic difference in RVO prevalence, and should not be expected to represent different ethnic groups outside the US. Other studies of multiple ethnic samples as a single study also did not have sufficient numbers of RVO cases to examine racial/ethnic differences by RVO subtypes. The higher prevalence of BRVO in some racial/ethnic groups may reflect different population distributions of RVO risk factors. For example, the prevalence of hypertension and uncontrolled hypertension is reported to be higher in Asians (Leenen et al., 2008)[23] and Hispanics (Read et al., 2007)[24] than in whites (Giles et al., 2007; Ostchega et al., 2008)[25,26].

Summarizing all available data on the prevalence rates of RVO worldwide, one may estimate that 14–19 million adults are affected by the disease worldwide. The prevalence of both BRVO and CRVO increases significantly with age but does not differ by gender. Possible racial/ethnic differences in the prevalence of RVO may reflect differences in the prevalence of vascular risk factors, particularly arterial hypertension, ethnic-related differences in the prevalence of glaucomatous optic neuropathy as the major ocular risk factor, or other unknown factors. Although population-based investigations revealed a significantly higher prevalence of BRVOs than of CRVOs, CRVOs cause considerably more visual burden.

Factors Associated with RVOs

In probably the largest study on associations between RVOs and other factors, Hayreh and colleagues investigated prospectively 1,090 consecutive patients with RVO, almost all of them Caucasians (Hayreh et al., 2001)[17]. They found that there was a significantly higher *prevalence of arterial hypertension* in BRVO compared with CRVO and hemicentral RVO. BRVO also had a significantly higher prevalence of peripheral vascular disease, venous disease, peptic ulcer, and other gastrointestinal disease compared with CRVO.

The proportion of patients with BRVO with cerebrovascular disease was also significantly greater than that of the combined group of patients with CRVO and patients with hemicentral RVO. There was no significant difference in the prevalence of any systemic disease between CRVO and hemicentral RVO. A significantly greater prevalence of arterial hypertension and diabetes mellitus was present in the ischemic CRVO compared with the nonischemic CRVO group. Similarly, arterial hypertension and ischemic heart disease were more prevalent in major BRVO than in macular BRVO.

Relative to the US white control population, the combined group of patients with CRVO and patients with hemicentral RVO had a higher prevalence of arterial hypertension, peptic ulcer, diabetes mellitus (in the ischemic type only), and thyroid disorder. The patients with BRVO showed a greater prevalence of arterial hypertension, cerebrovascular disease, chronic obstructive pulmonary disease, peptic ulcer, diabetes (in young patients only), and thyroid disorder compared with the US white control population.

A variety of systemic disorders may be present in association with different types of RVO and in different age groups, and their relative prevalence differs significantly, so that the common practice of generalizing about these disorders for an entire group of patients with RVO can be misleading. Apart from a routine medical evaluation, an extensive and expensive workup for systemic diseases seems unwarranted in the vast majority of patients with RVO (Hayreh et al., 2001)[17].

In a second study, the same author investigated hematological abnormalities associated with the various types of RVO (Hayreh et al., 2002)[27]. A variety of hematological abnormalities may be seen in association with different types of RVO but the routine, inexpensive hematological evaluation may usually be sufficient for RVO patients. Based on Hayreh's findings in the study and on literature review, the author additionally suggested that treatment with anticoagulants or platelet antiaggregating agents may adversely influence the visual outcome, without any evidence of a protective or beneficial effect. Similar findings were reported from other hospital-based studies (The Eye Disease Case-Control Study Group, 1993)[28], which underlined that CRVO patients display a cardiovascular risk profile. A decreased risk was observed with increasing levels of physical activity, increasing levels of alcohol consumption, and in women using postmenopausal estrogens.

Evidence gathered in population-based studies on associations between RVO and ocular and systemic factors confirms that RVOs are significantly associated with glaucomatous optic neuropathy and arterial hypertension, as shown in the Blue Mountains Eye Study, the Beaver Dam Eye Study and the Beijing Eye Study, to name only a few (Klein et al., 2000; Mitchell et al., 1996; Liu et al., 2007)[11,12,14]. Corresponding with the association with arterial hypertension, the studies also suggested an increased mortality for patients with RVOs and an age of less than 70 years (Cugati et al., 2007; Xu et al., 2007)[29,30].

Familial clustering of RVOs has been observed, yet the role of gene mutation in RVO remains uncertain (Girmens et al., 2008)[31]. It has remained unclear whether RVOs are associated with abnormalities of the blood clotting system, such as factor V Leiden, factor XII deficiency, glucose-6-phosphate dehydrogenase deficiency, decreased plasma homocysteine level, presence of anti-phospholipid antibodies, or intake of warfarin and aspirin (The Central Vein Occlusion Study Group, 1997; Glacet-Bernard et al., 1994;

Arsène et al., 2005; Kuhli et al., 2002; Kuhli et al., 2004; Pinna et al., 2007)[32–37].

Clinical Course

The natural history and prognosis of RVOs have been examined in only a few prospective studies (Koizumi et al., 2007)[38]. The natural history of CRVO has been examined in the Central Retinal Vein Occlusion Study (The Central Vein Occlusion Study Group, 1997)[32], a prospective cohort study with randomized clinical trials of specific subgroups of patients. It included 725 patients with CRVO who were observed for a 3-year follow-up every 4 months. Visual acuity outcome was largely dependent on initial acuity.

- Sixty-five percent of patients with initially good visual acuity (20/40 or better) maintained visual acuity in the same range at the end of the study.
- Patients with intermediate initial acuity (20/50 to 20/200) showed a variable outcome: 19% improved to better than 20/50, 44% stayed in the intermediate group, and 37% had final visual acuity worse than 20/200.
- Patients who had poor visual acuity at the first visit (<20/200) had an 80% chance of having a visual acuity less than 20/200 at the final visit, whether perfused or nonperfused initially.

In the first 4 months of follow-up, 81 (15%) of the 547 eyes with good perfusion developed ischemia. During the next 32 months of follow-up, an additional 19% of eyes were found to have developed ischemia yielding a total of 34% after 3 years. The development of nonperfusion or ischemia was most rapid in the first 4 months and progressed continuously throughout the entire duration of follow-up. When iris or angle neovascularization occurred, it was treated promptly with panretinal photocoagulation.

The strongest predictors of iris or angle neovascularization were visual acuity and the amount of nonperfusion seen by fluorescein angiography (FA). Of eyes initially categorized as nonperfused or indeterminate, 35% (61/176) developed iris or angle neovascularization, compared with 10% (56/538) of eyes initially categorized as perfused. Other risk factors were venous tortuosity, extensive retinal hemorrhage, and duration of less than 1 month. Neovascular glaucoma that was unsuccessfully managed with medical treatment developed in only 10 eyes. No eye was enucleated.

Thus, visual acuity at baseline is a strong predictor of visual acuity at 3 years for eyes with good baseline vision and eyes with poor baseline vision, but a poor predictor for intermediate acuities. Visual acuity is also a strong predictor for the development of iris and angle neovascularization, as is nonperfusion. During the course of follow-up, one third of the eyes with perfusion became ischemic. Some systemic factors have also been demonstrated to be associated with retinal ischemia, such as elevated hematocrit level, elevated fibrinogen, older age, and male gender (Glacet-Bernard et al., 1996)[39].

Some patients may present with pronounced perivenular whitening and abrupt visual loss. While the fundus shows minimal sign of venous obstruction, careful examination can reveal areas of retinal opacification in a perivenous pattern (fig. 3). These patients usually recover, even in cases with severe visual loss at presentation, often with residual microscotomas (Browning, 2002; Paques et al., 2003)[40,41]. Thus, in these patients the prognostic value of visual acuity at the initial examination may be questionable.

Another important aspect is duration of the disease. In some reports of the natural course, 26% of patients had transient macular edema with spontaneous resolution (Gutman, 1977)[42]. This fact might explain the relatively good results even in the control groups of some studies such as GENEVA, BRAVO, and CRUISE, in which patients with recent-onset macular edema due to RVO were included. In contrast, chronic macular edema is associated with poor visual prognosis and needs to be treated.

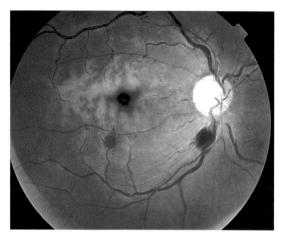

Fig. 3. Blue reflectance photograph of a patient with CRVO and perivenular whitening.

Diagnosis: Imaging and Functional Testing, Stages and Classifications

Clinical Signs
Patients with an RVO usually notice a painless loss in vision, which may affect parts of the whole visual field, depending on whether it is a BRVO or CRVO. If the drop in vision is experienced shortly after its development, the majority of the patients report they noticed the visual impairment in the morning (Hayreh et al., 1980)[43]. This may imply that the RVO occurred at night during sleep. Increasing pain is rarely the first symptom noticed by the patient. It can occur if a previously unnoticed ischemic RVO led to the development of iris neovascularization and neovascular glaucoma.

The ophthalmologic diagnosis of RVO is made primarily by conventional ophthalmoscopy. Recent RVOs are characterized by the presence of retinal edema, optic disk hyperemia or edema, scattered superficial or deep hemorrhages, cotton wool spots, and venous dilatation. Old RVOs are characterized by (occluded and) sheathed retinal veins, venous-venous collaterals, and intraretinal hard exudates.

The ophthalmoscopic examination allows the differentiation into CRVO and BRVO, and the subclassification into BRVO originating in the optic nerve head, and BRVO originating at arteriovenous crossings or limited to macular veinules (fig. 1, 2). In addition, the differentiation into ischemic RVOs (with large deep hemorrhage) and nonischemic RVOs (with mainly flame hemorrhage) is of high clinical importance, particularly with respect to the prognosis of the disease.

Slit lamp biomicroscopy of the anterior segment is mandatory for all patients with RVOs to detect iris neovascularization as early as possible. A vascular congestion of iris vessels may be considered as an early evidence of the presence of vasodilator factors released from the retina that precede in many patients the actual onset of iris neovascularization (Hayreh et al., 2005; Paques et al., 2004)[19,44].

Fluorescein Angiography
FA is the only examination which directly visualizes not only large retinal vessels but also the retinal macular capillary bed. FA both confirms the slowdown of retinal blood circulation and evaluates the effects of the vein obstruction on the capillary bed. FA is therefore the 'clue tool' for the diagnosis and prognosis of RVO, permitting the differentiation between the nonischemic type and the ischemic form (Hayreh, 1965; Coscas et al., 1978; Hayreh et al., 1990; Glacet-Bernard et al., 1996; Laatikainen et al., 1976)[1,3,8,39,45]. FA is essential in diagnosing RVO and before choosing the therapeutic option (fig. 4).

The confirmation of the RVO diagnosis is mainly related to the increase in the length of the retinal transit time, defined as the time between the first fluorescein appearance in the main retinal arteries and its appearance as a laminar flow in the main posterior veins. A transit time of less than 2–3 s is regarded as 'normal' and a longer time (more than 5 s) is considered 'delayed'. Nevertheless, the quantification of retinal transit time by FA is not significantly accurate because it depends on the rapidity of the antecubital intravenous injection and on the frequency of the frames.

However, video angiography using the scanning laser ophthalmoscope showed an improvement in the evaluation and the measurement of retinal circulation times, particularly important for the diagnosis of combined retinal occlusion, such as RVO associated with cilioretinal artery occlusion or combined retinal artery and vein occlusion.

FA also permits the localization and the qualitative evaluation of retinal capillary bed changes that includes either hyperpermeability and/or nonperfusion. Dilatation of retinal veins and capillaries, observed on the early frames of FA, is generally seen in all forms of RVO, with late leakage in the macular area and late staining at the level of the wall of the main posterior veins. Hyperpermeability can be more marked showing early and intense leakage from the macular capillary bed and collection of the dye on the late frames of FA in radially orientated pseudocystic cavities forming the typical cystoid macular edema with a 'petaloid pattern' (fig. 4, 5).

Capillary nonperfusion is most analyzable on the early frames of FA, at the arteriovenous time, before leakage. Macular nonperfusion is correlated with a bad visual prognosis and its diagnosis must be done in the pretherapeutic evaluation of a macular edema. Peripheral nonperfusion characterizes the ischemic forms, which are prone to ocular neovascularization (fig. 6). Sudden interruption of the blood flow can be observed giving the aspect of a dead tree, with late staining and/or leakage at the level of the wall of the vessels crossing over the ischemic area (Coscas et al., 1978)[3].

When retinal hemorrhages are numerous and deep, it can be impossible to assess the integrity of the retinal capillary bed. Extensive hemorrhagic RVO usually corresponds to ischemic RVO. The diagnosis of ischemic RVO is confirmed by clinical data such as severe and sudden loss in visual acuity, the presence of absolute central scotomas, and the iris and angle aspect.

FA is the easiest method to recognize the diverse types of RVO, not only perfused or nonperfused (and mixed types), but also to detect the different modalities in natural history [regression of the macular edema or progression to ischemic type (acutely or slowly)].

FA is the most effective method to determine the presence (or absence) of macular cystoid edema, its extension, persistence, or regression. Moreover, in BRVO, FA examination makes it easy to differentiate the cases threatening the macula and evaluate the extension of nonperfused capillary bed areas.

Optical Coherence Tomography
Optical coherence tomography (OCT) examination is widely used to detect changes in the retinal architecture of eyes affected by various macular diseases and to quantitatively measure retinal thickness (Catier et al., 2005)[46].

In RVO, OCT can display intraretinal cysts responsible for the increase in retinal thickness often associated with serous detachment of the neurosensory retina. The retinal cysts can be numerous and confluent, forming a large central cystoid space. Associated findings can be observed such as vitreous macular adherence, epiretinal membrane, hyperreflexivity of the posterior layer corresponding to atrophy or fibrosis of the retinal pigment epithelium, subretinal accumulation of material (fibrosis), lamellar macular hole, intraretinal lipid exudates, and intraretinal hemorrhage (fig. 4–6).

Recent studies have suggested that in BRVOs, visual function and recovery of vision is correlated with thickness of the central macula, and that is correlated with the integrity of the inner and outer segments of the photoreceptors in the fovea (Ota et al., 2008)[47].

Spectral domain OCT (SD-OCT) helps to quantify the amount of cystoid macular edema and supplies additional information, such as whether the accumulated fluid is located mostly within the retinal layers or additionally in the subretinal space (Shroff et al., 2008)[48]. Thanks to a better

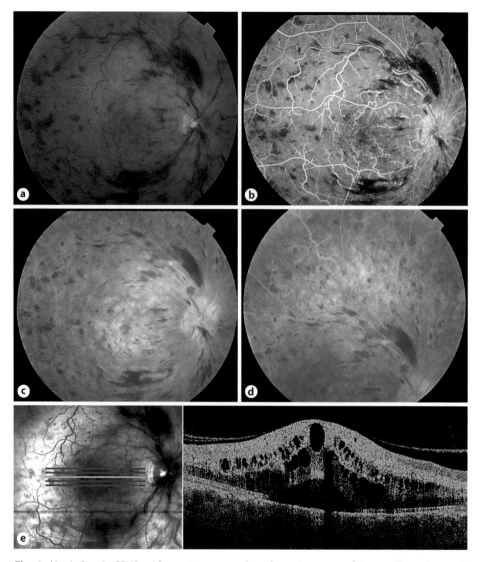

Fig. 4. Nonischemic CRVO with persistent macular edema (courtesy of Agnes Glacet-Bernard). **a** Color photography: well-perfused CRVO with flame-shaped hemorrhages. **b** FA displaying the slowdown of retinal blood circulation and dilation of the capillary bed, visible in the macular area. **c** On the late frame, fluorescein leakage is collected in pseudocystic cavities. **d** Peripheral retinal quadrants remained well-perfused. **e** SD-OCT: macular thickness was increased to 755 µm.

definition of the scans, SD-OCT can display the presence and integrity of the outer limiting membrane and of the inner and outer segments of the photoreceptors, which provides useful information for prognosis (fig. 4–6).

Additional Examinations

Additional diagnostic clues may be obtained by a modified type of ophthalmodynamometry (Hitchings et al., 1976; Jonas, 2003; Jonas, 2003; Jonas, 2003; Jonas, 2004)[49-53]. With this technique,

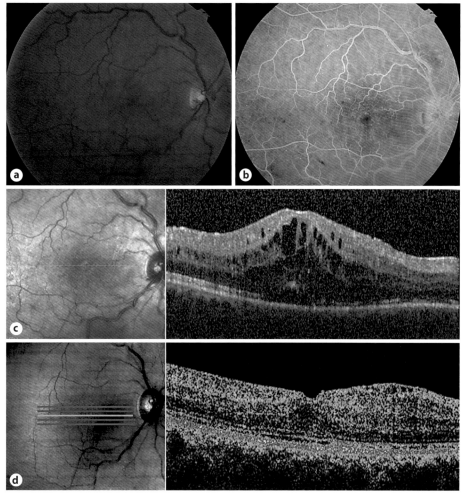

Fig. 5. Nonischemic CRVO with persistent macular edema (courtesy of Agnes Glacet-Bernard). **a** One year after the onset, fundus aspect returned grossly to normal. **b** FA showing persistent dilation of the capillary bed in the macular area. **c** SD-OCT (Spectralis): central macular thickness was 601 μm. **d** SD-OCT (Cirrus): 1 month after bevacizumab injection, macular edema completely disappeared.

the blood pressure in the central retinal vein can be assessed. Popular in the 1960s and 1970s, ophthalmodynamometry provided information about the diastolic and systolic blood pressure in the central retinal vessels or the ophthalmic artery. Due to marked limitations of the technique, the test was almost completely abandoned when

Doppler sonography allowed statements about the blood velocity through the carotid arteries.

The new Goldmann contact lens-associated ophthalmodynamometer device allows a direct visualization of the optic disk when manually asserting pressure onto the globe. In recent studies using this device, the ophthalmodynamometric

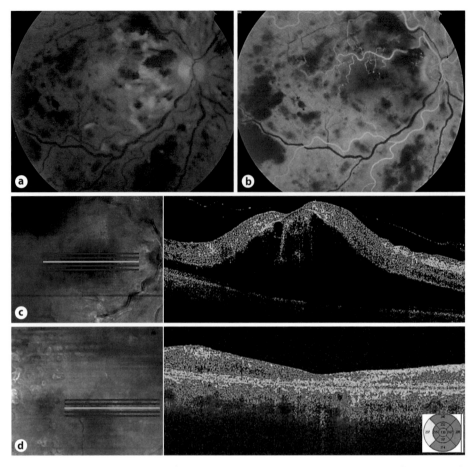

Fig. 6. Ischemic CRVO (courtesy of Agnes Glacet-Bernard). **a** Color photography of a CRVO with numerous cotton wool spots and deep hemorrhages. **b** FA displaying the slowdown of retinal blood circulation and widespread capillary nonperfusion. **c** OCT: macular thickness was dramatically increased up to more than 1,000 μm; a foveal detachment is visible. **d** Final OCT (16 months after the onset of the CRVO and after panretinal photocoagulation): macular atrophy. The photoreceptor layer is no longer visible. Central retinal thickness was 139 μm.

pressure measurements of the central retinal vein were significantly higher in eyes with retinal vein outflow disorders than in normal eyes (Harder et al., 2007; Jonas et al., 2007)[54,55]. In particular, ophthalmodynamometry allowed the differentiation between the ischemic type of CRVO versus the nonischemic type. The diastolic central retinal vein pressure was significantly higher in eyes with ischemic CRVO than in eyes with nonischemic

CRVO, in which it was significantly higher than in the eyes of a control group.

Using just a normal Goldmann contact lens without having the new device it was possible to show that the central retinal vein pressure was higher than the diastolic central retinal artery pressure in the majority of the eyes (7/7 or 100%) with an ischemic CRVO versus in a minority of the eyes (8/21 or 38%) with a nonischemic

CRVO (Jonas et al., 2007)[55]. Further studies may also address whether an increased central retinal vein pressure in asymptomatic eyes may indicate an increased risk for the eventual development of RVO. It may clinically be interesting particularly for the contralateral unaffected eyes.

Management

Treatment of Associated Conditions
Since the population-based studies mentioned above and multicenter prospective studies such as the Central Retinal Vein Occlusion Study have shown associations between RVOs and glaucoma and arterial hypertension (Klein et al., 2000; Mitchell et al., 1996; Wong et al., 2005)[11–13], any prevalent glaucoma and arterial hypertension should be excluded, or if present, treated accordingly.

It has remained unclear so far, whether a lowering of the intraocular pressure in the case of glaucoma patients or a better control of blood pressure in the case of patients with arterial hypertension is beneficial for the final visual outcome after RVOs.

Laser Photocoagulation

Central Retinal Vein Occlusion
In 1990, a prospective study of argon laser panretinal photocoagulation performed over a 10-year period in 123 eyes with ischemic CRVO was reported (Hayreh et al., 1990)[56]. It was found that when comparing the lasered eyes with the nonlasered eyes there was no statistically significant difference between the two groups in the incidence of angle neovascularization, neovascular glaucoma, retinal and/or optic disk neovascularization, vitreous hemorrhage, or in visual acuity. The study revealed, however, a statistically significant difference in the incidence of iris neovascularization between the two groups.

Consequently, the Central Retinal Vein Occlusion Study was conducted in the year 1997 (The Central Vein Occlusion Study Group, 1997)[32]. According to the results of the study, attention to visual acuity is a crucial element of the initial examination because it is an important indicator of final visual prognosis and neovascularization risk. A visual acuity worse than 20/200 is highly correlated with the presence and development of ischemia and neovascularization. The study suggested that at the patient's initial visit it would be important to perform a careful slit lamp examination and gonioscopy to evaluate any iris or anterior chamber angle neovascularization. If true neovascularization is already present, a panretinal laser photocoagulation should be considered. (In the rare clinical situation of simultaneous bilateral CRVOs, the possibility of hyperviscosity should be considered and diagnostically excluded.)

A follow-up schedule should be established depending on the duration and severity of the occlusion and the patient's circumstances.

- Patients with initial visual acuity less than 20/200 may be examined every month for the initial 6 months.
- Prognosis is mixed for patients with visual acuity between 20/50 and 20/200; either monthly or bimonthly follow-ups may be instituted initially (and possibly revised) depending on exactly where on the scale the patient's visual acuity falls, whether the CRVO is progressing or improving, and other factors.
- If visual acuity decreases at any time during follow-up to less than 20/200, it is likely that extensive nonperfusion has developed in the eye.
- If visual acuity is 20/40 or better, the patient may be asked to return every 1–2 months for 6 months, with precise examination of the macular area using FA and OCT.

A decrease in visual acuity may also be frequently associated with macular edema, persistent or recurrent, easily recognized with the help of FA and quantified in OCT examinations, during follow-up.

In 1995, The Central Retinal Vein Occlusion Study evaluated the efficacy of grid laser treatment on macular edema compared to a control group (The Central Retinal Vein Occlusion Study Group, 1995)[6]. Grid laser treatment clearly reduced angiographic evidence of macular edema compared to controls but visual acuity was not statistically improved in the treated group: after a 3-year follow-up, visual acuity improved spontaneously in 24% of the control group versus 27% after grid laser treatment. Nevertheless, grid laser treatment could be offered to young patients, even if no positive result but only a trend is shown in patients less than 60 years of age.

In conclusion, the first essential step in the management of CRVO is to determine the type of CRVO, since the prognosis, complications, visual outcome, and management of nonischemic and ischemic CRVO are different. Ocular neovascularization is a complication of ischemic CRVO only. (It is important to remember that the conventional prevalent use of a 10-disk area of retinal capillary obliteration is not a valid parameter to differentiate ischemic from nonischemic CRVO, or to predict ocular neovascularization.) The natural history of the disease with the possibility of a spontaneous improvement particularly in the nonischemic group, with macular edema, should not be mistaken for a beneficial effect of treatment in studies without a control group.

Branch Retinal Vein Occlusion
The Branch Vein Occlusion Study's multicenter, randomized, controlled clinical trial was designed to address questions regarding the management of complications of branch vein occlusion (The Branch Vein Occlusion Study Group, 1984; The Branch Vein Occlusion Study Group, 1986)[57,58].

With respect to the question whether grid argon laser photocoagulation was useful in improving visual acuity in eyes with BRVO and macular edema and vision reduced to 20/40 or worse, the study included 139 eyes, which were randomly assigned to either a treated group or an untreated control group with a mean follow-up of 3.1 years for all study eyes. The gain in visual acuity from baseline maintained for 2 consecutive visits was significantly greater in treated eyes (at least 2 Snellen lines). Grid laser photocoagulation was, therefore, recommended for patients with macular edema associated with BRVO who met the eligibility criteria of this study (visual acuity of 20/40 or less, persistent macular edema lasting for 4 months or longer, resorption of macular hemorrhages).

In 1993, another prospective study was reported on 271 eyes with major BRVO and ischemic hemicentral RVO, which either underwent scatter argon laser photocoagulation to the involved sector (n = 61 eyes) or remained untreated (n = 210 eyes) (Hayreh et al., 1993)[59]. This study concluded that argon laser photocoagulation treatment should be given only when neovascularization was seen and not otherwise, because in the latter case, the detrimental effects of laser coagulation might outweigh its beneficial effects. In the assessment of published studies on the effect of laser treatment on visual outcome of patients with RVO, every laser coagulation spot in the macular region led to a scotoma in the pericentral visual field.

Several other investigations were focused on the laser treatment of RVO (Arnarsson et al., 2000; Maár et al., 2004; Ohashi et al., 2004; Esrick et al., 2005; Parodi et al., 2006; Hayreh, 2003)[60–65]. Laser photocoagulation in a 'grid' pattern over the area, demonstrated as leaking by FA, remains the 'reference treatment for macular edema' due to BRVO. The Pascal® laser is useful for the comfort and safety of the patient, as it avoids overdosed or confluent impacts.

Ophthalmic: Surgical Treatment
Besides retinal laser coagulation, surgical treatment modalities have been reported for RVOs. For BRVO originating at arteriovenous crossings, a *sheathotomy* has been suggested to liberalize the retinal venule and the retinal arteriole from their

surrounding adventitious tissue at the crossing site (Opremcak et al., 1999; Shah et al., 2000; Le Rouic et al., 2001; Cahill et al., 2003; Fujii et al., 2003; Mason et al., 2004; Charbonnel et al., 2004; Yamaji et al., 2004; Yamamoto et al., 2004)[66–74]. Randomized trials with an untreated control group and a clear differentiation between the ischemic type of BRVO and the nonischemic type of BRVO have been limited. It may be questionable, therefore, whether the sheathotomy is recommended therapy for BRVOs originating at the arteriovenous crossing site. In most clinical sites, this surgical technique was not introduced or has been abandoned.

Radial neurotomy has been suggested as therapy for CRVO (Opremcak et al., 2001; García-Arumí et al., 2003; Weizer et al., 2003; Spaide et al., 2004; Arevalo et al., 2008)[75–79]. However, randomized prospective trials have not yet shown beneficial effects of radial neurotomy for the treatment of CRVO, so that it is unclear whether the technique should be recommended (Hayreh, 2002)[80]. Again, in most clinical sites, this surgical technique was not introduced or has been abandoned.

Another surgical technique which has been used for the treatment of RVOs is the *peeling of the inner limiting membrane* off the macula to reduce macular edema (Saika et al., 2001; García-Arumí et al., 2004; Mandelcorn et al., 2004; Radetzky et al., 2004; Nkeme et al., 2006; Kumagai et al., 2007; Kumagai et al., 2007; Berker et al., 2008; Oh et al., 2008; Arai et al., 2009; DeCroos et al., 2009; Lu et al., 2009; Uemura et al., 2009)[81–93]. In view of the risk of surgical complications (such as the development of iatrogenic peripheral retinal defects with secondary retinal detachment or a iatrogenic damage to the paracentral retina by the peeling of the inner limiting membrane), peeling of the inner limiting membrane may be reserved for clinical situations in which other modalities of treatment, namely the intravitreal injection of antiedematous (steroids) or anti-VEGF drugs, have failed in achieving a satisfactory improvement in vision, and in which the blood perfusion of the macula physiologically allows an increase in visual acuity.

The peeling of the inner limiting membrane of the retina is similar to the vitrectomy technique applied for diffuse diabetic macular edema associated with taut membranes (Lewis et al., 1992)[94]. The decrease in macular edema observed after vitrectomy could be the result of an increase in oxygen concentration in the macular area. Other hypotheses have been suggested to explain the positive effect of vitrectomy, such as a decompression from tangential tractions, removal of intravitreal proinflammatory and proangiogenic factors, collateral development stimulation, or specific Müller cell fibrosis (Mandelcorn et al., 2004; Stefánsson, 2009)[83,95].

The positive action of vitrectomy seems durable, which differs from intravitreal injection. The combination of surgery and intravitreal injection of steroids could permit a more rapid and lasting action (Nkeme et al., 2006)[85]. Another surgical technique consists of vitrectomy combined with an injection of tissue plasminogen activator into the retinal vein (Weiss, 1998; Weiss et al., 2001)[96,97]. This technique, however, has still not achieved a wide distribution and application.

Ophthalmic: Intravitreal Drug

Intravitreal Steroids (Triamcinolone, Fluocinolone, Dexamethasone)
Intravitreal triamcinolone acetonide has been increasingly used in studies for treatment of various intraocular proliferative, edematous, and neovascular diseases, such as diffuse diabetic macular edema, proliferative diabetic retinopathy, neovascular glaucoma, persistent pseudophakic cystoid macular edema, CRVO (Greenberg et al., 2002; Jonas et al., 2002; Park et al., 2003)[98–100] and in other clinical situations. Systemic and local side effects reported include cataract, secondary ocular hypertension leading in some patients to secondary chronic open-angle glaucoma, and postinjection infectious endophthalmitis (Wingate

et al., 1999; Bakri et al., 2003; Benz et al., 2003; Jonas et al., 2003; Jonas et al., 2003; Jonas et al., 2004)[101–106].

Due to its antiedematous and antiangiogenic effects, as shown in experimental investigations and clinical studies (Ishibashi et al., 1985; Wilson et al., 1992; Antoszyk et al., 1993; Penfold et al., 2001; Penfold et al., 2002)[107–111], *intravitreal triamcinolone acetonide* has additionally been used in studies on RVOs (Jonas et al., 2002; Bashshur et al., 2004; Ip et al., 2004; Jonas et al., 2004; Karacorlu et al., 2004; Karacorlu et al., 2005; Cekiç et al., 2005, Cekiç et al., 2005; Jonas et al., 2005; Jonas et al., 2005; Jonas et al., 2005; Lee et al., 2005; Chen et al., 2006; Goff et al., 2006; Gregori et al., 2006; Jonas, 2006; Ramezani et al., 2006; Bhavsar et al., 2007; Hirano et al., 2007; Jonas et al., 2007; Karacorlu et al., 2007; Pathai, 2007; Cakir et al., 2008; Chung et al., 2008; Park et al., 2008; Parodi et al., 2008; Patel et al., 2008; Riese et al., 2008; Roth et al., 2008; Cheng et al., 2009; Gewaily and Greenberg, 2009; McAllister et al., 2009; Scott et al., 2009; Wang et al., 2009; Wu et al., 2009)[112–146].

Although randomized trials on the intravitreal use of triamcinolone in particular and of steroids in general as treatment of RVO have been missing until recently, the available literature strongly suggests an anti-edematous effect of intravitreal triamcinolone and an associated improvement in vision. Due to the limited duration of the intraocular availability of triamcinolone, the visual improvement is limited in its duration. It may depend on the dosage of triamcinolone used.

Recently, new prospective double-masked randomized trials have been published presenting leading knowledge on the intravitreal use of steroids for treatment of RVOs (Scott et al., 2009; Scott et al., 2009; Scott et al., 2009)[144,147,148]. The Standard Care versus Corticosteroid for Retinal Vein Occlusion (SCORE) study's multicenter clinical trial of 411 participants compared the efficacy and safety of 1-mg and 4-mg doses of preservative-free intravitreal triamcinolone with standard care (grid photocoagulation in eyes without dense macular hemorrhage and deferral of photocoagulation until hemorrhage clears in eyes with dense macular hemorrhage) for eyes with vision loss associated with macular edema secondary to BRVO. The drug used in this trial was prepared as a sterile, preservative-free, single-use, intravitreal injection (Trivaris®; Allergan, Inc., Irvine, Calif., USA) in 1-mg and 4-mg doses, in a volume of 0.05 ml. The main outcome measure was the gain in visual acuity letter score of 15 or more from baseline to month 12. Twenty-nine, 26, and 27% of the participants achieved the primary outcome in the standard care, 1-mg and 4-mg groups, respectively. None of the pairwise comparisons between the 3 groups was statistically significant at month 12. The rates of elevated intraocular pressure and cataract were similar for the standard care and 1-mg groups, but higher in the 4-mg group.

The study group concluded that there was no difference identified in visual acuity at 12 months for the standard care group compared with the triamcinolone groups; however, rates of adverse events (particularly elevated intraocular pressure and cataract) were highest in the 4-mg group.

The authors inferred that 'grid photocoagulation as applied in the SCORE study remained the standard care for patients with vision loss associated with macular edema secondary to BRVO who have characteristics similar to participants in the SCORE-BRVO trial. Grid photocoagulation should remain the benchmark against which other treatments are compared in clinical trials for eyes with vision loss associated with macular edema secondary to BRVO'. One may, however, also consider the limitation of the study. Central visual acuity and the paracentral visual field both contribute to the quality of vision. Paracentral laser coagulation in contrast to intravitreal triamcinolone leads to paracentral visual field defects. Since the paracentral visual field or reading ability was not examined, the conclusions of the SCORE-BRVO study may be valid for the outcome parameter of central visual acuity, however, it may remain questionable whether the results also refer to the quality of vision in general.

As mentioned in the natural course section, it is important to consider the *duration of the edema*. In the subgroup analysis in the SCORE-BRVO trial, patients with a duration of less than 3 months showed a trend to have more benefit with usual care. However, among those patients that had a macular edema of more than 3 months' duration 34% in the 4-mg group showed a gain in visual acuity letter score of 15 or more, versus 15% in the photocoagulation group. According to the authors, these numbers were not significant but show the importance of the duration of the edema at the time of analyzing the results of the different trials, which may differ in the baseline characteristics. In the SCORE-BRVO trial, more than 50% of the patients had a macular edema with a duration of less than 3 months. If approximately 25% of patients with BRVO have a transient edema as a natural course (Gutman, 1977)[42], it is possible that in the SCORE-BRVO study approximately 12% of patients had transient macular edema with spontaneous resolution.

With respect to CRVO, the results of the SCORE-CRVO study differed from the findings in the SCORE-BRVO study. In the SCORE-CRVO study (Ip et al., 2009)[149], 271 participants with macular edema secondary to perfused CRVO were included. Seven, 27, and 26% of participants achieved the primary outcome (i.e., gain in visual acuity letter score of 15 or more from baseline to month 12) in the observation, 1-mg, and 4-mg groups, respectively. The odds of achieving the primary outcome were 5.0 times greater in the 1-mg group than in the observation group (p = 0.001) and 5.0 times greater in the 4-mg group than in the observation group (p = 0.001). There was no difference identified between the 1-mg and 4-mg groups (p = 0.97). The rates of elevated intraocular pressure and cataract were similar for the observation and 1-mg groups, but higher in the 4-mg group.

The study group concluded that intravitreal triamcinolone was superior to observation for treating vision loss associated with macular edema secondary to CRVO in patients who had characteristics similar to those in the SCORE-CRVO trial. The 1-mg dose had a safety profile superior to that of the 4-mg dose. The authors suggested that intravitreal triamcinolone in a 1-mg dose, following the retreatment criteria applied in the SCORE study, should be considered for up to 1 year and possibly 2 years for patients with characteristics similar to those in the SCORE-CRVO trial. The formulation used in this study (Trivaris®) is not currently available.

Dexamethasone has been used for a long time as a potent corticosteroid that decreases inflammatory mediators implicated in macular edema. Due to its anti-edematous and anti-angiogenic effects, intravitreal dexamethasone has been used in studies on RVOs. Previous data suggest fewer side effects than for other corticosteroids. Because of the short half-life of intravitreal injections of dexamethasone, an intravitreal dexamethasone implant (Ozurdex) was developed to deliver sustained levels of dexamethasone to the back of the eye, in a 6-month, randomized, controlled, clinical trial on macular edema associated with RVO, the GENEVA study.

The objective of the GENEVA study was to evaluate an intravitreal dexamethasone drug delivery system (Ozurdex®) in patients with vision loss due to macular edema associated with RVO. The study design includes 2 identical, randomized, prospective, multicenter, masked, sham-controlled, parallel groups. Phase 3 clinical trials were conducted in 2 periods of 6 months each.

In the double-masked, initial treatment phase, patients were randomly assigned (1:1:1) to receive either a 350-μg or a 700-μg dexamethasone implant, or to receive sham treatment (needleless applicator). In the open-label phase (2nd injection), patients received a 700-μg dexamethasone implant.

The primary endpoint was the time to achieve a ≥15-letter (3 Snellen lines) improvement in best-corrected visual acuity (BCVA) and key secondary endpoints included BCVA over the 6-month trial, central retinal thickness measured by OCT, and safety. To be eligible for the study, the patients had to be >18 years of age, have a >34- and <68-letter improvement in BCVA (20/200 to 20/50), and a macular edema with the following characteristics: (1) involvement of the fovea; (2) due to either BRVO or CRVO; (3) duration of macular edema of 6 weeks to 12 months for BRVO; (4) duration of macular edema of 6 weeks to 9 months for CRVO; (5) visual acuity decrease due to edema, and (6) retinal thickness of ≥300 μm in the central 1-mm macula subfield.

The percentage of patients with BRVO or CRVO was similar in the 3 groups with about two thirds of BRVO patients (68.1% of BRVO patients for the dexamethasone 700-μg group) and one third of CRVO patients in each group (39.1% of CRVO patients for the dexamethasone 700-μg group). Duration of macular edema was similar in each group with about 15% of patient with a macular edema of <3 months' duration, 50% with a macular edema duration between 3 and 6 months, and 30% with a macular edema duration >6 months (16.4% of the patients <3 months, 51.3% between 3 and 6 months and 32.3% >6 months). Only 1.2% of patients in the dexamethasone 700-μg group and 1% of patient in the dexamethasone 350-μg group discontinued because of an ocular adverse event. It is noteworthy that only 15% of patients had macular edema of less than 3 months' duration in comparison to more than 50% in the SCORE-BRVO trial, 51.5–53.8% in the BRAVO trial, and 51.5–61.5% in the CRUISE trial. This might affect the results and create difficulties when comparing trials, since spontaneous resolution is higher among those trials in which a large number of patients have a short duration of the macular edema.

The proportion of patients achieving at least a 15-letter or 10-letter improvement from baseline BCVA was significantly greater in the dexamethasone 700-μg group than in the sham group from day 30 through day 90. The greatest response was seen at day 60:

- 29% of patients in the dexamethasone 700-μg group achieved at least a 15-letter improvement from baseline as compared with 11% in the sham group;
- 51% of patients in the dexamethasone 700-μg group achieved at least a 10-letter improvement from baseline as compared with 26% in the sham group;
- statistical differences between the dexamethasone groups and the sham group were no longer seen at day 180 in an analysis of all patients.

The difference in mean change in BCVA from baseline between the dexamethasone 700-μg group and the sham group was statistically significant: (1) at all time points for all patients; (2) at all time points for BRVO patients, and (3) at days 30, 60, and 90 for CRVO patients. The main difference between the BRVO and CRVO subgroups was in the sham treatment group. Among patients with BRVO in the sham group, mean BCVA slowly improved over the course of the study. In contrast, mean BCVA slowly declined to below baseline levels among CRVO patients in the sham group.

Mean change from baseline in BCVA was similar following a second treatment with dexamethasone 700 or 350 μg. Patients who had received sham treatment in the initial treatment phase demonstrated a lower mean change from baseline in BCVA after receiving open-label treatment than patients who had received dexamethasone 700 or 350 μg during the initial treatment phase.

The percentage of patients in the dexamethasone groups reaching an intraocular pressure of ≥35 mm Hg (about 2–3% of the patients at day 60), ≥25 mm Hg (about 15% of the patients at day 60), and ≥10 mm Hg (about 15% of the patients at day 60) peaked at day 60 and returned to baseline by day 180. After 12 months (2 injections of dexamethasone), only 1.2% of the patients (n = 4) had an intraocular pressure procedure and 0.9% of patients (n = 3) a cataract surgery (for the 700-μg/700-μg group, patients injected twice). Adverse events in the initial treatment whose maximum severity increased during the open-label extension were reported for 2.6% of the patients (700-μg/700-μg group).

In summary, 2 identical, randomized, prospective, multicenter, masked, sham-controlled, parallel-group, phase 3 clinical trials showed a statistically significant effect and a rapid action, with a maximum effect at day 60 and a decrease of the effect beginning at day 90 but still persistent at day 180. The 2nd injection is effective, with an even slightly better effect than after the 1st injection. No adverse events were related to the injection, with a low cataract rate and low rates of persistent intraocular pressure increases. These results suggest that this slow-release device for the intraocular dexamethasone delivery could be considered as a first-choice therapy in both BRVO and CRVO retinal diseases.

Intravitreal Anti-VEGF Drugs
Bevacizumab. Since the landmark study on the intravitreal use of bevacizumab for treatment of exudative age-related macular degeneration (Rosenfeld et al., 2005)[150] bevacizumab has become a medication used worldwide for patients affected by various neovascular intraocular diseases including RVOs (Iturralde et al., 2006; Jaissle et al., 2006; Rosenfeld et al., 2006; Spandau et al., 2006; Costa et al., 2007; Matsumoto et al., 2007; Rabena et al., 2007)[151–157]. Most of the studies published so far agree that bevacizumab and ranibizumab appear to have improved vision in patients with RVOs. Since these studies were mostly case series studies without a randomized control group, they must be taken as an indication, not as evidence, for the usefulness of the therapy. In addition, the majority of the studies failed to clearly differentiate between the nonischemic and the ischemic type of RVOs. Randomized controlled trials will be required as final proof for the useful application of anti-VEGF drugs.

Ranibizumab, Pegaptanib. Related to bevacizumab, the effect of *ranibizumab* and *pegaptanib* on macular edema in eyes with RVOs has been reported in several studies (Campochiaro et al., 2008; Pieramici et al., 2008; Spaide et al., 2009; Wroblewski et al., 2009)[158–161]. These studies all report a reduction in macular edema after the intravitreal injection of the anti-VEGF drugs. The first multicenter, randomized study on the effect of anti-VEGF therapy in the treatment of RVO was designed to evaluate the efficacy of pegaptanib sodium. The results have been reported at the Congress of the European Vitreo-Retinal Society in 2006. Patients with visual loss due to macular edema secondary to CRVO were randomly assigned to sham injection, 0.3 or 1 mg of pegaptanib sodium. The group treated with 1 mg pegaptanib sodium showed a higher rate of visual gain superior to 5 letters and a lower rate of loss of 15 letters or more than the control group (p < 0.05 and p < 0.01, respectively). There was a difference of 13 letters in the change in visual acuity between the control group (sham injections) and the group treated with 1 mg pegaptanib sodium.

Ranibizumab. CRUISE and BRAVO are two phase 3 studies of Lucentis (ranibizumab injection) in macular edema due to RVO. The preliminary results at 6 months from both trials were presented at the Retina Congress Meeting in October 2009. BRAVO is a multicenter, randomized, double-masked, sham injection-controlled phase 3 study of 397 patients designed to assess the safety and efficacy profile of Lucentis in macular edema secondary to BRVO. Patients were randomized into 3 groups: (1) standard care with grid laser treatment; (2) intravitreal injection of 0.5 mg ranibizumab, and (3) both grid laser treatment and intravitreal injection of 0.3 or 0.5 mg ranibizumab. CRUISE is a multicenter, randomized, double-masked, sham injection-controlled phase 3 study designed to assess the safety and efficacy profile of Lucentis. The study includes 392 patients with macular edema secondary to CRVO. Patients were randomized into 2 groups: sham injection and intravitreal injection of 0.3 or 0.5 mg ranibizumab. In both studies, patients received monthly intravitreal injections during the first 6 months, and between month 6 and month 12. Evaluations have to determine if retreatment is needed. The preliminary results at 6 months showed in both studies that the treated groups had better visual recovery than control groups. In the BRAVO study, 55% of patients who received 0.3 mg of Lucentis and 61% who received 0.5 mg of Lucentis had their vision improved by 15 letters or more compared to 29% of patients receiving sham injections and grid laser treatment. In the CRUISE study, 46% of patients given 0.3 mg of Lucentis and 48% given 0.5 mg of Lucentis had their vision improved by 15 letters or more compared to 17% of patients receiving sham injections. The results at the final follow-up of 12 and 24 months are expected later. More than half the patients had a short duration of the macular edema, i.e. 51.5–53.8% in the BRAVO trial and 51.5–61.5% in CRUISE.

Systemic Therapy
Several studies have suggested a beneficial effect of hemodilution as a therapy of the early phase of RVOs. Hemodilution is expected to prevent the slowdown of blood circulation and its complications by dramatically lowering blood viscosity. Some randomized studies have been published on the topic showing a statistically significant difference between treated and nontreated patients (Hansen et al., 1989; Hansen et al., 1989; Wolf et al., 1994; Hattenbach et al., 1999; Glacet-Bernard et al., 2001)[162–166].

These monocenter studies were conducted in the 1980s and 1990s, and used different treatment protocols. Prospective multicenter studies are now under way with a new method of hemodilution and erythroapheresis, and are expected to answer the question whether or not hemodilution should be recommended for therapy of RVOs.

Prevention
Only a few studies have addressed the prevention of a recurrence of an RVO in the same eye or the development of an RVO in the contralateral eye. So far, none of these studies have shown

any benefit. In particular, thrombocyte aggregation inhibitors and anticoagulant drugs were not shown to be of benefit (Koizumi et al., 2007; McIntosh et al., 2007)[38,167].

Potential Future Developments
Future developments will include new intraocular drug delivery systems, such as the dexamethasone posterior-segment drug delivery system (Ozurdex®) for intraocular delivery of steroids (Kuppermann et al., 2007; Williams et al., 2009)[168,169] which has already shown positive results for treatment of macular edema due to other reasons.

Other future developments are combination treatments of steroids with anti-VEGF drugs, slow-release devices for the intraocular steroid delivery (Ramchandran et al., 2008)[170], and addressing aspects of retinal protection and reopening of occluded retinal capillaries (Otani et al., 2004; Harris et al., 2006; Smith, 2006; Jonas et al., 2008; Jonas et al., 2009; Ma et al., 2009)[171–176].

Conclusion

RVOs belong to the most frequently encountered retinal vascular diseases in all ethnic groups. If the macula is involved, central visual acuity drops, depending on the amount of foveal edema and macular ischemia. It is essential to differentiate between the nonischemic type, which has a relatively good prognosis without treatment, and the ischemic type, which has a relatively poor prognosis. Known risk factors for RVOs include systemic arterial hypertension and glaucomatous optic neuropathy.

Generally vision can be improved as much as it was decreased by macular edema. The amount of vision loss due to capillary nonperfusion cannot currently be markedly increased. Recent case series studies and prospective randomized trials have suggested that intravitreal steroids (triamcinolone, fluocinolone, dexamethasone in a slow-release device) and intravitreal anti-VEGF drugs (bevacizumab, ranibizumab, pegaptanib) may at least temporarily reduce foveal edema and correspondingly improve visual function. Duration of edema is also crucial. Some patients may have transient macular edema with spontaneous visual acuity recovery. Alternatively, when macular edema is persistent the earlier the treatment the better the chances of visual response.

Since most studies, particularly those on the use of retinal laser coagulation, performed so far have addressed mainly central visual acuity and have not taken into account the pericentral visual field, and since pericentral laser coagulation in contrast to an intravitreal drug therapy deteriorates the pericentral visual field, the clinical value of a pericentral laser treatment in comparison with intravitreal drug therapy has remained unclear.

A preventive therapy to avoid a recurrence of RVOs or the development of an RVO in the contralateral eye has not yet been shown.

Key Messages

- The diagnosis of macular edema from RVO is now facilitated by OCT, which allows retinal thickness to be quantified, and is a useful tool to evaluate the treatment.
- FA remains essential to differentiate perfused macular edema from ischemic macular edema, which is often a contraindication for treatment.
- Grid laser photocoagulation remains the reference treatment for macular edema from BRVO.
- In CRVO, intravitreal injections of steroids or antiangiogenic drugs seem to demonstrate a benefit compared to the natural course. Ongoing studies are expected to confirm these preliminary results.
- Some patients may have transient macular edema with spontaneous visual acuity recovery, but when macular edema is persistent, the earlier the treatment the better the chances of visual response.

References

1 Hayreh SS: Occlusion of the central retinal vessels. Br J Ophthalmol 1965;49: 626–645.
2 Hayreh SS: An experimental study of the central retinal vein occlusion. Trans Ophthalmol Soc UK 1964;84:586–595.
3 Coscas G, Dhermy P: Occlusions veineuses rétiniennes. Paris, Masson, 1978, pp 283–346.
4 Hayreh SS: Classification of central retinal vein occlusion. Ophthalmology 1983;90:458–474.
5 The Central Vein Occlusion Study. Baseline and early natural history report. Arch Ophthalmol 1993;111:1087–1095.
6 The Central Vein Occlusion Study Group M report. Evaluation of grid pattern photocoagulation for macular edema in central vein occlusion. Ophthalmology 1995;102:1425–1433.
7 The Central Vein Occlusion Study Group N report. A randomized clinical trial of early panretinal photocoagulation for ischemic central vein occlusion. Ophthalmology 1995;102:1434–1444.

8 Hayreh SS, Klugman MR, Beri M, Kimura AE, Podhajsky P: Differentiation of ischemic from non-ischemic central retinal vein occlusion during the early acute phase. Graefes Arch Clin Exp Ophthalmol 1990;228:201–217.
9 Coscas G, Gaudric A: Natural course of nonaphakic cystoid macular edema. Surv Ophthalmol 1984;28(Suppl):471–484.
10 Liebreich R: Ueber die Farbe des Augenhintergrundes. Albrecht Von Graefes Arch Ophthalmol 1855;1:333–358.
11 Klein R, Klein BE, Moss SE, Meuer SM: The epidemiology of retinal vein occlusion: the Beaver Dam Eye Study. Trans Am Ophthalmol Soc 2000;98:133–141.
12 Mitchell P, Smith W, Chang A: Prevalence and associations of retinal vein occlusion in Australia. The Blue Mountains Eye Study. Arch Ophthalmol 1996;114:1243–1247.

13 Wong TY, Larsen EK, Klein R, et al: Cardiovascular risk factors for retinal vein occlusion and arteriolar emboli: the Atherosclerosis Risk in Communities & Cardiovascular Health studies. Ophthalmology 2005;112:540–547.
14 Liu W, Xu L, Jonas JB: Vein occlusion in Chinese subjects. Ophthalmology 2007;114:1795–1796.
15 Cheung N, Klein R, Wang JJ, et al: Traditional and novel cardiovascular risk factors for retinal vein occlusion: the multiethnic study of atherosclerosis. Invest Ophthalmol Vis Sci 2008;49:4297–4302.
16 Lim LL, Cheung N, Wang JJ, et al: Prevalence and risk factors of retinal vein occlusion in an Asian population. Br J Ophthalmol 2008;92:1316–1319.
17 Hayreh SS, Zimmerman B, McCarthy MJ, Podhajsky P: Systemic diseases associated with various types of retinal vein occlusion. Am J Ophthalmol 2001; 131:61–77.

18 O'Mahoney PR, Wong DT, Ray JG: Retinal vein occlusion and traditional risk factors for atherosclerosis. Arch Ophthalmol 2008;126:692–699.

19 Hayreh S: Prevalent misconceptions about acute retinal vascular occlusive disorders. Prog Retin Eye Res 2005;24:493–519.

20 McIntosh R, Mohamed Q, Saw S, Wong T: Interventions for branch retinal vein occlusion. Ophthalmology 2006;114:835–854.

21 Mohamed Q, McIntosh R, Saw S, Wong T: Interventions for central retinal vein occlusion: an evidence-based systematic review. Ophthalmology 2006;114:507–519.

22 Rogers S, McIntosh RL, Cheung N, et al: The prevalence and number of people with retinal vein occlusion: pooled data from population-based studies from the US, Europe, Australia and Asia. Ophthalmology 2010;117:313–319.e1.

23 Leenen FH, Dumais J, McInnis NH, et al: Results of the Ontario survey on the prevalence and control of hypertension. CMAJ 2008;178:1441–1449.

24 Read JG, Gorman BK: Racial/ethnic differences in hypertension and depression among US adult women. Ethn Dis 2007;17:389–396.

25 Giles T, Aranda JMJ, Suh DC, et al: Ethnic/racial variations in blood pressure awareness, treatment, and control. J Clin Hypertens 2007;9:345–354.

26 Ostchega Y, Hughes JP, Wright JD, et al: Are demographic characteristics, health care access and utilization, and comorbid conditions associated with hypertension among US adults? Am J Hypertens 2008;21:159–165.

27 Hayreh SS, Zimmerman MB, Podhajsky P: Hematological abnormalities associated with various types of retinal vein occlusion. Graefes Arch Clin Exp Ophthalmol 2002;240:180–196.

28 The Eye Disease Case-Control Study Group. Risk factors for branch retinal vein occlusion. Am J Ophthalmol 1993;116:286–296.

29 Cugati S, Wang JJ, Knudtson MD, et al: Retinal vein occlusion and vascular mortality: pooled data analysis of 2 population-based cohorts. Ophthalmology 2007;114:520–524.

30 Xu L, Liu W, Wang Y, Yang H, Jonas JB: Retinal vein occlusions and mortality. The Beijing Eye Study. Am J Ophthalmol 2007;144:972–973.

31 Girmens JF, Scheer S, Heron E, Sahel JA, Tournier-Lasserve E, Paques M: Familial central retinal vein occlusion. Eye 2008;22:308–310.

32 The Central Vein Occlusion Study Group. Natural history and clinical management of central retinal vein occlusion. Arch Ophthalmol 1997;115:486–491.

33 Glacet-Bernard A, Bayani N, Chretien P, Cochard C, Lelong F, Coscas G: Antiphospholipid antibodies in retinal vascular occlusions. A prospective study of 75 patients. Arch Ophthalmol 1994;112:790–795.

34 Arsène S, Delahousse B, Regina S, Le Lez ML, Pisella PJ, Gruel Y: Increased prevalence of factor V Leiden in patients with retinal vein occlusion and under 60 years of age. Thromb Haemost 2005;94:101–106.

35 Kuhli C, Scharrer I, Koch F, Ohrloff C, Hattenbach LO: Factor XII deficiency: a thrombophilic risk factor for retinal vein occlusion. Am J Ophthalmol 2004;137:459–464.

36 Kuhli C, Hattenbach LO, Scharrer I, Koch F, Ohrloff C: High prevalence of resistance to APC in young patients with retinal vein occlusion. Graefes Arch Clin Exp Ophthalmol 2002;240:163–168.

37 Pinna A, Carru C, Solinas G, Zinellu A, Carta F: Glucose-6-phosphate dehydrogenase deficiency in retinal vein occlusion. Invest Ophthalmol Vis Sci 2007;48:2747–2752.

38 Koizumi H, Ferrara DC, Bruè C, Spaide RF: Central retinal vein occlusion case-control study. Am J Ophthalmol 2007;144:858–863.

39 Glacet-Bernard A, Coscas G, Chabanel A, Zourdani A, Lelong F, Samama MM: Prognostic factors for retinal vein occlusion: prospective study of 175 cases. Ophthalmology 1996;103:551–560.

40 Browning DJ: Patchy ischemic retinal whitening in acute central retinal vein occlusion. Ophthalmology 2002;109:2154–2159.

41 Paques M, Gaudric A: Perivenous macular whitening during central retinal vein occlusion. Arch Ophthalmol 2003;121:1488–1491.

42 Gutman FA: Macular edema in branch retinal vein occlusion: prognosis and management. Trans Am Acad Ophthalmol Otolaryngol 1977;83:488–495.

43 Hayreh SS, Hayreh MS: Hemi-central retinal vein occlusion. Pathogenesis, clinical features, and natural history. Arch Ophthalmol 1980;98:1600–1609.

44 Paques M, Girmens JF, Riviere E, Sahel J: Dilation of the minor arterial circle of the iris preceding rubeosis iridis during retinal vein occlusion. Am J Ophthalmol 2004;138:1083–1086.

45 Laatikainen L, Kohner EM: Fluorescein angiography and its prognostic significance in central retinal vein occlusion. Br J Ophthalmol 1976;60:411–418.

46 Catier A, Tadayoni R, Paques M, Erginay A, Haouchine B, Gaudric A, Massin P: Characterization of macular edema from various etiologies by optical coherence tomography. Am J Ophthalmol 2005;140:200–206.

47 Ota M, Tsujikawa A, et al: Integrity of foveal photoreceptor layer in central retinal vein occlusion. Retina 2008;28:1502–1508.

48 Shroff D, Mehta DK, et al: Natural history of macular status in recent-onset branch retinal vein occlusion: an optical coherence tomography study. Int Ophthalmol 2008;28:261–268.

49 Hitchings RA, Spaeth GL: Chronic retinal vein occlusion in glaucoma. Br J Ophthalmol 1976;60:694–699.

50 Jonas JB: Reproducibility of ophthalmodynamometric measurements of the central retinal artery and vein collapse pressure. Br J Ophthalmol 2003;87:577–579.

51 Jonas JB: Ophthalmodynamometric assessment of the central retinal vein collapse pressure in eyes with retinal vein stasis or occlusion. Graefes Arch Clin Exp Ophthalmol 2003;241:367–370.

52 Jonas JB: Central retinal artery and vein pressure in patients with chronic open-angle glaucoma. Br J Ophthalmol 2003;87:949–951.

53 Jonas JB: Ophthalmodynamometric determination of the central retinal vessel collapse pressure correlated with systemic blood pressure. Br J Ophthalmol 2004;88:501–504.

54 Harder B, Jonas JB: Frequency of spontaneous pulsations of the central retinal vein in normal eyes. Br J Ophthalmol 2007;91:401–402.

55 Jonas JB, Harder B: Ophthalmodynamometric differences between ischemic versus non-ischemic retinal vein occlusion. Am J Ophthalmol 2007;143:112–116.

56 Hayreh SS, Klugman MR, Podhajsky P, Servais GE, Perkins ES: Argon laser pan-retinal photocoagulation in ischemic central retinal vein occlusion. A 10-year prospective study. Graefes Arch Clin Exp Ophthalmol 1990;228:281–296.

57 The Branch Vein Occlusion Study Group. Argon laser photocoagulation for macular edema in branch vein occlusion. Am J Ophthalmol 1984;98:271–282.

58 The Branch Vein Occlusion Study Group. Argon laser scatter photocoagulation for prevention of neovascularization and vitreous hemorrhage in branch vein occlusion. A randomized clinical trial. Arch Ophthalmol 1986;104:34–41.

59 Hayreh SS, Rubenstein L, Podhajsky P: Argon laser scatter photocoagulation in treatment of branch retinal vein occlusion. A prospective clinical trial. Ophthalmologica 1993;206:1–14.

60 Arnarsson A, Stefánsson E: Laser treatment and the mechanism of edema reduction in branch retinal vein occlusion. Invest Ophthalmol Vis Sci 2000; 41:877–879.

61 Maár N, Luksch A, Graebe A, Ergun E, Wimpissinger B, Tittl M, Vécsei P, Stur M, Schmetterer L: Effect of laser photocoagulation on the retinal vessel diameter in branch and macular vein occlusion. Arch Ophthalmol 2004;122: 987–991.

62 Ohashi H, Oh H, Nishiwaki H, Nonaka A, Takagi H: Delayed absorption of macular edema accompanying serous retinal detachment after grid laser treatment in patients with branch retinal vein occlusion. Ophthalmology 2004;111:2050–2056.

63 Esrick E, Subramanian ML, Heier JS, Devaiah AK, Topping TM, Frederick AR, Morley MG: Multiple laser treatments for macular edema attributable to branch retinal vein occlusion. Am J Ophthalmol 2005;139:653–657.

64 Parodi MB, Spasse S, Iacono P, Di Stefano G, Canziani T, Ravalico G: Subthreshold grid laser treatment of macular edema secondary to branch retinal vein occlusion with micropulse infrared (810 nanometer) diode laser. Ophthalmology 2006;113:2237–2242.

65 Hayreh SS: Management of central retinal vein occlusion. Ophthalmologica 2003;217:167–188.

66 Opremcak EM, Bruce RA: Surgical decompression of branch retinal vein occlusion via arteriovenous crossing sheathotomy: a prospective review of 15 cases. Retina 1999;19:1–5.

67 Shah GK, Sharma S, Fineman MS, Federman J, Brown MM, Brown GC: Arteriovenous adventitial sheathotomy for the treatment of macular edema associated with branch retinal vein occlusion. Am J Ophthalmol 2000;129:104–106.

68 Le Rouic JF, Bejjani RA, Rumen F, Caudron C, Bettembourg O, Renard G, Chauvaud D: Adventitial sheathotomy for decompression of recent onset branch retinal vein occlusion. Graefes Arch Clin Exp Ophthalmol 2001;239:747–751.

69 Cahill MT, Kaiser PK, Sears JE, Fekrat S: The effect of arteriovenous sheathotomy on cystoid macular oedema secondary to branch retinal vein occlusion. Br J Ophthalmol 2003;87:1329–1332.

70 Fujii GY, de Juan E Jr, Humayun MS: Improvements after sheathotomy for branch retinal vein occlusion documented by optical coherence tomography and scanning laser ophthalmoscope. Ophthalmic Surg Lasers Imaging 2003;34:49–52.

71 Mason J 3rd, Feist R, White M Jr, Swanner J, McGwin G Jr, Emond T: Sheathotomy to decompress branch retinal vein occlusion: a matched control study. Ophthalmology 2004;111:540–545.

72 Charbonnel J, Glacet-Bernard A, Korobelnik JF, Nyouma-Moune E, Pournaras CJ, Colin J, Coscas G, Soubrane G: Management of branch retinal vein occlusion with vitrectomy and arteriovenous adventitial sheathotomy, the possible role of surgical posterior vitreous detachment. Graefes Arch Clin Exp Ophthalmol 2004;242:223–228.

73 Yamaji H, Shiraga F, Tsuchida Y, Yamamoto Y, Ohtsuki H: Evaluation of arteriovenous crossing sheathotomy for branch retinal vein occlusion byfluorescein videoangiography and image analysis. Am J Ophthalmol 2004;137:834–841.

74 Yamamoto S, Saito W, Yagi F, Takeuchi S, Sato E, Mizunoya S: Vitrectomy with or without arteriovenous adventitial sheathotomy for macular edema associated with branch retinal vein occlusion. Am J Ophthalmol 2004;138:907–914.

75 Opremcak EM, Bruce RA, Lomeo MD, Ridenour CD, Letson AD, Rehmar AJ: Radial optic neurotomy for central retinal vein occlusion: a retrospective pilot study of 11 consecutive cases. Retina 2001;215:408–415.

76 García-Arumí J, Boixadera A, Martinez-Castillo V, Castillo R, Dou A, Corcostegui B: Chorioretinal anastomosis after radial optic neurotomy for central retinal vein occlusion. Arch Ophthalmol 2003;121: 1385–1391.

77 Weizer JS, Stinnett SS, Fekrat S: Radial optic neurotomy as treatment for central retinal vein occlusion. Am J Ophthalmol 2003;136:814–819.

78 Spaide RF, Klancnik JM Jr, Gross NE: Retinal choroidal collateral circulation after radial optic neurotomy correlated with the lessening of macular edema. Retina 2004;243:356–359.

79 Arevalo JF, Garcia RA, Wu L, et al, Pan-American Collaborative Retina Study Group: Radial optic neurotomy for central retinal vein occlusion: results of the Pan-American Collaborative Retina Study Group (PACORES). Retina 2008;288:1044–1052.

80 Hayreh SS: Radial optic neurotomy for central retinal vein occlusion. Retina 2002;226:827.

81 Saika S, Tanaka T, Miyamoto T, Ohnishi Y: Surgical posterior vitreous detachment combined with gas/air tamponade for treating macular edema associated with branch retinal vein occlusion: retinal tomography and visual outcome. Graefes Arch Clin Exp Ophthalmol 2001;239:729–732.

82 García-Arumí J, Martinez-Castillo V, Boixadera A, Blasco H, Corcostegui B: Management of macular edema in branch retinal vein occlusion with sheathotomy and recombinant tissue plasminogen activator. Retina 2004;24:530–540.

83 Mandelcorn MS, Nrusimhadevara RK: Internal limiting membrane peeling for decompression of macular edema in retinal vein occlusion: a report of 14 cases. Retina 2004;24:348–355.

84 Radetzky S, Walter P, Fauser S, Koizumi K, Kirchhof B, Joussen AM: Visual outcome of patients with macular edema after pars plana vitrectomy and indocyanine green-assisted peeling of the internal limiting membrane. Graefes Arch Clin Exp Ophthalmol 2004;242:273–278.

85 Nkeme J, Glacet-Bernard A, Gnikpingo K, Zourdani A, Mimoun G, Mahiddine H, Gkoritsa A, Tchamo A, Coscas G, Soubrane G: Surgical treatment of persistent macular edema in retinal vein occlusion. J Fr Ophthalmol 2006;29: 808–814.

86 Kumagai K, Furukawa M, Ogino N, Uemura A, Larson E: Long-term outcomes of vitrectomy with or without arteriovenous sheathotomy in branch retinal vein occlusion. Retina 2007;27:49–54.

87 Kumagai K, Furukawa M, Ogino N, Larson E, Uemura A: Long-term visual outcomes after vitrectomy for macular edema with foveal hemorrhage in branch retinal vein occlusion. Retina 2007;27:584–588.

88 Berker N, Batman C: Surgical treatment of central retinal vein occlusion. Acta Ophthalmol 2008;86:245–252.

89 Oh IK, Kim S, Oh J, Huh K: Long-term visual outcome of arteriovenous adventitial sheathotomy on branch retinal vein occlusion induced macular edema. Korean J Ophthalmol 2008;22:1–5.

90 Arai M, Yamamoto S, Mitamura Y, Sato E, Sugawara T, Mizunoya S: Efficacy of vitrectomy and internal limiting membrane removal for macular edema associated with branch retinal vein occlusion. Ophthalmologica 2009;223: 172–176.

91 DeCroos FC, Shuler RK Jr, Stinnett S, Fekrat S: Pars plana vitrectomy, internal limiting membrane peeling, and panretinal endophotocoagulation for macular edema secondary to central retinal vein occlusion. Am J Ophthalmol 2009;147: 627–633.e1.

92 Lu N, Wang NL, Wang GL, Li XW, Wang Y: Vitreous surgery with direct central retinal artery massage for central retinal artery occlusion. Eye 2009;23:867–872.

93 Uemura A, Yamamoto S, Sato E, Sugawara T, Mitamura Y, Mizunoya S: Vitrectomy alone versus vitrectomy with simultaneous intravitreal injection of triamcinolone for macular edema associated with branch retinal vein occlusion. Ophthalmic Surg Lasers Imaging 2009;40:6–12.

94 Lewis H, Abrams GW, Blumenkranz MS, Campo RV: Vitrectomy for diabetic macular traction and edema associated with posterior hyaloidal traction. Ophthalmology 1992;99:753–759.

95 Stefánsson E: Physiology of vitreous surgery. Graefes Arch Clin Exp Ophthalmol 2009;247:147–163.

96 Weiss JN: Treatment of central retinal vein occlusion by injection of tissue plasminogen activator into a retinal vein. Am J Ophthalmol 1998;126:142–144.

97 Weiss JN, Bynoe LA: Injection of tissue plasminogen activator into a branch retinal vein in eyes with central retinal vein occlusion. Ophthalmology 2001;108:2249–2257.

98 Greenberg PB, Martidis A, Rogers AH, Duker JS, Reichel E: Intravitreal triamcinolone acetonide for macular oedema due to central retinal vein occlusion. Br J Ophthalmol 2002;86:247–248.

99 Jonas JB, Kreissig I, Degenring RF: Intravitreal triamcinolone acetonide as treatment of macular oedema in central retinal vein occlusion. Graefes Arch Clin Exp Ophthalmol 2002;240:782–783.

100 Park CH, Jaffe GJ, Fekrat S: Intravitreal triamcinolone acetonide in eyes with cystoidmacular edema associated with central retinal vein occlusion. Am J Ophthalmol 2003;136:419–425.

101 Wingate RJ, Beaumont PE: Intravitreal triamcinolone and elevated intraocular pressure. Aust NZ J Ophthalmol 1999;27:431–432.

102 Bakri SJ, Beer PM: The effect of intravitreal triamcinolone acetonide on intraocular pressure. Ophthalmic Surg Lasers Imaging 2003;34:386–390.

103 Benz MS, Murray TG, Dubovy SR, Katz RS, Eifrig CW: Endophthalmitis caused by *Mycobacterium chelonae* abscessus after intravitreal injection of triamcinolone. Arch Ophthalmol 2003;121:271–273.

104 Jonas JB, Kreissig I, Degenring RF: Endophthalmitis after intravitreal injection of triamcinolone acetonide. Arch Ophthalmol 2003;121:1663–1664.

105 Jonas JB, Kreissig I, Degenring R: Intraocular pressure after intravitreal injection of triamcinolone acetonide. Br J Ophthalmol 2003;87:24–27.

106 Jonas JB, Bleyl U: Morphallaxia-like ocular histology after intravitreal triamcinolone acetonide. Br J Ophthalmol 2004;88: 839–840.

107 Ishibashi T, Miki K, Sorgente N, Patterson R, Ryan SJ: Effects of intravitreal administration of steroids on experimental subretinal neovascularization in the subhuman primate. Arch Ophthalmol 1985;103:708–711.

108 Wilson CA, Berkowitz BA, Sato Y, Ando N, Handa JT, de Juan E Jr: Treatment with intravitreal steroid reduces blood-retinal barrier breakdown due to retinal photocoagulation. Arch Ophthalmol 1992;110:1155–1159.

109 Antoszyk AN, Gottlieb JL, Machemer R, Hatchell DL: The effects of intravitreal triamcinolone acetonide on experimental pre-retinal neovascularization. Graefes Arch Clin Exp Ophthalmol 1993;231:34–40.

110 Penfold PL, Wong JG, Gyory J, Billson FA: Effects of triamcinolone acetonide on microglial morphology and quantitative expression of MHC-II in exudative age-related macular degeneration. Clin Experiment Ophthalmol 2001;29:188–192.

111 Penfold PL, Wen L, Madigan MC, King NJ, Provis JM: Modulation of permeability and adhesion molecule expression by human choroidal endothelial cells. Invest Ophthalmol Vis Sci 2002;43: 3125–3130.

112 Jonas JB, Kreissig I, Degenring RF: Intravitreal triamcinolone acetonide as treatment of macular edema in central retinal vein occlusion. Graefes Arch Clin Exp Ophthalmol 2002;240:782–783.

113 Bashshur ZF, Ma'luf RN, Allam S, Jurdi FA, Haddad RS, Noureddin BN: Intravitreal triamcinolone for the management of macular edema due to nonischemic central retinal vein occlusion. Arch Ophthalmol 2004;122:1137–1140.

114 Ip MS, Gottlieb JL, Kahana A, Scott IU, Altaweel MM, Blodi BA, Gangnon RE, Puliafito CA: Intravitreal triamcinolone for the treatment of macular edema associated with central retinal vein occlusion. Arch Ophthalmol 2004;122:1131–1136.

115 Jonas JB, Degenring R, Kamppeter B, Kreissig I, Akkoyun I: Duration of the effect of intravitreal triamcinolone acetonide as treatment of diffuse diabetic macular edema. Am J Ophthalmol 2004;138:158–160.

116 Karacorlu M, Ozdemir H, Karacorlu S: Intravitreal triamcinolone acetonide for the treatment of central retinal vein occlusion in young patients. Retina 2004;24:324–327.

117 Karacorlu M, Ozdemir H, Karacorlu SA: Resolution of serous macular detachment after intravitreal triamcinolone acetonide treatment of patients with branch retinal vein occlusion. Retina 2005;25:856–860.

118 Cekiç O, Chang S, Tseng JJ, Barile GR, Weissman H, Del Priore LV, Schiff WM, Weiss M, Klancnik JM Jr: Intravitreal triamcinolone treatment for macular edema associated with central retinal vein occlusion and hemiretinal vein occlusion. Retina 2005;25:846–850.

119 Cekiç O, Chang S, Tseng JJ, Barile GR, Del Priore LV, Weissman H, Schiff WM, Ober MD: Intravitreal triamcinolone injection for treatment of macular edema secondary to branch retinal vein occlusion. Retina 2005;25:851–855.

120 Jonas JB, Akkoyun I, Kamppeter B, Kreissig I, Degenring RF: Branch retinal vein occlusion treated by intravitreal triamcinolone acetonide. Eye 2005;19:65–71.

121 Jonas JB, Akkoyun I, Kamppeter B, Kreissig I, Degenring RF: Intravitreal triamcinolone acetonide for treatment of central retinal vein occlusion. Eur J Ophthalmol 2005;15:751–758.

122 Jonas JB, Kreissig I, Degenring R: Intravitreal triamcinolone acetonide for treatment of intraocular proliferative, exudative, and neovascular diseases. Prog Retin Eye Res 2005;24:587–611.

123 Lee H, Shah GK: Intravitreal triamcinolone as primary treatment of cystoid macular edema secondary to branch retinal vein occlusion. Retina 2005;25:551–555.

124 Chen SD, Sundaram V, Lochhead J, Patel CK: Intravitreal triamcinolone for the treatment of ischemic macular edema associated with branch retinal vein occlusion. Am J Ophthalmol 2006;141:876–883.

125 Goff MJ, Jumper JM, Yang SS, Fu AD, Johnson RN, McDonald HR, Ai E: Intravitreal triamcinolone acetonide treatment of macular edema associated with central retinal vein occlusion. Retina 2006;26:896–901.

126 Gregori NZ, Rosenfeld PJ, Puliafito CA, Flynn HW Jr, Lee JE, Mavrofrides EC, Smiddy WE, Murray TG, Berrocal AM, Scott IU, Gregori G: One-year safety and efficacy of intravitreal triamcinolone acetonide for the management of macular edema secondary to central retinal vein occlusion. Retina 2006;26:889–895.

127 Jonas JB: Intravitreal triamcinolone acetonide: a change in a paradigm. Ophthalmic Res 2006;38:218–245.

128 Ramezani A, Entezari M, Moradian S, Tabatabaei H, Kadkhodaei S: Intravitreal triamcinolone for acute central retinal vein occlusion; a randomized clinical trial. Graefes Arch Clin Exp Ophthalmol 2006;244:1601–1606.

129 Bhavsar AR, Ip MS, Glassman AR, DRCRnet and the SCORE Study Groups: The risk of endophthalmitis following intravitreal triamcinolone injection in the DRCRnet and SCORE clinical trials. Am J Ophthalmol 2007;144:454–456.

130 Hirano Y, Sakurai E, Yoshida M, Ogura Y: Comparative study on efficacy of a combination therapy of triamcinolone acetonide administration with and without vitrectomy for macular edema associated with branch retinal vein occlusion. Ophthalmic Res 2007;39:207–212.

131 Jonas JB, Rensch F: Decreased retinal vein diameter after intravitreal triamcinolone for retinal vein occlusions. Br J Ophthalmol 2007;91:1711–1712.

132 Karacorlu M, Karacorlu SA, Ozdemir H, Senturk F: Intravitreal triamcinolone acetonide for treatment of serous macular detachment in central retinal vein occlusion. Retina 2007;27:1026–1030.

133 Pathai S: Intravitreal triamcinolone acetonide for treatment of persistent macular oedema in branch retinal vein occlusion. Eye 2007;21:255–256.

134 Cakir M, Dogan M, Bayraktar Z, Bayraktar S, Acar N, Altan T, Kapran Z, Yilmaz OF: Efficacy of intravitreal triamcinolone for the treatment of macular edema secondary to branch retinal vein occlusion in eyes with or without grid laser photocoagulation. Retina 2008;28:465–472.

135 Chung EJ, Lee H, Koh HJ: Arteriovenous crossing sheathotomy versus intravitreal triamcinolone acetonide injection for treatment of macular edema associated with branch retinal vein occlusion. Graefes Arch Clin Exp Ophthalmol 2008;246:967–974.

136 Park SP, Ahn JK: Changes of aqueous vascular endothelial growth factor and interleukin-6 after intravitreal triamcinolone for branch retinal vein occlusion. Clin Experiment Ophthalmol 2008;36:831–835.

137 Parodi MB, Iacono P, Ravalico G: Intravitreal triamcinolone acetonide combined with subthreshold grid laser treatment for macular oedema in branch retinal vein occlusion: a pilot study. Br J Ophthalmol 2008;92:1046–1050.

138 Patel PJ, Zaheer I, Karia N: Intravitreal triamcinolone acetonide for macular oedema owing to retinal vein occlusion. Eye 2008;22:60–64.

139 Riese J, Loukopoulos V, Meier C, Timmermann M, Gerding H: Combined intravitreal triamcinolone injection and laser photocoagulation in eyes with persistent macular edema after branch retinal vein occlusion. Graefes Arch Clin Exp Ophthalmol 2008;246:1671–1676.

140 Roth DB, Cukras C, Radhakrishnan R, Feuer WJ, Yarian DL, Green SN, Wheatley HM, Prenner J: Intravitreal triamcinolone acetonide injections in the treatment of retinal vein occlusions. Ophthalmic Surg Lasers Imaging 2008;39:446–454.

141 Cheng KC, Wu WC, Lin CJ: Intravitreal triamcinolone acetonide for patients with macular oedema due to central retinal vein occlusion in Taiwan. Eye 2009;23:849–857.

142 Gewaily D, Greenberg PB: Intravitreal steroids versus observation for macular edema secondary to central retinal vein occlusion. Cochrane Database Syst Rev 2009;1:CD007324.

143 McAllister IL, Vijayasekaran S, Chen SD, Yu DY: Effect of triamcinolone acetonide on vascular endothelial growth factor and occludin levels in branch retinal vein occlusion. Am J Ophthalmol 2009;147:838–846.

144 Scott IU, Ip MS, VanVeldhuisen PC, et al, SCORE Study Research Group: A randomized trial comparing the efficacy and safety of intravitreal triamcinolone with standard care to treat vision loss associated with macular edema secondary to branch retinal vein occlusion: the Standard Care vs Corticosteroid for Retinal Vein Occlusion (SCORE) study report 6. Arch Ophthalmol 2009;127:1115–1128.

145 Wang L, Song H: Effects of repeated injection of intravitreal triamcinolone on macular oedema in central retinal vein occlusion. Acta Ophthalmol 2009;87:285–289.

146 Wu WC, Cheng KC, Wu HJ: Intravitreal triamcinolone acetonide vs bevacizumab for treatment of macular oedema due to central retinal vein occlusion. Eye 2009;23:2215–2222.

147 Scott IU, VanVeldhuisen PC, Oden NL, Ip MS, Blodi BA, Jumper JM, Figueroa M, SCORE Study Investigator Group: SCORE Study report 1: baseline associations between central retinal thickness and visual acuity in patients with retinal vein occlusion. Ophthalmology 2009; 116:504–512.

148 Scott IU, Blodi BA, Ip MS, Vanveldhuisen PC, Oden NL, Chan CK, Gonzalez V, SCORE Study Investigator Group: SCORE Study Report 2: interobserver agreement between investigator and reading center classification of retinal vein occlusion type. Ophthalmology 2009;116:756–761.

149 Ip MS, Scott IU, VanVeldhuisen PC, Oden NL, Blodi BA, Fisher M, Singerman LJ, Tolentino M, Chan CK, Gonzalez VH, SCORE Study Research Group: A randomized trial comparing the efficacy and safety of intravitreal triamcinolone with observation to treat vision loss associated with macular edema secondary to central retinal vein occlusion: the Standard Care vs Corticosteroid for Retinal Vein Occlusion (SCORE) study report 5. Arch Ophthalmol 2009;127: 1101–1114.

150 Rosenfeld PJ, Moshfeghi AA, Puliafito CA: Optical coherence tomography findings after an intravitreal injection of bevacizumab (Avastin) for neovascular age-related macular degeneration. Ophthalmic Surg Lasers Imaging 2005;36: 331–335.

151 Iturralde D, Spaide RF, Meyrele CB, et al: Intravitreal bevacizumab (Avastin) treatment of macular edema in central retinal vein occlusion: a short-term study. Retina 2006;26:279–284.

152 Jaissle GB, Ziemssen F, Petermeier K, et al: Bevacizumab zur Therapie des sekundären Makulaödems nach venösen Gefässverschlüssen. Ophthalmologe 2006;103:471–475.

153 Rosenfeld PJ, Fung AE, Pulifito CA: Optical coherence tomography findings after an intravitreal injection of bevacizumab (Avastin) for macular edema from central retinal vein occlusion. Ophthalmic Surg Lasers Imaging 2006;36: 336–339.

154 Spandau UH, Ihloff AK, Jonas JB: Intravitreal bevacizumab treatment of macular oedema due to central retinal vein occlusion. Acta Ophthalmol 2006;84:555–556.

155 Costa RA, Jorge R, Calucci D, et al: Intravitreal bevacizumab (Avastin) for central and hemicentral retinal vein occlusions: IBeVO study. Retina 2007;27:141–149.

156 Matsumoto Y, Freund KB, Peiretti E, et al: Rebound macular edema following bevacizumab (Avastin) therapy for retinal venous occlusive disease. Retina 2007;27:426–431.

157 Rabena MD, Pieramici DJ, Castellarin AA, et al: Intravitreal bevacizumab (Avastin) in the treatment of macular edema secondary to branch retinal vein occlusion. Retina 2007;27:419–425.

158 Campochiaro PA, Hafiz G, Shah SM, Nguyen QD, Ying H, Do DV, Quinlan E, Zimmer-Galler I, Haller JA, Solomon SD, Sung JU, Hadi Y, Janjua KA, Jawed N, Choy DF, Arron JR: Ranibizumab for macular edema due to retinal vein occlusions: implication of VEGF as a critical stimulator. Mol Ther 2008;16:791–799.

159 Pieramici DJ, Rabena M, Castellarin AA, Nasir M, See R, Norton T, Sanchez A, Risard S, Avery RL: Ranibizumab for the treatment of macular edema associated with perfused central retinal vein occlusions. Ophthalmology 2008;115:e47–e54.

160 Spaide RF, Chang LK, Klancnik JM, Yannuzzi LA, Sorenson J, Slakter JS, Freund KB, Klein R: Prospective study of intravitreal ranibizumab as a treatment for decreased visual acuity secondary to central retinal vein occlusion. Am J Ophthalmol 2009;147:298–306.

161 Wroblewski JJ, Wells JA 3rd, Adamis AP, Buggage RR, Cunningham ET Jr, Goldbaum M, Guyer DR, Katz B, Altaweel MM, Pegaptanib in Central Retinal Vein Occlusion Study Group: Pegaptanib sodium for macular edema secondary to central retinal vein occlusion. Arch Ophthalmol 2009;127:374–380.

162 Hansen LL, Wiek J, Schade M, Müller-Stolzenburg N, Wiederholt M: Effect and compatibility of isovolaemic haemodilution in the treatment of ischaemic and non-ischaemic central retinal vein occlusion. Ophthalmologica 1989;199:90–99.

163 Hansen LL, Wiek J, Wiederholt M: A randomised prospective study of treatment of non-ischaemic central retinal vein occlusion by isovolaemic haemodilution. Br J Ophthalmol 1989;73:895–899.

164 Wolf S, Arend O, Bertram B, Remky A, Schulte K, Wald KJ, Reim M: Hemodilution therapy in central retinal vein occlusion. One-year results of a prospective randomized study. Graefes Arch Clin Exp Ophthalmol 1994;232:33–39.

165 Hattenbach LO, Wellermann G, Steinkamp GW, Scharrer I, Koch FH, Ohrloff C: Visual outcome after treatment with low-dose recombinant tissue plasminogen activator or hemodilution in ischemic central retinal vein occlusion. Ophthalmologica 1999;2136:360–366.

166 Glacet-Bernard A, Zourdani A, et al: Effect of isovolemic hemodilution in central retinal vein occlusion. Graefes Arch Clin Exp Ophthalmol 2001;239: 909–914.

167 McIntosh RL, Mohamed Q, Saw SM, Wong TY: Interventions for branch retinal vein occlusion: an evidence-based systematic review. Ophthalmology 2007;114:835–854.

168 Kuppermann BD, Blumenkranz MS, Haller JA, Williams GA, Weinberg DV, Chou C, Whitcup SM, Dexamethasone DDS Phase II Study Group: Randomized controlled study of an intravitreous dexamethasone drug delivery system in patients with persistent macular edema. Arch Ophthalmol 2007;125:309–317.

169 Williams GA, Haller JA, Kuppermann BD, Blumenkranz MS, Weinberg DV, Chou C, Whitcup SM, Dexamethasone DDS Phase II Study Group: Dexamethasone posterior-segment drug delivery system in the treatment of macular edema resulting from uveitis or Irvine-Gass syndrome. Am J Ophthalmol 2009;1476:1048–1054.

170 Ramchandran RS, Fekrat S, Stinnett SS, Jaffe GJ: Fluocinolone acetonide sustained drug delivery device for chronic central retinal vein occlusion: 12-month results. Am J Ophthalmol 2008;146: 285–291.

171 Otani A, Dorrell MI, Kinder K, Otero FJ, Schimmel P, Friedlander M: Rescue of retinal degeneration by intravitreally injected adult bone marrow-derived lineage-negative hematopoietic stem cells. J Clin Invest 2004;114:765–774.

172 Harris JR, Brown GA, Jorgensen M, Kaushal S, Ellis EA, Grant MB, Scott EW: Bone marrow-derived cells home to and regenerate retinal pigment epithelium after injury. Invest Ophthalmol Vis Sci 2006;47:2108–2113.

173 Smith LE: Bone marrow-derived stem cells preserve cone vision in retinitis pigmentosa. J Clin Invest 2006;114:755–757.

174 Jonas JB, Witzens-Harig M, Arseniev L, Ho AD: Intravitreal autologous bone marrow derived mononuclear cell transplantation. A feasibility report. Acta Ophthalmol 2008;86:225–226.

175 Jonas JB, Witzens-Harig M, Arseniev L, Ho AD: Intravitreal autologous bone-marrow-derived mononuclear cell transplantation. Acta Ophthalmol 2009, E-pub ahead of print.

176 Ma K, Xu L, Zhang H, Zhang S, Pu M, Jonas JB: Effect of brimonidine on retinal ganglion cell survival in an optic nerve crush model. Am J Ophthalmol 2009;147:326–331.

Prof. Jost Jonas
Universitäts-Augenklinik
Theodor-Kutzer-Ufer 1–3
DE–68167 Mannheim (Germany)
E-Mail jost.jonas@augen.ma.uni-heidelberg.de

Coscas G (ed): Macular Edema.
Dev Ophthalmol. Basel, Karger, 2010, vol 47, pp 136–147

Cystoid Macular Edema in Uveitis

Marc D. de Smet[a–c] · Annabelle A. Okada[d]

[a]Retina and Inflammatory Diseases Unit, Center for Specialized Ophthalmology, Clinique de Montchoisi, Lausanne, Switzerland; [b]Department of Ophthalmology, University of Amsterdam, Amsterdam, The Netherlands; [c]Department of Ophthalmology, Ghent State University, Ghent, Belgium; [d]Department of Ophthalmology, Kyorin University, Tokyo, Japan

Abstract

Macular edema is a major cause of morbidity in uveitis patients. Inflammatory mediators act on the integrity of the blood ocular barrier and on the function of the RPE pump. Chronicity leads to irreversible changes and is reported to cause up to 30% of permanent visual loss in uveitis patients. Assessing the presence and severity of edema with appropriate investigational techniques (Spectral domain OCT, and angiography) help to determine its reversibility and define a therapeutic strategy wherein intraocular steroids play a key role while RPE pump stimulators and surgery are restricted to more severe disease or the presence of tractional syndromes.

Copyright © 2010 S. Karger AG, Basel

Inflammation is involved in all forms of macular edema. However, the mechanisms by which inflammation contributes to macular edema vary from one etiology to the next. If one only considers for example surgically induced inflammation versus endogenous inflammation, significant differences are already evident. Prostaglandins play a significant role, particularly in anterior segment surgery, and are potent inducers of vascular leakage in the macular area (Pournaras et al., 2008)[1].

The use of topical and systemic nonsteroidal agents has a major impact on the incidence and severity of postsurgical inflammation but is much less likely to influence macular edema due to endogenous uveitis (Foster et al., 1989)[2]. This chapter will limit itself to discussing macular edema arising as a result of endogenous uveitis, its etiology and management.

Epidemiology

A number of epidemiological studies and retrospective series have clearly identified macular edema as one of the most serious long-term complications of chronic uveitis. The prevalence among uveitis patients is between 20 and 30% (Rothova et al., 1996; Rothova, 2007; Lardenoye et al., 2006)[3–5]. It is a major cause of permanent vision loss, as about 35% of patients with uveitis who have vision less than 0.1 (6/60) have macular edema. It is also common in children where it is the third most common cause of low vision (de Boer et al., 2003)[6]. In a large multicenter survey taken in the United States, the prevalence increases with chronicity of the disease. It is reported to be 17% at year 1, increasing to 30% by year 5 (Smith et al., 2009)[7].

Macular edema develops typically in patients with posterior uveitis, but it can be seen in patients with isolated anterior segment inflammation, in particular HLA-B27-related uveitic syndromes (Lardenoye et al., 2006)[5]. Among the posterior pole entities with the highest prevalence of cystoid macular edema are birdshot retinochoroidopathy, sarcoidosis, and Behçet disease, which have a prevalence of 60% or higher in patients with disease of more than 1 year's duration (Lardenoye et al., 2006; Monnet et al., 2007; Johnson, 2009)[5,8,9]. Significant vision impairment in patients with infectious etiologies such as acute retinal necrosis or toxoplasmosis also occurs, but the incidence is less at 15–20% of cases.

Chronic macular edema has a significant impact on the quality of life of these patients, affecting their ability to read and their function in society (Kiss et al., 2006; Hazel et al., 2000)[10,11]. It is important to remember that in comparison to other causes of macular edema, this tends to occur in a younger population, often between 30 and 50 years of age.

Pathophysiology

Several factors contribute to the development of macular edema. The exact trigger varies among patients and is based on their background, associated diseases, and the nature of their inflammation. Perpetuation also requires a constellation of factors in which the balance of forces of passive permeability of fluid into the retina (due to breakdown of the blood-ocular barrier) is greater than the active transport of fluid out of the macular area. In this fine balance, release and diffusion of inflammatory mediators, vascular incompetence, dysfunction of the retinal pigment epithelium (RPE) pump, and mechanical forces all play a role.

In the normal eye, the volume and composition of the extracellular compartment is regulated by endothelial tight junctions from the retinal capillaries (the inner retinal barrier), those of the RPE (the outer retinal barrier), and by the pump function of RPE cells. Intraretinal fluid accumulates when there is loss of integrity of one of these barriers combined with dysfunction in the RPE pump.

Early cystoid changes on optical coherence tomography (OCT) tend to occur either at the level of the outer retina (primary RPE dysfunction) or within the plexiform layers (vascular dysfunction) (Markomichelakis et al., 2005; Catier et al., 2005)[12,13] (fig. 1). Serous exudative detachments of the macula occur frequently (Tran et al., 2008)[14]. Such detachments are of no prognostic significance for vision as opposed to the situation in diabetic macular edema. This probably results from an early impairment of the RPE pump caused by inflammatory mediators before structural damage to the RPE or retina has occurred.

Retinal vascular hyperpermeability is influenced by a number of mediators. A direct inhibition of nitric oxide, tumor necrosis factor α, and vascular endothelial growth factors can lead to partial resolution of macular edema (Acharya et al., 2009; Markomichelakis et al., 2005)[15,16]. Other important factors include prostaglandins, leukotrienes, cytokines IP-10 and IL-6 (van Kooij et al., 2006; Probst et al., 2004; Curnow et al., 2005)[17–19]. Vascular leakage also results from endothelial cell damage as a result of leukostasis mediated by adhesion molecules, and nitric oxide (Leal et al., 2007)[20].

The inherent vascular competence of the retina influences the ease with which macular edema develops during an inflammatory episode. Leakage is amplified by factors that increase retinal blood flow such as vasodilatation, increased intraluminal pressure, and increased blood flow.

Hence, patients with concurrent cardiovascular disease, hypertension, diabetes, or hyperlipidemia have an increased risk of developing macular edema and when present it tends to be more persistent (van Kooij et al., 2004)[21]. Smoking is also an independent risk factor in intermediate uveitis, as it is in other associated disease states (Lin et al., 2010; Thorne et al., 2008; Kramer et al., 2008)[22–24]. Leakage from the optic nerve, which is often present in uveitis, may also contribute to the development of persistent macular edema (Pruett et al., 1974; van Kooij et al., 2008)[25,26].

Finally, tractional stress by perifoveal vitreous attachments may cause deformational macular

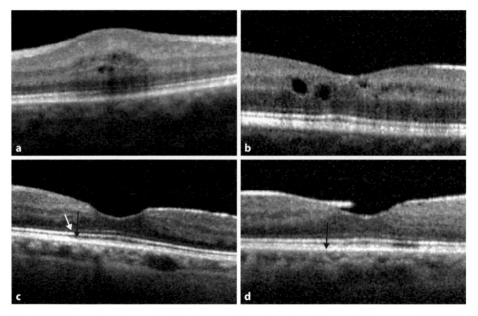

Fig. 1. Early macular edema develops in one of two locations. Commonly, it appears in the inner plexiform layer (**a, b**). In certain pathologies that more affect the choroid and choriocapillaris, changes are more prominent in the outer segments. In a patient with birdshot retinochoroidopathy, the outer segments are disrupted (**c**) and small cystic spaces in the outer plexiform layer are seen (white arrow). Vision was 0.25. In the contralateral eye (**d**), vision was 1.0. The outer segment layer is intact in the foveal area (red arrow).

thickening and cystoid space formation (often more superficial in location).

As will be discussed later in the chapter, resolving one or more of the elements contributing to inflammatory macular edema can lead to its subsidence. Homeostasis may be restored and sustained, particularly when structural damage has not yet occurred. Early diagnosis and therapy are therefore thought to be critical in the management of this disorder.

Diagnostics

When severe enough, uveitic macular edema is visible by biomicroscopy as a constellation of cystoid spaces of various sizes located in the foveal area. Often the cystic spaces are not easily seen

due to the presence of media opacities. RPE stippling or hyperpigmentation develops as the edema becomes more chronic and may be an indication of present or past macular edema. Its presence, however, is an indication that vision recovery is less likely.

For most patients, fluorescein angiography and OCT are the preferred examination. The latter is particularly useful in identifying associated pathologies such as macular detachment and vitreomacular traction, which otherwise would not be seen (Markomichelakis et al., 2005)[27].

Fluorescein Angiography
Retinal vascular integrity and the extent of inflammation in the retina and optic nerve can be determined by using fluorescein angiography. In the arteriovenous phase, the integrity of the

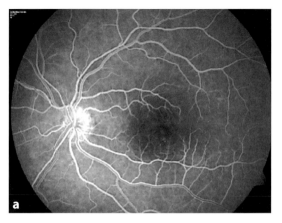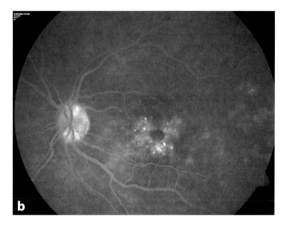

Fig. 2. a Early arterovenous phase in a patient with a history of intermediate uveitis in a quiescent phase. There is enlargement of the foveal avascular zone and dropout of the microvasculature in the macular area. **b** In the venous phase, the cystoid spaces are largely limited to the area of vascular incompetence, indicating that much of the process is due to an ischemic process. Optic nerve disk hyperfluorescence is also present as well as some dispersed diffuse microvascular leakages but not localized in the foveal area.

perifoveal vascular network can be assessed as well as the location and extent of vascular leakage. Leakage can be present on the basis of localized ischemia or on the basis of inflammation (fig. 2, 3). Inflammation generally causes a more diffuse microvascular leakage, though it may be patchy in nature, but is not limited to the area surrounding the foveal avascular zone or areas of nonperfusion (Forooghian et al., 2009)[28].

The frames taken in the venous phase provide information on the extent and severity of diffuse microvascular leakage originating from either the retina and/or the RPE (fig. 3, 4), as well as providing an indication of large vessel involvement. Optic disk leakage and hyperfluorescence can be assessed in late frames and is often present in chronic macular edema (Pruett et al., 1974; van Kooij et al., 2008; Gürlü et al., 2007)[25,26,29]. Optic disk hyperfluorescence was present in 66% of patients with quiescent intermediate uveitis of which 24% had macular edema (Gürlü et al., 2007)[29].

In some cases of macular edema with mainly an RPE dysfunction, inflammation may be localized more in the choroidal than in the retinal circulation. In such cases, the extent of inflammation will

be better assessed by indocyanine green (Tugal-Tutkun et al., 2008)[30]. While attempts were made in the past to assess the severity of edema by judging the height of the cystic spaces on stereoscopic angiograms, the information provided on angiography was mainly qualitative (Nussenblatt et al., 1987)[31]. A correlation exists between the extent of dye leakage and visual acuity, but it is not of sufficient significance for use in therapeutic decisions (Tran et al., 2008)[14].

Optical Coherence Tomography
OCT provides reliable cross-sectional images of the retina and is useful to study retinal pathology. Studies using time domain OCT were able show a negative correlation between visual acuity and central macular thickness (Markomichelakis et al., 2005)[27]. Macular thickness, however, was poorly correlated with the likelihood of vision recovery (Tran et al., 2008)[14]. The structural characteristics of the edema, however, in particular the presence of cystoid versus diffuse edema, had prognostic significance, as the former was associated with a higher probability of vision improvement after treatment (Tran et al., 2008)[14].

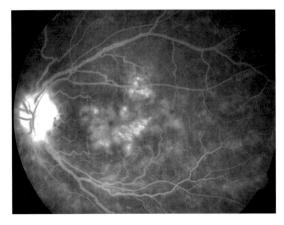 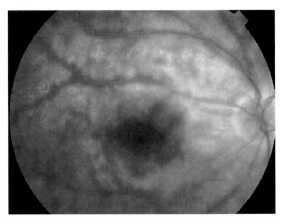

Fig. 3. Late-phase angiogram in a patient with birdshot retinochoroidopathy. Diffuse macular edema is present. An intact foveal avascular zone is visible even in this late stage. There is diffuse microvascular leakage. The major vessels are largely competent, while the optic nerve is significantly hyperfluorescent.

Fig. 4. Late frame from the fluorescein angiogram of a patient with birdshot retinochoroidopathy showing diffuse microvascular leakage. The vascular incompetence is located in the retina capillaries as well as the RPE.

The presence of a macular detachment did not impact visual recovery, but correcting for its presence on the macular thickness maps did lead to an improved correlation between thickness and vision in the cystoid edema group.

Spectral domain systems have allowed us to better visualize the area between the inner photoreceptor junction and the RPE (Kiernan et al., 2009)[32]. This has helped us realize the importance of the outer retina in assessing inflammatory macular edema and the potential for vision recovery (fig. 5). The presence of a line corresponding to the junction between the inner and outer photoreceptor segments – even if present as a discontinuous line – is associated with a potential for vision recovery, while its absence is an indication of a poor prognosis (Monnet et al., 2007; Roesel et al., 2009)[8,33].

Studies done using simultaneous microperimetry and OCT reveal that the areas with inner segment/outer segment disruption have a low stimulus response irrespective of the retinal thickness (fig. 6). Inversely, microperimetry may be an interesting adjunct to assess the potential for visual recovery when the inner segment/outer segment interface is not visible due to the intensity of edema (Vujosevic et al., 2006)[34].

Clinical Course and Management

While there are no guidelines or consensus on when and how inflammatory macular edema should be treated, certain tenants are generally accepted. Macular edema associated with active inflammation requires immediate treatment. Therapy should be instituted when macular edema impairs vision. It should also be considered to treat subclinical forms of edema particularly when these have been associated in prior inflammation flare-ups with a drop in vision.

The approach used depends on the laterality of disease, its response to therapy, and the side effects of the proposed medication, if prolonged treatment is required.

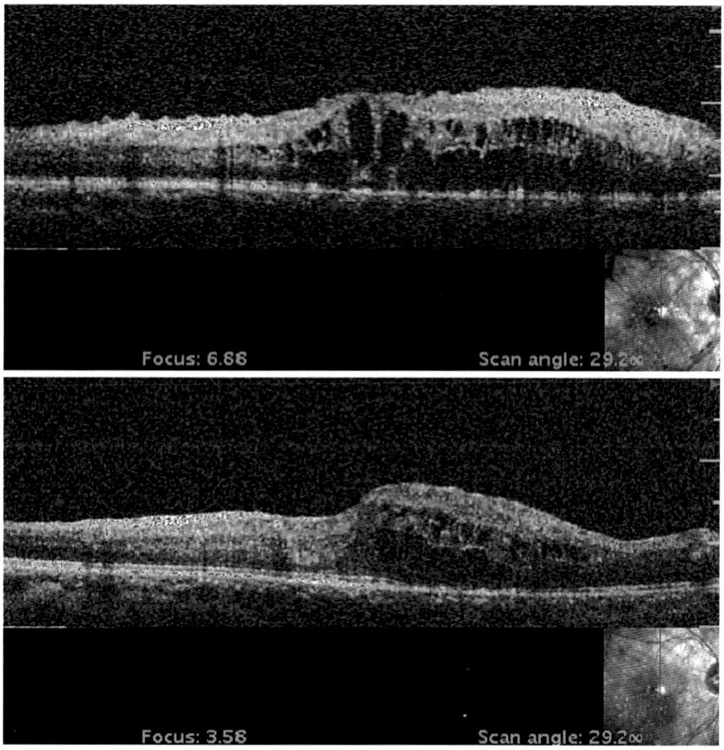

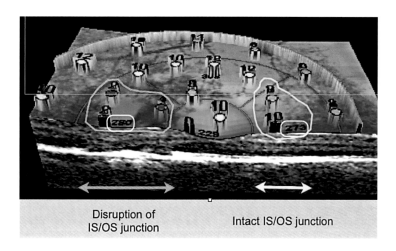

Fig. 5. Spectral domain OCT showing a case of diffuse edema pretreatment and posttreatment with intravitreal triamcinolone. The vision prior to the injection was 0.05, which improved to 0.5, 2 months following the injection of steroids. The cystoid edema, located mainly in the foveal area resolved, while in the area with diffuse edema, retinal thickness only decreased slightly. The junction between the inner and outer photoreceptors is clearly visible in the lower panel in the macular area but is also distinguishable in the upper panel as a discontinuous line.

Fig. 6. Simultaneous OCT and microperimetry showing that in the area with inner segment/outer segment (IS/OS) junction disruption stimulus response is absent. This is true irrespective of the retinal thickness in the specific location.

Anti-Inflammatory Medication

Management of inflammatory macular edema should start with an attempt to treat the underlying cause. Control of inflammation will often lead to resolution of the edema, provided the cause is mainly inflammatory and not due to macular ischemia or associated with macular atrophy (Forooghian et al., 2009)[28]. Here the therapeutic approach depends on prior response to immuno-suppressive agents and the etiology (Jabs et al., 2001; Mochizuki et al., 1994)[35,36].

Oral corticosteroids are good first-choice agents, due to their broad spectrum of action. They provide a more rapid and sustained response than sub-Tenon injections with regard to resolution of macular edema (Rhen et al., 2005; Venkatesh et al., 2007)[37,38]. Due to the numerous systemic side effects associated with the use of steroids, however, they should be tapered quickly to a dose equivalent or less than 5 mg/day. Patients should not be maintained on higher doses of steroids for more than 3 months.

Most *systemic immunomodulators* require a certain amount of time to achieve their biologic effect, i.e. up to 8 weeks for methotrexate and mycophenolic acid (Vujosevic et al., 2006)[34]. As these agents are being introduced, control of inflammation may be achieved by systemic or local administration of steroids as will be discussed more extensively below.

Biologic agents have received considerable attention in the last few years due to their potency and selectivity. Certain agents such as anti-tumor necrosis factor α can lead to a dramatic reduction in vascular leakage over the span of a few days. They can also quickly lead to a significant reduction in macular edema (Markomichelakis et al., 2004; Hale et al., 2006)[39,40].

Anti-tumor necrosis factor antibodies are expensive and may cause serious and even life-threatening side effects, hence their use should be limited to cases that have failed other therapies and when adequate monitoring by internal medicine specialists is possible.

Interferon α$_{2a}$ was initially proposed as a treatment of Behçet disease. With a high rate of remission (Kötter et al., 2004; Kötter et al., 1998; Tugal-Tutkun et al., 2006)[41–43], and a potent regulator of monocytes, it leads to resolution of macular edema in chronic uveitis patients who were unresponsive to more conventional treatments (Deuter et al., 2006; Bodaghi et al., 2007; Plskova et al.,

2007)[44–46]. Side effects are quite frequent and patients must be warned of their occurrence when they are placed on this medication (Bodaghi et al., 2007; Plskova et al., 2007)[45,46]. Combining the treatment with steroids may allow for a more tapered approach with a lowered systemic dose and better tolerance (Bodaghi et al., 2007)[45]. Response to interferon therapy can be delayed by up to 2 months.

Local Steroid Delivery
Local delivery of corticosteroids is one of the preferred approaches to treat uniocular disease or to bridge the time gap between the initiation of a new immunomodulator and its biologic effect. For posterior uveitis, topical delivery is rarely sufficient. They should be given using a periocular approach (orbital floor or sub-Tenon delivery) or by direct intraocular injection (Cunningham et al., 2008; Sallam et al., 2008; Okada et al., 2003)[47–49]. For a rapid response, intraocular injection is the preferred mode. Corticosteroids can also be used as a therapeutic challenge to determine if macular edema is responsive to therapy and to judge the overall ocular response to anti-inflammatory medication.

When present, the response will not persist. It will taper within 2–3 months in a nonvitrectomized eye, and within a month in most vitrectomized eyes (Schindler et al., 1982; Beer et al., 2003)[50,51]. There are also significant side effects reported including cataract formation, glaucoma, and endophthalmitis, which limit repeatability (Kok et al., 2005; Yamamoto et al., 2008; Maca et al., 2009)[52–54]. Steroid use is the most frequent cause of ocular hypertension in uveitis patients (66%). In these patients, however, the pressure rise is usually responsive to topical therapy with fewer patients requiring filtering surgery, as compared to patients developing glaucoma for other reasons (Sallam et al., 2009)[55]. The risk of ocular hypertension increases with repeated steroid use, particularly in younger individuals and in those who demonstrated a pressure rise after the first intravitreal administration (Inatani et al., 2008)[56].

Endophthalmitis rates are generally reported to be between 0.2 and 0.8% for intravitreous injections (Scott et al., 2007)[57]. These can be minimized by thorough cleansing of the ocular adnexa, avoiding injections in eyes with blepharitis or eyelid inflammation, and adequate attention to an aseptic technique (Bhavsar et al., 2009; Bhavsar et al., 2007)[58,59]. Single-use instruments and custom packs further help to reduce the risk of infection, as are single-use injection devices or syringes. Pseudo-endophthalmitis as was seen with the use of Kenalog® is rare to nonexistent with preservative-free preparations. It was characterized by a quiet eye, with a white hypopyon but characteristically without fibrin in the anterior chamber (Chen et al., 2004)[60]. Pain was variable, but vision was not significantly decreased.

Sub-Tenon injections are in this perspective a safer approach as it avoids intraocular delivery (Byun et al., 2009)[61]. For an optimal intraocular effect, however, it must be placed adjacent to the eye. When adequately positioned the effect will progressively manifest itself. According to several nonrandomized case series, the effect on vision and macular thickness is similar to intraocular delivery at 3 months. Adequate placement is challenging, as only about 30% are in the correct location (contiguous with the sclera and close to the macula), and absorption through the scleral wall may be variable (Thomas et al., 2006)[62]. To facilitate placement, either the use of the Nozik technique is recommended (Nozik et al., 1972)[63], or the use of an episcleral cannula inserted through Tenon's capsule into the appropriate location (Okada et al., 2003)[49].

The disadvantages of both intraocular and sub-Tenon approaches are their limited duration of action, inherent risk of infection, and the uncertainty of placement. These can potentially be overcome by implanting a slow-release device in the eye. Two solutions have been proposed: the fluocinolone implant (Retisert®) or a self-degrading device (Ozurdex™).

Sustained-Release Steroid Therapy

The HURON study evaluated Ozurdex in a 26-week, randomized, sham-controlled clinical trial in noninfectious intermediate or posterior uveitis patients. Dexamethasone (DEX) has 25 times the potency of cortisol and appears to have a better safety profile for ocular tissues. While triamcinolone in cell viability assays was shown to be toxic to in vitro preparations of RPE and retinal cells, this does not appear to be the case with DEX (Narayanan et al., 2006; Chung et al., 2007; Spitzer et al., 2008)[64–66].

In the HURON trial, 229 patients were randomized to a DEX 700 µg implant, a DEX 350 µg implant, or sham injection on a 1:1:1 randomization. Ninety-three percent or more of patients completed the study. Baseline characteristics were similar in all groups, with roughly 80% of patients having intermediate uveitis. In all groups, the mean vitreous haze score was 2. The primary endpoint (clearance of vitreous haze) at 8 weeks was reached in 45% of patients with a DEX 700 µg implant. It reached statistical significance compared to sham injection by week 8, and was sustained to week 12. Improvements in vision were statistically significant for DEX 700 µg at all time points starting at week 3. Intraocular pressure increases were noted, more frequently in the higher DEX implant group, but these responded to medical therapy and were nonsustained. None of the patients had an intraocular pressure above 25 mm Hg at week 26. At week 26, 17% of patients with a DEX 700 µg implant, 8% of patients with a DEX 350 µg implant, and 9% of sham-injected patients were on anti-glaucoma medication. The safety profile and ease of injection make it an interesting alternative to triamcinolone, as it appears to avoid – at least in the short term – many of the complications related to the use of intraocular steroids.

The fluocinolone implant (Retisert) uses a 0.59-mg drug pellet, which is slowly released over a 36-month period (Driot et al., 2004; Jaffe et al., 2006)[67,68]. The interim report of a randomized trial comparing a 0.59-mg with a 2.1-mg implant on

278 patients revealed that 87% of patients had stabilized or improved vision at 34 weeks (Pearson et al., 2006)[69]. Vision improvement was usually due to a reduction in cystoid macular edema. Patients required significantly less systemic medication, but over half of the patients required pressure-lowering medication, and by the 34-week time point, 5.8% of patients had required glaucoma surgery. Cataract progression was noted in 20% of patients and 10% of eyes required surgery. In a multicenter trial for diabetic macular edema, by the third year, 28% of eyes required glaucoma filtering surgery, and 95% of those eyes entering the study as phakic eyes required surgery (Hsu, 2007; Galor et al., 2007)[70,71]. Additional complications can be seen including transient hypotony, exposed struts requiring resuturing, the development of vitreous veils, and the development of cytomegalovirus in a non-AIDS patient (Ufret-Vincenty et al., 2007; Taban et al., 2008)[72,73]. Reimplantation after the initial implant has run out is associated with continued control of inflammation and a further increase in the risk of glaucoma (Whitcup et al., 1996)[74].

RPE Pump Stimulators

Certain patients have an insufficient response to anti-inflammatory medication. Inflammation may cause a diminution in the fluid pump function of the RPE, which can be either transient or permanent. In addition, cumulated insults from repeated inflammatory episodes can lead to chronic vascular incompetence, which the RPE pump is unable to match. In these cases, stimulation of the pump function of the remaining RPE cells may lead to resolution – partial or complete – of the macular edema. Diamox can lead to macular edema resolution in about 1/3 of patients, but the effect is not sustained and often insufficient to prevent recurrence with even mild inflammatory flare-ups (Whitcup et al., 1996; Shilling et al., 2005; Guez-Crosier et al., 1992)[74-76]. It is also associated with significant possible side effects, particularly in the elderly, including muscle cramps, itching, lightheadedness, and electrolyte imbalances. Therefore, its chronic use should be avoided if possible.

Another approach involves the stimulation of growth hormone receptors present within RPE cells resulting in an increased pump function. A few studies have shown that the use of octreotide or other somatostatin analogs can lead to a reduction in macular edema. This is often associated with a reduction in the need for adjunctive anti-inflammatory medication (Missotten et al., 2007; Papadaki et al., 2005; Kuijpers et al., 1998)[77-79]. The mechanism of action is through an enhanced apical-basal fluid transport through the RPE. The initial response is observed within a mean of about 3 months of continuous treatment (Missotten et al., 2007)[77]. The medication can be discontinued in some patients after several months of use (12–24 months), but recurrences are frequent. A positive response, however, is usually seen upon reintroduction of the growth hormone analog (Missotten et al., 2007; Papadaki et al., 2005)[77,78].

Surgical Therapy

Careful review of OCT images from patients with uveitic macular edema revealed that an epiretinal membrane was present in 40% (Hazel et al., 2000)[11], and frank macular traction was present in 10%. A number of case series have shown that the elimination of macular traction leads to an improvement in vision. When surgery is performed late in the course of disease, the improvement is only transient in nature. If it is done in a timely fashion, at a time when response to medical therapy is still present but requires ever-increasing doses of medication, it can lead to a sustained improvement in vision, and often to a reduced need for pharmacotherapy. Surgery should not be seen as a cure as it does not influence the underlying disease, but it can minimize the sequelae of repeated inflammatory episodes.

The surgical approach includes adequate control of the inflammation preoperatively. If manipulation of the iris or uvea is anticipated, judicious use of nonsteroidal anti-inflammatory medication can reduce the intensity and severity of postoperative inflammation. Surgery should be performed to minimize trauma. Using small-gauge surgery may promote a more rapid recovery with minimal inflammation, provided hypotony is avoided. For macular edema, the main objective is to relieve traction. Peeling of the posterior hyaloid membrane, while often performed to avoid the development of a pucker, must be weighed against the risk of causing a macular hole in eyes with severe macular edema. Peeling the circumfoveal retina while leaving the fovea intact may prevent the development of a hole while removing traction.

References

1 Pournaras CJ, Rungger-Brändle E, Riva CE, et al: Regulation of retinal blood flow in health and disease. Prog Retin Eye Res 2008;27:284–330.

2 Foster CS, Fong LP, Singh G: Cataract surgery and intraocular lens implantation in patients with uveitis. Ophthalmology 1989;96:281–288.

3 Rothova A, Suttorp-van Schulten MSA, Terffers WF, Kijlstra A: Causes and frequency of blindness in patients with intraocular inflammatory disease. Br J Ophthalmol 1996;80:332–336.

4 Rothova A: Inflammatory cystoid macular edema. Curr Opin Ophthalmol 2007;18:487–492.

5 Lardenoye CWTA, van Kooij B, Rothova A: Impact of macular edema on visual acuity in uveitis. Ophthalmology 2006;113:1446–1449.

6 de Boer J, Wulffraat N, Rothova A: Visual loss in uveitis of childhood. Br J Ophthalmol 2003;87:879–884.

7 Smith JA, Mackensen F, Sen HN, et al: Epidemiology and course of disease in childhood uveitis. Ophthalmology 2009;116:1544–1551.

8 Monnet D, Levinson RD, Holland GN, et al: Longitudinal cohort study of patients with birdshot chorioretinopathy. 3. Macular imaging at baseline. Am J Ophthalmol 2007;144:818–828.

9 Johnson MW: Etiology and treatment of macular edema. Am J Ophthalmol 2009;147:11–21.

10 Kiss CG, Barisani-Asenbauer T, Maca S, et al: Reading performance of patients with uveitis-associated cystoid macular edema. Am J Ophthalmol 2006;142:620–624.e1.

11 Hazel A, Petre K, Armstrong RA: Visual function and subjective quality of life compared in subjects with acquired macular disease. Invest Ophthalmol Vis Sci 2000;41:1309–1315.

12 Markomichelakis NN, Halkiadais I, Pantelia E, et al: Patterns of macular edema in patients with uveitis. Qualitative and quantitative assessment using optical coherence tomography. Ophthalmology 2005;111:946–953.

13 Catier A, Tadayoni R, Paques M, et al: Characterization of macular edema from various etiologies by optical coherence tomography. Am J Ophthalmol 2005;140:200–206.

14 Tran THC, de Smet MD, Bodaghi B, et al: Uveitic macular oedema: correlation between optical coherence tomography patterns with visual acuity and fluorescein angiography. Br J Ophthalmol 2008;92:922–927.

15 Acharya NR, Hong KC, Lee SM: Ranibizumab for refractory uveitis-related macular edema. Am J Ophthalmol 2009;148:303–309.

16 Markomichelakis NN, Theodossiadis PG, Sfikakis PP: Regression of neovascular age-related macular degeneration following infliximab therapy. Am J Ophthalmol 2005;139:537–540.

17 van Kooij B, Rothova A, Rijkers GT, de Groot-Mijnes JDF: Distinct cytokine and chemokine profiles in the aqueous of patients with uveitis and cystoid macular edema. Am J Ophthalmol 2006;142:192–194.

18 Probst K, Fijnheer R, Rothova A: Endothelial cell activation and hypercoagulability in ocular Behçet's disease. Am J Ophthalmol 2004;137:850–857.

19 Curnow SJ, Falciani F, Durrani OM, et al: Multiplex bead immunoassay analysis of aqueous humor reveals distinct cytokine profiles in uveitis. Invest Ophthalmol Vis Sci 2005;46:4251–4259.

20 Leal E, Manivannan A, Hosoya K, et al: Inducible nitric oxide synthase isoform is a key mediator of leukostasis and blood-reinal barrier breakdown in diabetic retinopathy. Invest Ophthalmol Vis Sci 2007;48:5257–5265.

21 van Kooij B, Fijnheer R, Roest M, Rothova A: Trace microalbuminuria in inflammatory cystoid macular edema. Am J Ophthalmol 2004;138:1010–1015.

22 Lin P, Loh AR, Margolis TP, et al: Cigarette smoking as a risk factor for uveitis. Ophthalmology 2010;117:585–590.

23 Thorne JE, Daniel E, Jabs DA, et al: Smoking as a risk factor for cystoid macular edema complicating intermediate uveitis. Am J Ophthalmol 2008;145:841–846.

24 Kramer CK, de Azevedo MJ, da Costa Rodrigues T, et al: Smoking habit is associated with diabetic macular edema in type 1 diabetes mellitus patients. J Diabetes Complications 2008;22:430.

25 Pruett R, Brockhurst RJ, Letts N: Fluorescein angiography of peripheral uveitis. Am J Ophthalmol 1974;77:448–453.

26 van Kooij B, Probst K, Fijnheer R, et al: Risk factors for cystoid macular oedema in patients with uveitis. Eye 2008;22:256–260.

27 Markomichelakis NN, Halkiadais I, Pantelia E, Peponis V, Patelis A, Theodossiadis P, Theodossiadis G: Patterns of macular edema in patients with uveitis. Qualitative and quantitative assessment using optical coherence tomography. Ophthalmology 2005;111:946–953.

28 Forooghian F, Yeh S, Faia LJ, Nussenblatt RB: Uveitis foveal atrophy. Arch Ophthalmol 2009;127:179–186.

29 Gürlü VP, Alimgil ML, Esgin H: Fluorescein angiographic findings in cases with intermediate uveitis in the inactive phase. Can J Ophthalmol 2007;42:107–109.

30 Tugal-Tutkun I, Herbort CP, Khairallah M, The Angiographic Scoring for Uveitis Working Group (ASUWOG): Scoring of dual fluorescein and ICG inflammatory angiographic signs for the grading of posterior segment inflammation (dual fluorescein and ICG angiographic scoring system for uveitis). Int Ophthalmol 2008, E-pub ahead of print.

31 Nussenblatt RB, Kaufman SC, Palestine AG, et al: Macular thickening and visual acuity. Measurement in patients with cystoid macular edema. Ophthalmology 1987;94:1134–1139.

32 Kiernan DF, Hariprasad SM, Chin EK, et al: Prospective comparison of cirrus and stratus optical coherence tomography for quantifying retinal thickness. Am J Ophthalmol 2009;147:267–275.

33 Roesel M, Henschel A, Heinz C, et al: Fundus autofluorescence and spectral domain optical coherence tomography in uveitis macular edema. Graefes Arch Clin Exp Ophthalmol 2009;247:1685–1689.

34 Vujosevic S, Midena E, Pilotto E, et al: Diabetic macular edema: correlation between microperimetry and optical coherence tomography findings. Invest Ophthalmol Vis Sci 2006;47:3044–3051.

35 Jabs DA, Rosenbaum JT: Guidelines for the use of immunosuppressive drugs in patients with ocular inflammatory disorders: recommendations of an expert panel. Am J Ophthalmol 2001;131:679.

36 Mochizuki M, de Smet MD: Use of immunosuppressive agents in ocular diseases. Prog Retin Eye Res 1994;13:479–506.

37 Rhen T, Cidlowski JA: Antiinflammatory action of glucocorticoids – new mechanisms for old drugs. N Engl J Med 2005;353:1711–1723.

38 Venkatesh P, Abhas Z, Garg S, Vohra R: Prospective optical coherence tomographic evaluation of the efficacy of oral and posterior subtenon corticosteroids in patients with intermediate uveitis. Graefes Arch Clin Exp Ophthalmol 2007;245:59–67.

39 Markomichelakis NN, Theodossiadis PG, Pantalia E, et al: Infliximab for chronic cystoid macular edema associated with uveitis. Am J Ophthalmol 2004;138:648–650.

40 Hale S, Lightman S: Anti-TNF therapies in the management of acute and chronic uveitis. Cytokine 2006;33:231–237.

41 Kötter I, Günaydin I, Zierhut M, Stübiger N: The use of interferon αin Behçet disease: review of the literature. Semin Arthritis Rheum 2004;33:320–325.

42 Kötter I, Eckstein AK, Stübiger N, Zierhut M: Treatment of ocular symptoms of Behçet's disease with interferon α_{2a}: a pilot study. Br J Ophthalmol 1998;82:488–494.

43 Tugal-Tutkun I, Güney-Tefekli E, Urancioglu M: Results of interferon-α therapy in patients with Behçet uveitis. Graefes Arch Clin Exp Ophthalmol 2006;244:1692–1695.

44 Deuter CME, Kötter I, Günaydin I, et al: Interferon-2A: a new treatment option for long lasting refractory cystoid macular edema in uveitis? Retina 2006;26:786–791.

45 Bodaghi B, Gendron G, Wechsler B, et al: Efficacy of interferon αin the treatment of refractory and sight threatening uveitis: a retrospective monocentric study of 45 patients. Br J Ophthalmol 2007;91:335–359.

46 Plskova J, Greiner K, Forrester JV: Interferon-α as an effective treatment for noninfectious posterior uveitis and panuveitis. Am J Ophthalmol 2007;144:55–61.

47 Cunningham MA, Edelman JL, Kaushal S: Intravitreal steroids for macular edema: the past, the present, and the future. Surv Ophthalmol 2008;53:139–149.

48 Sallam A, Comer RM, Chang JH, et al: Short-term safety and efficacy of intravitreal triamcinolone acetonide for uveitic macular edema in children. Arch Ophthalmol 2008;126:200–205.

49 Okada AA, Wakabayashi T, Morimura Y, et al: Trans-tenon's retrobulbar triamcinolone infusion for the treatment of uveitis. Brit J Ophthalmol 2003;87:1–4.

50 Schindler RH, Chandler D, Thresher R, Machemer R: The clearance of intravitreal triamcinolone acetonide. Am J Ophthalmol 1982;93:415–417.

51 Beer PM, Bakri SJ, Singh RJ, et al: Intraocular concentration and pharmacokinetics of triamcinolone acetonide after a single intravitreal injection. Ophthalmology 2003;110:681–686.

52 Kok H, Lau C, Maycock N, et al: Outcome of intravitreal triamcinolone in uveitis. Ophthalmology 2005;112:1916.

53 Yamamoto Y, Komatsu T, Koura Y, et al: Intraocular pressure elevation after intravitreal or posterior sub-tenon triamcinolone acetonide injection. Can J Ophthalmol 2008;43:42–47.

54 Maca SM, Abela-Formanek C, Kiss CG, et al: Intravitreal triamcinolone for persistent cystoid macular oedema in eyes with quiescent uveitis. Clin Experiment Ophthalmol 2009;37:389–396.

55 Sallam A, Sheth HG, Habot-Wilner Z, Lightman S: Outcome of raised intraocular pressure in uveitic eyes with and without a corticosteroid-induced hypertensive response. Am J Ophthalmol 2009;148:207–213.

56 Inatani M, Iwao K, Kawaji T, et al: Intraocular pressure elevation after injection of triamcinolone acetonide: a multicenter retrospective case-control study. Am J Ophthalmol 2008;145:676–681.

57 Scott IU, Flynn HW Jr: Reducing the risk of endophthalmitis following intravitreal injections. Retina 2007;27:10–12.

58 Bhavsar AR, Googe JM Jr, Stockdale CR, et al: Risk of endophthalmitis after intravitreal drug injection when topical antibiotics are not required: the diabetic retinopathy clinical research network laser-ranibizumab-triamcinolone clinical trials. Arch Ophthalmol 2009;127:1581–1583.

59 Bhavsar AR, Ip MS, Glassman AR: The risk of endophthalmitis following intravitreal triamcinolone injection in the DRCRnet and SCORE clinical trials. Am J Ophthalmol 2007;144:454–456.

60 Chen SDM, Lochhead J, McDonald B, Patel CK: Pseudohypopyon after intravitreal triamcinolone injection for the treatment of pseudophakic cystoid macular oedema. Br J Ophthalmol 2004;88:843–844.

61 Byun YS, Park Y-H: Complications and safety profile of posterior subtenon injection of triamcinolone acetonide. J Ocul Pharmacol Ther 2009;25:159–162.

62 Thomas ER, Wang J, Ege E, et al: Intravitreal triamcinolone acetonide concentration after subtenon injection. Am J Ophthalmol 2006;142:860–861.

63 Nozik RA: Periocular injection of steroids. Trans Am Acad Ophthalmol Otolaryngol 1972;76:695–705.

64 Narayanan R, Mungcal JK, Kenney MC, et al: Toxicity of triamcinolone acetonide on retinal neurosensory and pigment epithelial cells. Invest Ophthalmol Vis Sci 2006;47:722–728.

65 Chung H, Hwang JJ, Koh JY, et al: Triamcinolone acetonide-mediated oxidative injury in retinal cell culture: comparison with dexamethasone. Invest Ophthalmol Vis Sci 2007;48:5742–5749.

66 Spitzer MS, Yoeruek E, Kaczmarek RT, et al: Sodium hyaluronate gels as a drug-release system for corticosteroids: release kinetics and antiproliferative potential for glaucoma surgery. Acta Ophthalmol 2008;86:842–848.

67 Driot JY, Novack GD, Rittenhouse KD, et al: Ocular pharmacokinetics of fluocinolone acetonide after Retisert intravitreal implantation in rabbits over a 1-year period. J Ocul Pharmacol Ther 2004;20:269–275.

68 Jaffe GJ, Martin D, Callanan D, et al: Fluocinolone acetonide implant (Retisert) for noninfectious posterior uveitis: thirty-four-week results of a multicenter randomized clinical study. Ophthalmology 2006;113:1020–1027.

69 Pearson P, Leavy B, Comstock T, Fluocinolone Acetonide Implant Study Group: Fluocinolone acetonide intravitreal implant to treat diabetic macular edema: 3-year results of a multicenter clinical trial (E-abstract). Invest Ophthalmol Vis Sci 2006;47:5442.

70 Hsu J: Drug delivery methods for posterior segment disease. Curr Opin Ophthalmol 2007;18:235–239.

71 Galor A, Margolis R, Kaiser PK, Lowder CY: Vitreous band formation and the sustained-release, intravitreal fluocinolone (Retisert) implant. Arch Ophthalmol 2007;125:836–838.

72 Ufret-Vincenty RL, Singh RP, Lowder CY, Kaiser PK: Cytomegalovirus retinitis after fluocinolone acetonide (Retisert™) implant. Am J Ophthalmol 2007;143:334–335.

73 Taban MM, Lowder CYMDP, Kaiser PKM: Outcome of fluocinolone acetonide implant Retisert™ reimplantation for chronic noninfectious posterior uveitis. Retina 2008;28:1280–1288.

74 Whitcup SM, Csaky KG, Podgor MJ, et al: A randomized, masked, cross-over trial of acetazolamide for cystoid macular edema in patients with uveitis. Ophthalmology 1996;103:1054–1062.

75 Schilling H, Heiligenhaus A, Laube T, et al: Long-term effect of acetazolamide treatment of patients with uveitic chronic cystoid macular edema is limited by persisting inflammation. Retina 2005;25:182–188.

76 Guex-Crosier Y, Othenin-Girard P, Herbort CP: Traitement différencié de l'oedème maculaire cystoide inflammatoire postopératoire et secondaire aux uvéites. Klin Monbl Augenheilkd 1992;200:367–373.

77 Missotten T, van Laar JAM, van der Loos TL, et al: Octreotide long-acting repeatable for the treatment of chronic macular edema in uveitis. Am J Ophthalmol 2007;144:838–843.

78 Papadaki T, Zacharopoulos I, Iaccheri B, et al: Somatostatin for uveitic cystoid macular edema (CME). Ocul Immunol Inflamm 2005;13:469–470.

79 Kuijpers RWAM, Baarsma S, van Hagen PM: Treatment of cystoid macular edema with octreotide. N Engl J Med 1998;338:624–626.

Marc D. de Smet, MDCM, PhD, FRCSC
Department of Ophthalmology
University of Amsterdam, Meibergdreef 9
NL–1105 AZ Amsterdam (The Netherlands)
E-Mail mddesmet1@mac.com

Chapter 9

Coscas G (ed): Macular Edema.
Dev Ophthalmol. Basel, Karger, 2010, vol 47, pp 148–159

Postsurgical Cystoid Macular Edema

Anat Loewenstein · Dinah Zur

Department of Ophthalmology, Tel Aviv Medical Center, Tel Aviv University, Tel Aviv, Israel

Abstract

Cystoid macular edema (CME) is a primary cause of reduced vision following both cataract and successful vitreoretinal surgery. The incidence of clinical CME following modern cataract surgery is 0.1–2.35%. Preexisting conditions such as diabetes mellitus and uveitis as well as intraoperative complications can raise the risk of developing CME postoperatively. The etiology of CME is not completely understood. Prolapsed or incarcerated vitreous and postoperative inflammatory processes have been proposed as causative agents. Pseudophakic CME is characterized by poor postoperative visual acuity. Fluorescein angiography is indispensable in the workup of CME, showing the classical perifoveal petaloid staining pattern and late leakage of the optic disk. Optical coherence tomography is a useful diagnostic tool, which displays cystic spaces in the outer nuclear layer. The most important differential diagnoses include age-related macular degeneration and other causes of CME such as diabetic macular edema. Most cases of pseudophakic CME resolve spontaneously. The value of prophylactic treatment is doubtful. First-line treatment of postsurgical CME should include topical nonsteroidal anti-inflammatory drugs and corticosteroids. Oral carbonic anhydrase inhibitors can be considered complementary. In cases of resistant CME, periocular or intraocular corticosteroids present an option. Antiangiogenic agents, though experimental, should be considered for nonresponsive persistent CME. Surgical options should be reserved for special indications.

Definition and Epidemiology

Cystoid macular edema (CME) is a primary cause of reduced vision following both cataract and successful vitreoretinal surgeries.[a] CME remains a distressing problem after cataract (Gass et al., 1966; Irvine, 1976)[1,2] and other ocular surgeries such as neodymium:yttrium-aluminum-garnet (Nd:YAG) capsulotomy, penetrating keratoplasty, scleral buckling, filtering procedures, and panretinal photocoagulation (Shimura et al., 2009)[3]. Its etiology is not completely understood (Rossetti et al., 2000)[4].

Although the introduction of phacoemulsification has led to a significant decrease in postoperative CME, and in spite of the fact that the accompanying visual loss is usually self-limiting, the condition remains a therapeutic challenge to ophthalmologists, especially when it persists for several months. Possible explanations for the variation

---

[a] Usually named Irvine-Gass syndrome, CME could more appropriately be named Hruby-Irvine-Gass Syndrome, since Irvine did not notice the foregoing biomicroscopic observations of K. Hruby.

in reported CME incidence are differences in surgical techniques, rates of surgical complications, and methods of diagnostic assessment.

The incidence of clinical CME following modern cataract surgery is reported as 0.1–2.35% (Henderson et al., 2007)[5]. Angiographic CME is much more frequent with incidence assessments, although variable, reaching 70% in some studies (Flach, 1998)[6].

Pathology and Pathophysiology

Histopathological Features
Histopathological specimens of CME following cataract surgery display retinal capillary dilation, serous fluid in the outer plexiform and inner nuclear layer, and inflammatory cells in the iris-ciliary perivascular complex (Neal et al., 2005)[7].

Intraretinal accumulation of fluid causes formation of perifoveal cysts, which may combine to larger cysts and give rise to lamellar holes. In severe cases, the edema involves most of the retinal layers.

Pathophysiology
There is considerable alteration in the protein composition of the vitreous fluid after cataract extraction as compared to phakic eyes. The following modifications of the retinal microenvironment may contribute to the development of retinal disease (Hruby, 1985)[8]:

(1) vitreous traction on the macula;

(2) vitreous incarceration in the wound;

(3) vitreous uveal traction;

(4) inflammation (the role of prostaglandins and other inflammatory mediators released during surgical trauma and causing increased vascular permeability; cyclooxygenase expression);

(5) light damage.

Direct macular traction from vitreous prolapse, incarcerated iris, or vitreous has been proposed as being responsible for the development of CME. The presence of fine strands of vitreous connecting the detached posterior vitreous face and the macular area support this theory (Tolentino et al., 1965)[9].

Other theories suggest that inflammation and increased levels of intraocular prostaglandins after cataract surgery are a cause of CME. The association of severe anterior ocular inflammation and postsurgical CME accords with this thesis (Rossetti et al., 2000)[4]. Following cataract surgery, inflammatory mediators (prostaglandins, cytokines, and other vasopermeability factors) disrupt the blood-retinal barrier, increasing permeability of the perifoveal capillaries and resulting in fluid accumulation in the perifoveal retina (Miyake et al., 2002)[10].

The occasional accumulation of subretinal fluid indicates a disruption of normal apposition between the retinal pigment epithelium and photoreceptors, in contrast to the usual disruption of cell-cell contacts within the retina.

Phototoxicity has been suggested as another cause of CME. Light from the operating microscope was thought to increase the proportion of relatively short wavelength light entering the eye and subsequently releasing prostaglandin and advancing CME. Such a mechanism for the development of CME, however, has been disproved (Iliff, 1985)[11].

Risk Factors

Identifying risk factors for postsurgical CME is crucial for prevention and adequate treatment. Systemic diseases, intraoperative complications, and preexisting ocular conditions influence the development of CME.

Systemic Factors
Diabetes mellitus promotes the development of CME even in the absence of diabetic retinopathy. In a large cost analysis study of almost 140,000 patients, diabetes increased CME incidence rates from 1.73 to 3.05% (Schmier et al., 2007)[12].

Systemic hypertension apparently increases the incidence of postsurgical CME (Flach,1998)[6].

Furthermore, it is a risk factor for retinal vein occlusion, which itself increases CME.

Complicated Surgery

Advancement in surgical techniques has significantly reduced the rate of CME over the last decades. Intracapsular cataract extraction was much more frequently associated with CME than extracapsular cataract extraction. Now, pseudo- or aphakic CME occurs primarily in patients following uncomplicated surgery.

Still, certain surgical complications raise the risk of CME. Rupture of the posterior capsule, as well as secondary capsulotomy, including YAG capsulotomy, are associated with a higher rate of CME. Remarkably, a well-designed study showed an increase in angiographic CME but no significant difference in vision following capsulotomy (Kraff et al., 1984)[13].

Vitreous loss increases the prevalence of CME by 10–20%. Vitreous to the wound prolongs CME and can be associated with a poorer prognosis (Flach, 1998)[6]. Iris incarceration, an additional risk factor for CME, may have a more important association with poor vision in patients with chronic postsurgical CME than with other intraoperative complications. Specific intraocular lenses (IOLs) are associated with increased occurrence of CME. A meta-analysis of Flach et al. showed that the prevalence of CME is highest with implantation of an iris-fixated IOL. Anterior chamber IOLs raise the risk more than posterior chamber IOLs.

Review of patients with CME following pars plana vitrectomy for retained lens fragments revealed that 8% of eyes with a sulcus-fixated posterior chamber IOL implanted at cataract extraction and 46% of eyes with aphakia or an anterior chamber IOL developed CME (Cohen et al., 2006)[14].

Preexisting Conditions

In patients with uveitis, CME is the most important cause for poor visual outcome following cataract surgery, especially in the long term. Implantation of an IOL in cases of anterior and intermediate uveitis is controversial. Preoperative diabetic retinopathy considerably increases the risk of onset and the persistence of CME (Iliff, 1985)[11]. A history of retinal vein occlusion and epiretinal membrane (ERM) also predict development of CME (Henderson et al., 2007)[5]. Caution is advised since ERM can induce macular edema without cataract surgery, and CME itself is associated with generation of ERM.

The topical use of latanoprost in glaucoma patients has been reported in association with pseudophakic CME (Warwar et al., 1998)[15]. A randomized controlled study investigated the effects of latanoprost on the blood-aqueous barrier and onset of angiographic CME in early postoperative pseudophakia (Miyake et al., 2002)[10]. Latanoprost was shown to enhance the disruption of the blood-aqueous barrier. Patients treated with latanoprost and fluorometholone developed significantly more CME and showed a greater amount of flare than patients treated with latanoprost and diclofenac. Pseudophakic and aphakic CME in patients treated with prostaglandin analogues usually resolves after discontinuation of treatment and therapy with nonsteroidal anti-inflammatory drugs (NSAIDs).

The above conditions may compromise the integrity of the blood-retinal barrier and boost inflammatory activity.

Diagnosis

Clinical Findings

The most frequent sign of CME is poor postoperative visual acuity. Onset of clinically significant CME is generally 4–12 weeks after surgery, and reaches its peak at 4–6 weeks postoperatively. Hence, patients may complain of impaired vision after an initial postoperative period of improved vision. Less common complaints are positive central scotoma, metamorphopsia, low-grade

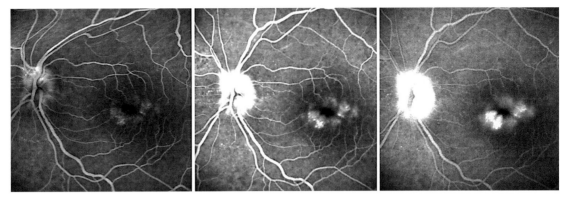

Fig. 1. FA of a patient with postsurgical CME. Note petaloid hyperfluorescence, which increases in size and intensity accumulating in a cystoid manner and late staining of the optical nerve.

eye redness, photophobia, and ocular irritation. Reduced contrast sensitivity is also an early sign of diabetic macular edema that may present in CME.

In biomicroscopy, the loss of foveal depression is the most common sign of CME. The perifoveal area appears yellow xanthophyllic colored. Intraretinal cystoid spaces can be detected. Small splinter retinal hemorrhages may appear as well. In about 10% of the cases, ERMs are present. Optic nerve head swelling is frequently seen.

In cases of chronic CME, the cystoid spaces fuse to foveal cysts. These patients have worse visual acuity and worse prognosis.

Imaging

Fluorescein Angiography
Clinical examination was shown to miss the diagnosis of CME in 5–10% of cases (Tolentino et al., 1965)[9]. Fluorescein angiography (FA) is highly valuable for diagnosing CME, especially in uncertain cases. In the early phase of FA, capillary dilation and leakage from small perifoveal capillaries are visible. In later phases, pooling in the outer plexiform layer results in the classic perifoveal 'petaloid' staining pattern.

Another common sign is late leakage and staining of the optic nerve due to capillary leakage (Arciere et al., 2005)[16]. Improvement in CME correlates with decreased optic nerve staining.

In severe CME, cystoid spaces may have a honeycomb appearance in FA, which correlates with large cystoid spaces, extending outside the immediate perifoveal region (fig. 1).

Optical Coherence Tomography
Optical coherence tomography (OCT) is a useful supplemental tool for detecting postsurgical CME (fig. 2). In correlation with histological findings, OCT displays cystic spaces in the outer nuclear layer of the central macula. The peak incidence of CME, when detected by OCT, is 4 weeks after cataract surgery. Foveal thickness was found to increase significantly and correlate with decreased visual acuity, whereas control groups of pseudophakic eyes without CME showed only a minimal increase in foveal thickness and improvement in visual acuity. In the future, the application of OCT to diagnose postsurgical CME is sure to increase.

Regardless, FA is indispensable for the diagnosis of CME from other causes.

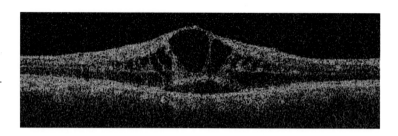

Fig. 2. OCT of a patient with CME following cataract surgery. Note cystic spaces of the macula, subretinal fluid, and significantly increased foveal thickness.

Functional Testing (Electrophysiology)
In electrophysiologic studies – for scientific use rather than for clinical use – aphakic CME is characterized by reduced amplitudes of oscillatory potentials with normal a-wave and b-wave responses.

Stages

Angiographic CME
Angiographic CME is defined as the presence of fluorescein leakage in FA. It is classified by 4 levels: in level 1, the edema is less than 360° perifoveal; in level 2, minimal but 360° perifoveal edema is seen; level 3 is associated with moderate perifoveal edema, and level 4 is characterized by severe perifoveal edema.

Angiographic CME is mostly asymptomatic. Decreased visual acuity does not correlate with the extension of leakage. Therefore, the grading system has little clinical importance (Tolentino et al., 1965)[9].

Clinical CME
Clinically significant macular edema presents with decreased vision and is diagnosed by biomicroscopy.

The exact relationship between angiographic CME and clinically significant CME is uncertain. Patients with clinically significant CME may have a chronic form of angiographic CME. Otherwise, both may be separate conditions on a histologic or pathophysiologic level – not differentiable using conventional FA.

Classification

The following classifications are used:
(a) acute: acute CME appears within 4 months of surgery;
(b) late onset: late onset occurs after more than 4 months postoperatively;
(c) chronic: chronic CME lasts more than 6 months;
(d) recurrent.

Differential Diagnosis

Differentiation between postsurgical CME and other ocular pathologies has important implications for treatment. Conversely, several ocular and systemic diseases are themselves associated with CME.

It is important to distinguish macular edema, a common cause of poor visual outcome following cataract surgery in diabetic patients, from diabetic macular edema. Frequently, preexisting diabetic macular edema worsens considerably after surgery. The clinical presentation of diabetic macular edema is accompanied by microaneurysms, intraretinal hemorrhages, and lipid deposits. FA is helpful for differential diagnosis. Diabetic macular edema presents with diffuse leakage that may not be localized only at the foveal area. Since disk leakage is absent in diabetic macular edema, its presence should raise suspicion for postsurgical CME (Arciere et al., 2005)[16].

In acute retinal vein occlusion, biomicroscopy shows intraretinal hemorrhages and edema according to the distribution of the affected vein. CME can accompany these findings. FA shows delayed venous filling and increasing leakage of dye. In some cases, hypofluorescent areas of retinal ischemia may be present at the periphery. Again, retinal vein occlusion itself is predictive of the development of postsurgical CME.

CME also occurs as a component of hypertensive retinopathy. A history of chronic systemic hypertension and additional signs such as cotton wool spots, retinal hemorrhages, hyperemic optic disk, and exudates are also present.

Preexisting ERM is a risk factor for developing postsurgical CME. Secondary ERM, which can occur after every vitreoretinal procedure, may be confused with CME. Both conditions present with decreased vision and metamorphopsia. In ERM, biomicroscopy reveals an irregular light reflex or thickening of the macula, distortion of blood vessels, and retinal wrinkling, which is best seen in red-free light. FA may be an auxiliary tool in detecting the extent of vessel distortion and the associated leakage of dye.

Retinitis pigmentosa presenting with nyctalopia is also associated with CME. Onset is generally during the third decade, an untypical age for cataract surgery. CME occurs relatively late in the course of this disease and is usually accompanied by the typical signs in fundus examination.

Age-related macular degeneration is the most common cause of choroidal neovascularization and mostly affects the same age group as cataracts. Choroidal neovascularization can be mistaken for postsurgical CME. Exudative maculopathy caused by choroidal neovascularization presents with intraretinal and subretinal hemorrhages, retinal pigment epithelium detachments,

and hard exudates, which are not found in postoperative CME. Furthermore, it is important to distinguish postsurgical CME from CME caused by occult choroidal neovascularization. In FA, occult choroidal neovascularization is seen with gradually increasing irregular hyperfluorescence and leakage of dye from the retinal pigment epithelium in the late phase. An elevated area of hyperfluorescence marks the region of the fibrovascular retinal pigment epithelium detachment. Disk leakage does not appear in occult choroidal neovascularization.

Macular edema is sometimes a component of radiation retinopathy. A history of ocular or facial radiotherapy should prompt this differential diagnosis when diagnosing postsurgical CME.

Management

Angiographic CME does not necessarily portend a poor visual outcome (fig. 3). Most cases of postoperative CME resolve spontaneously, with only a 1–3% incidence of clinical persistence (angiographic CME with visual acuity of 20/40 or less, 6 or more months after cataract surgery) (Solomon, 1995)[17].

Available therapeutic interventions, both for prophylaxis and for treatment of CME, are based on theories regarding the pathogenesis of the condition. Studies testing the efficacy of these interventions have generally not been well designed or conducted, and results have been inconsistent. Thus, there is no widely accepted technique to treat chronic CME.

Most treatment strategies have concentrated on inflammation or vitreous traction as the hypothetical etiology. The goal of treatment is to decrease the macular edema and thereby increase visual acuity.

Prophylaxis (Topical NSAIDs)
Prophylactic medical intervention has demonstrated effectiveness in preventing angiographic

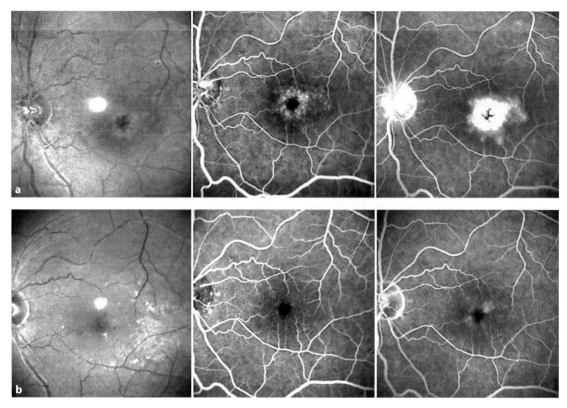

Fig. 3. a Fluorescein angiogram showing the classical petaloid appearance of CME (visual acuity 20/80). **b** The same patient after treatment with topical corticosteroids (visual acuity 20/25). Note almost complete resolution of macular hyperfluorescence and no staining of the optical nerve.

CME but is inconclusive in preventing clinically diagnosed CME or loss of vision. From their meta-analysis published in 1998, Rosetti et al. (Rossetti et al., 1998)[18] concluded that prophylactic intervention was beneficial for both angiographically diagnosed and clinically diagnosed CME.

Medical prophylaxis also appears to protect against loss of vision in patients undergoing cataract surgery. Cataract surgery has changed considerably over the past 15 years. Outcomes and complication rates for intracapsular extraction differ greatly from modern extracapsular extraction and phacoemulsification. Variations in procedures undoubtedly affect complications, including CME incidence.

Bias may also explain variations in incidence rates. Nonrandomized trials reported the highest incidence rates. Exaggerated treatment effects in nonrandomized studies are usually attributed to unintentional or intentional bias in reporting. Such an interpretation may also be applicable here. Though a number of studies demonstrated the effectiveness of topical NSAIDs in preventing angiographic CME, a statistically significant effect over more than 1 year was not proven. Furthermore, long-term visual advantage from prophylactic treatment remains doubtful.

Conventional Medical Treatment

NSAIDs Inhibiting Cyclooxygenase
A number of studies have investigated the therapeutic value of cyclooxygenase inhibitors for postsurgical CME (Peterson et al., 1992)[19]. Topical administration of NSAIDs shows better ocular penetration than systemic administration and achieves higher aqueous levels. Furthermore, there are fewer adverse effects.

Some studies found a positive effect for ketorolac tromethamine on visual acuity. Rho reported improvement of CME in 90% of patients after 6 months, with no difference between those treated with diclofenac and with ketorolac (Rho, 2003)[20].

A large prospective double-masked study examined the prophylactic and therapeutic effect of topical indomethacin on the incidence of CME following cataract surgery. While the incidence of angiographic CME was significantly higher in the placebo-treated patients, there was no significant difference in visual outcome (Kraff et al., 1984)[13].

In prescribing NSAIDs for CME, one should be aware of the 'on-off' phenomena, occurring with cessation and resumption of treatment (Rossetti et al., 1998)[18].

Steroids (Topical, Periocular, Intraocular, Systemic)
Well-controlled studies of the efficacy of steroids for prophylaxis and treatment of CME are lacking. In 1981, Stern et al. described a series of 49 patients who developed CME following intracapsular cataract extraction with iris-fixated IOL (Stern et al., 1981)[21]. They showed a positive response to systemic corticosteroids. In this, as in other retrospective studies, the impact of spontaneous resolution on visual improvement is unclear. Furthermore, systemic corticosteroids are not an accepted treatment due to their severe adverse effects.

Periocular corticosteroids have been proposed for CME resistant to topical medication. A comparison between retrobulbar and sub-Tenon injections showed no significant differences for visual improvement and elevation of intraocular pressure. (Thach et al., 1997)[22].

Heier et al. found that for acute CME, therapy combining topical ketorolac and prednisolone is superior to either treatment alone (Heier et al., 2000)[23]. Patients in the ketorolac group improved by 1.6 Snellen lines, the prednisolone group by 1.1 lines, and patients administered a combination treatment by 3.8 lines with a quicker response.

Intravitreal triamcinolone acetonide has been used successfully to treat macular edema associated with conditions such as retinal vein occlusion, uveitis, and diabetic maculopathy (Ip et al., 2004; Kok et al., 2005)[24,25]. Some case series have also described a beneficial effect in pseudophakic CME (Jonas et al., 2003; Boscia et al., 2005)[26,27].

Recently, a retrospective case series review of 21 eyes (20 patients) showed that following an intravitreal injection of 4 mg triamcinolone for postoperative CME, the mean logarithm of the minimum angle of resolution visual acuity decreased significantly from 0.53 to 0.33 at 1 month after injection ($p < 0.001$). At the latest review, 43% of eyes had improved Snellen visual acuity by 2 or more lines and 86% by 1 or more lines compared to baseline. The remaining 14% had reduced Snellen visual acuity compared to baseline. In the postinjection period, 33% of eyes developed an intraocular pressure of 22 mm Hg or higher and all responded well to short-term topical agents (Conway et al., 2003)[28].

Carbonic Anhydrase Inhibitors
The aim of treatment of macular edema with acetazolamide is improvement of the pumping function of the retinal pigment epithelium, to reduce intraretinal fluid, and improve vision. Furthermore, carbonic anhydrase inhibitors induce acidification of the subretinal space and thereby increase fluid resorption from the retina

through the retinal pigment epithelium into the choroid.

Acetazolamide demonstrated effectiveness in treating macular edema caused by uveitis or resulting from inherited outer retinal diseases such as retinitis pigmentosa but not in treating primary retinal vascular disorders (Farber et al., 1994; Grover et al., 2006)[29,30]. Case reports documenting the effect of acetazolamide on postsurgical CME are encouraging (Catier et al., 2005)[31]. One describes a positive effect on CME following scleral buckling (Weene, 1992)[32].

Close follow-up of patients treated with carbonic anhydrase inhibitors is important due to the potentially adverse effects such as nausea, dizziness, and paresthesia.

Experimental Medical Treatment
(Antiangiogenic Agents)
Vascular endothelial growth factor is a crucial mediator in postoperative CME, in addition to its role as mediator in the onset of inflammatory macular edema. Bevacizumab, a monoclonal antibody against all isoforms of vascular endothelial growth factor, has been used off-label to treat various neovascular eye diseases. Spitzer et al. showed in a series of 16 eyes that single or repeat injection of intravitreal bevacizumab did not improve visual acuity in patients with postoperative CME (Spitzer et al., 2008)[33]. A slight anatomical improvement on OCT did not translate into functional improvement.

Laser Treatment (Vitreolysis)
Vitreous incarceration in the cataract incision wound complicates CME and prolongs its healing. Nd:YAG laser has shown promising results for such cases (Steinert et al., 1989)[34]. Interpretation of these results, however, has been difficult for several reasons: since anti-inflammatory drops were often prescribed after laser treatment, the therapeutic effect could have been a combination of both Nd:YAG laser and anti-inflammatory drops. These studies had no control groups. Moreover,

treatment was started early and spontaneous regression may have interfered.

Though an advantage of YAG laser vitreolysis is avoidance of invasive surgery, severe complications, such as elevation of intraocular pressure and retinal detachment, may present (Schmier et al., 2007)[12].

Grid laser photocoagulation was described as a therapeutic option in a few patients with mixed results (Lardenoye et al., 1998)[35]. Controlled clinical trials investigating its efficacy and safety have yet to be conducted.

Surgical Treatments (Vitrectomy, IOL Replacement)
The rationale for performing vitrectomy in postsurgical CME is removal of vitreous adhesions and inflammatory mediators in the vitreous and greater access of topical steroids to the posterior pole.

Aphakic CME has become less important. A large multicenter prospective, randomized, controlled study investigated the efficacy of vitrectomy in patients with chronic aphakic CME and vitreous incarceration to the corneoscleral wound (Fung, 1985)[36]. The group that underwent vitrectomy demonstrated visual improvement. However, treatment of this group and not the control group with corticosteroids may have influenced the results. Since spontaneous resolution of CME in patients with a visual acuity of 20/80 or better is almost 30%, surgery was performed only in cases with lower and long-standing decreased vision. The pars plana approach seemed superior to the limbal approach.

In a retrospective study of 24 patients with chronic pseudophakic CME and vitreous adhesions, or iris capture of the IOL unresponsive to medical treatment, who underwent vitrectomy (Harbour et al., 1995)[37], the mean visual improvement was 4.7 Snellen lines. The presence of an anterior or posterior chamber IOL was irrelevant. Postoperative visual improvement was not related to the time interval between cataract surgery and vitrectomy. It is noteworthy that patients received corticosteroids after vitrectomy.

Vitreous incarceration due to cataract surgery is a relatively uncommon complication. Well-designed studies of visual improvement following vitrectomy are lacking. In any case, current opinion does not consider surgery as a first-line treatment for postoperative CME due to other reasons such as severe potential operative complications and the high spontaneous resolution rate of CME. Still, in cases unresponsive to medical treatment for more than 1 and less than 2 years, vitrectomy may present an alternative.

Former types of IOLs were more frequently associated with CME due to particular technical and anatomical properties. Small-scale studies showed a slight visual benefit after removal or replacement of the lens (Shepard, 1979)[38]. Improved quality of modern IOLs has considerably diminished their impact on CME development over recent decades. In cases of postsurgical CME and coexisting problems that can be attributed to the presence of the IOL (i.e., pseudobullous keratopathy, chronic inflammation), removal or exchange of the IOL still presents a therapeutic option (Price et al., 1990)[39].

Prevention

Surgical Technique in Primary Surgery
Atraumatic surgery is a primary means of preventing CME. Some operative factors significantly influence the development of CME. Extracapsular cataract extraction reduces the risk compared to intracapsular cataract extraction. Posterior chamber IOL should be preferred to anterior chamber IOL. Iris clip lenses are associated with the highest risk of all IOLs. Special care should be taken to keep the posterior capsule intact.

Prophylaxis-Preventive NSAIDs
NSAIDs were reported beneficial in preventing CME – with limitations – regarding long-term

visual outcome. Ketorolac and diclofenac demonstrated equal safety and effectiveness in controlling inflammation after uncomplicated cataract surgery and implantation of the IOL (Rho, 2003)[20].

Key Messages

Ways to Prevent Postsurgical CME
Prevention of postsurgical CME starts with a thorough preoperative evaluation of the patient to identify treatable risk factors and preexisting anatomic conditions that can complicate cataract surgery. Patients with known preexisting conditions or complicated surgery should be followed up closely postoperatively for early detection of CME.

Explicit recommendations for prophylactic treatment are not relevant due to a lack of well-founded information. Currently, medical prophylaxis is not approved for normal eyes without previous problems. In patients who experienced postoperative CME in the fellow eye, or in cases of complicated operations, prophylactic treatment should be considered and offered for a period of 1 month after surgery.

Main Treatment Modalities of CME
First-line treatment of postsurgical CME should include topical NSAIDs and corticosteroids. Oral carbonic anhydrase inhibitors can be considered complementary. In cases of resistant CME, periocular or intraocular corticosteroids present an option. Antiangiogenic agents, though experimental, should be considered for nonresponsive persistent CME. Surgical options should be reserved for special indications.

Best Sequential Management

We propose the following flow chart for best sequential management:

(1) Topical NSAIDs × 4/d + topical cortico-steroids × 4/day (+ acetazolamide?);
(2) periocular corticosteroid;
(3) intravitreal triamcinolone (possibly intra-venous antiangiogenic agents);

(4) vitreous incarceration → consider surgery;
(5) persistent inflammatory reaction → consid-er IOL removal or vitrectomy.

References

1 Gass JD, Norton EW: Fluorescein studies of patients with macular edema and papilledema following cataract extrac-tion. Trans Am Ophthalmol Soc 1966;64:232–249.
2 Irvine AR: Cystoid maculopathy. Surv Ophthalmol 1976;21:1–17.
3 Shimura M, Yasuda K, Nakazawa T et al: Panretinal photocoagulation induces pro-inflammatory cytokines and macu-lar thickening in high-risk proliferative diabetic retinopathy. Graefes Arch Clin Exp Ophthalmol 2009;247:1617–1624.
4 Rossetti L, Autelitano A: Cystoid macu-lar edema following cataract surgery. Opin Ophthalmol 2000;11:65–72.
5 Henderson BA, Kim JY, Ament CS: Clin-ical pseudophakic cystoid macular edema. Risk factors for development and duration after treatment. J Cataract Refract Surg 2007;33:1550–1558.
6 Flach AJ: The incidence, pathogenesis and treatment of cystoid macular edema following cataract surgery. Trans Am Ophthalmol Soc 1998;96:557–634.
7 Neal RE, Bettelheim FA, Lin C, Winn KC, Garland JS, Zigler JS: Alterations in human vitreous humour following cata-ract extraction. Exp Eye Res 2005;80:337–347.
8 Hruby K: The first description of the Irvine syndrome. Klin Monatsbl Augen-heilkd 1985;187:549–550.
9 Tolentino Fl, Schepens CL: Edema of the posterior pole after cataract extraction: a biomicroscopic study. Arch Ophthalmol 1965;74:781–786.
10 Miyake K, Ibaraki N: Prostaglandins and cystoid macular edema. Surv Ophthal-mol 2002;47(suppl 1):S203–S218.
11 Iliff WJ: Aphakic cystoid macular edema and the operating microscope: is there a connection? Trans Am Ophthalmol Soc 1985;83:476–500.
12 Schmier JK, Halpern MT, Covert DW, et al: Evaluation of costs for cystoid macu-lar edema among patients after cataract surgery. Retina 2007;27:621–628.

13 Kraff MC, Sanders DR, Jampol LM, et al: Effect of primary capsulotomy with ext-racapsular surgery on the incidence of pseudophakic cystoid macular edema. Am J Ophthalmol 1984;96:166–170.
14 Cohen SM, Davis A, Cukrowski C: Cystoid macular edema after pars plana vitrec-tomy for retained lens fragments. J Cata-ract Refract Surg 2006;32:1521–1526.
15 Warwar RE, Bullock JD, Ballal D: Cystoid macular edema and anterior uveitis associated with latanoprost use. Experi-ence and incidence in a retrospective review of 94 patients. Ophthalmology 1998;105:263–268.
16 Arciere ES, Santana A, Rocha FN: Blood-aqueous barrier changes after the use of prostaglandin analogues in patients with pseudophakia and aphakia. Arch Oph-thalmol 2005;123:186–192.
17 Solomon LD: Efficacy of topical flur-biprofen and indomethacin in prevent-ing pseudophakic cystoid macular edema. Flurbiprofen-CME Study Group I. J Cataract Refract Surg 1995;21:73–81.
18 Rossetti L, Chaudhwi H, Dickersin K: Medical prophylaxis and treatment of cystoid macular edema after cataract surgery. The Results of a Meta-Analysis. Ophthalmology 1998;105:397–405.
19 Peterson M, Yoshizumi MO, Hepler R, et al: Topical indomethacin in the treat-ment of chronic cystoid macular edema. Graefes Arch Clin Exp Ophthalmol 1992;230:401–405.
20 Rho DS: Treatment of acute pseudopha-kic cystoid macular edema: diclofenac versus ketorolac. J Cataract Refract Surg 2003;29:2378–2384.
21 Stern AL, Taylor DM, Dalburg LA, et al: Pseudophakic cystoid maculopathy: a study of 50 cases. Ophthalmology 1981;88:942–946.
22 Thach AB, Dugel PU, Flindall RJ, et al: A comparison of retrobulbar versus sub-Tenon's corticosteroid therapy for cys-toid macular edema refractory to topical medications. Ophthalmology 1997;104:2003–2008.

23 Heier JS, Topping TM, Baumann W, et al: Ketorolac versus prednisolone versus combination therapy in the treatment of acute pseudophakic cystoid macular edema. Ophthalmology 2000;107:2034–2038, discussion 2039.
24 Ip MS, Gottlieb JL, Kahana A, et al: Intravitreal triamcinolone for treatment of macular edema associated with cen-tral retinal vein occlusion. Arch Oph-thalmol 2004;122:1131–1136.
25 Kok H, Lan C, Maycock N, McCluskey P, Lightman S: Outcome of intravitreal triamcinolone in uveitis. Ophthalmology 2005;112:1916–1921.
26 Jonas JB, Kreissing I, Segenring RF: Intravitreal triamcinolone acetonide for pseudophakic cystoid macular edema. Am J Ophthalmol 2003:136:384–386.
27 Boscia F, Furino C, Dammacco R, Ferreri P, Sborgia L, Sborgia C: Intravitreal tri-amcinolone acetonide in refractory pseudophakic cystoid macular edema: functional and anatomic results. Eur J Ophthalmol 2005;15:89–95.
28 Conway MD, Canakis C, Livir-Rallatos C, Peyman GA: Intravitreal triamcino-lone acetonide for refractory chronic pseudophakic cystodi macular edema. J Cataract Refract Surg 2003;29:27–33.
29 Farber MD, Lam S, Tessler HH, et al: Reduction of macular oedema by aceta-zolamide in patients with chronic irido-cyclitis: a randomised prospective cross-over study. Br J Ophthalmol 1994;78:4–7.
30 Grover S, Apushkin MA, Fishman GA: Topical dorzolamide for the treatment of cystoid macular edema in patients with retinitis pigmentosa. Am J Ophthalmol 2006;141:850–858.
31 Catier A, Tadayoni R, Massin P, et al: Advantages of acetazolamide associated with anti-inflammatory medications in postoperative treatment of macular edema. J Fr Ophtalmol 2005;28:1027–1031.

32 Weene LE: Cystoid macular edema after scleral buckling responsive to acetazolamide. Ann Ophthalmol 1992;24:423–424.

33 Spitzer MS, Ziemssen F, Yoeruek E, et al: Efficacy of intravitreal bevacizumab in treating postoperative pseudophakic cystoid macular edema. J Cataract Refract Surg 2008;34:70–75.

34 Steinert RF, Wasson PJ: Neodymium:YAG laser anterior vitreolysis for Irvine-Gass cystoid macular edema. J Cataract Refract Surg 1989;15:304–307.

35 Lardenoye CWTA, van Schooneveld MJ, Treffers WF, et al: Grid laser photocoagulation for macular oedema in uveitis or the Irvine-Gass syndrome. Br J Ophthalmol 1998;82:1013–1016.

36 Fung WE: Vitrectomy for chronic aphakic cystoid macular edema. Results of a national, collaborative, prospective, randomized investigation. Ophthalmology 1985;92:1102–1111.

37 Harbour JW, Smiddy WE, Rubsamen PE, et al: Pars plana vitrectomy for chronic pseudophakic cystoid macular edema. Am J Ophthalmol 1995;120:302–307.

38 Shepard DD: The fate of eyes from which intraocular lenses have been removed. Ophthalmic Surg 1979;10:58–60.

39 Price FW Jr, Whitson WE: Natural history of cystoid macular edema in pseudophakic bullous keratopathy. J Cataract Refract Surg 1990;16:163–169.

Prof. Anat Loewenstein
Department of Ophthalmology, Tel Aviv Medical Center
Sackler Faculty of Medicine, Tel Aviv University
6 Weizmann St.
Tel Aviv 64239 (Israel)
E-Mail anatl@tasmc.health.gov.il

Coscas G (ed): Macular Edema.
Dev Ophthalmol. Basel, Karger, 2010, vol 47, pp 160–167

Retinitis Pigmentosa and Other Dystrophies

José Sahel[a,b] · Sébastien Bonnel[a] · Sarah Mrejen[b] · Michel Paques[a,b]

[a]Department of Ophthalmology of the Foundation Rothschild, and [b]Department of Ophthalmology, Quinze-Vingts Hospital and the Vision Institute, Pierre et Marie Curie University Paris 6, Paris, France

Abstract

Retinitis pigmentosa (RP) is an inherited retinal degeneration that affects predominantly peripheral visual fields. Macular edema may cause additional central visual acuity decrease. Fluorescein angiography and/or optical coherence tomography detect the presence of macular edema in 10–20% of RP patients. Macular edema can manifest at any stage of the disease and may be unilateral or bilateral. In X-linked forms, macular edema is very rare. The origin of macular edema in RP patients still remains poorly understood. The possible pathophysiological role of autoantibodies has been suggested (retinal, carbonic anhydrase, and enolase antibodies). Drug therapy is the primary treatment for macular edema in patients with RP. Systemic carbonic anhydrase inhibitors, such as oral acetazolamide or topical dorzolamide, still are the mainstay of initial therapy. If cystoid macular edema is refractory to acetazolamide, intravitreal corticosteroid injections could be administered. Intravitreal anti-vascular endothelial growth factor therapy has also been used in cases of macular edema persistence after oral acetazolamide therapy, though with uncertain results. Vitrectomy can also be proposed, but its role is not clear yet. Autoimmune retinopathies (AIRs) are a group of rare diseases characterized by acute or subacute progressive vision loss and are thought to be mediated by autoantibodies specific to retinal antigens. The AIRs encompass paraneoplastic syndromes, such as cancer-associated retinopathy and melanoma-associated retinopathy, and a larger group of AIRs that have similar clinical and immunological findings but without underlying malignancy. These diseases may also be complicated by macular edema.

Retinitis pigmentosa (RP) is one of the most common forms of inherited retinal degeneration. It displays extensive clinical and genetic variations and leads to progressive blindness with variable onset.

Factors of Visual Acuity Decrease and Retinitis Pigmentosa

RP is a degenerative process of the retina that primarily affects the rod photoreceptors and the retinal pigment epithelium. Although rod photoreceptors are thought to be the main target of the disease, there is histological and functional evidence for cone photoreceptor damage that seems to develop secondarily to rod degeneration (Sahel et al., 2001)[1]. Most of the forms of RP are caused by mutations in genes coding for proteins restricted to rod photoreceptors (Travis, 1998)[2]. Cone survival, however, appears to depend on the presence of rod photoreceptors, even if they are not functional (Mohand-Said et al., 2000; Leveillard et al., 2004)[3,4]. Accordingly, the survival of cone receptors can be a promising target for development of future therapeutic options in useful visual acuity (VA) gain.

As RP progresses, symptoms worsen. One of the earliest symptoms of RP is difficulty in seeing at night (nyctalopia or night blindness), which is due to rod degeneration. Later in the disease course, a reduction in the peripheral visual field also develops, resulting in loss of central vision in some cases. The rate of central VA loss depends on the mutated gene, the type of mutation, and modifying factors (i.e., genetic and environmental interactions). Depending on the transmission mode, central vision loss appears at the age of 20–30 years in X-linked forms, at the age of 20–40 years in autosomal recessive forms, and at the age of 60 years in autosomal dominant forms. In particular cases, such as sector RP, VA can remain intact.

It is extremely important to note that in addition to the underlying degenerative pathology, other causes for decrease of the central VA in patients with RP can potentially exist (e.g. macular edema, epiretinal membrane, and posterior subcapsular cataract). In these cases, the VA can improve with treatment.

Among the possible complications that may decrease the central VA in RP patients, we will focus our attention on the occurrence of cystoid macular edema (CME). CME may cause fast VA decrease in patients with good central vision despite abnormal visual field.

Retinitis Pigmentosa and Macular Edema

Epidemiology and Natural Course
Fluorescein angiography detects the presence of CME in 10–20% of RP patients (Fishman et al., 1977; Pruett, 1983; Heckenlively, 1987)[5–7]. Advances in in vivo optical imaging technologies, such as optical coherence tomography (OCT), have permitted more sensitive detection of CME (in about 20–50% of patients with RP), even in cases with no diffusion on angiography (Hirakawa et al., 1999; Adackapara et al., 2008; Hajali et al., 2008)[8–10].

CME can manifest at any stage of the disease and may be unilateral or bilateral. Interestingly, in the late stages of the degenerative pathology, CME seems less likely to appear. There are no differences in the prevalence of CME that are associated with the inheritance pattern (autosomal dominant, recessive, and sporadic forms) (Hajali et al., 2009)[11]. Nevertheless, in X-linked forms, CME is very rare.

The high rate of macular edema that can be detected by OCT shows the importance of this type of investigation in case of VA decline. The indications for treatment of macular edema will be discussed later. Another point which must be kept in mind during OCT analysis is the imperfect correlation between retinal thickness and VA.

Physiopathology
Numerous hypotheses have been proposed to explain the origin of CME in various pathologies, including mechanical traction on the vitreoretinal interface (as in epiretinal membrane or vitreoretinal traction syndrome), retinal toxicity, and release of proinflammatory factors [e.g. cytokines (as in uveitis) or proangiogenic factors (as in patients with diabetes or venous occlusion)].

These mechanisms are implicated in a bloodretinal barrier breakdown and accumulation of liquid localized in the outer plexiform layer that may lead to development of CME. Other factors, such as vascular endothelial growth factor or interleukin-6, also seem to play an important role in CME formation. At present, no correlation between the mechanisms underlying the formation of CME and its chronicity has been established.

In RP, the origin of CME still remains poorly understood. The possible pathophysiological role of some antibodies has been proposed (retinal, carbonic anhydrase, and enolase antibodies) (Heckenlively et al., 1996)[12]. We suggest that loss of retinoschisin levels secondary to photoreceptor loss should be considered as a mechanism. Other authors proposed that anomaly in the polarity of the pigment epithelium cells may result in a defective absorption of liquid in the outer neuroretina. (Cox et al., 1988)[13].

Further studies are needed to understand CME physiopathology in patients with RP.

Clinical Diagnosis

When facing a patient with RP who presents a VA decrease that is neither explained by formation of a cataract nor by retinal degeneration, the ophthalmologist must consider the presence of CME. For the diagnosis of CME, a macular contact lens should be used. This will reveal thickening of the macular profile and cystoid cavities of variable size. Detection of diffuse macular edema is more difficult. When performing fundus examination, posterior hyaloid and retinal vessels must be carefully examined in order to establish the differential diagnosis.

Diagnosis and follow-up of macular edema have become easier with the introduction of OCT. This tool is critical to make the distinction between the evolution of RP as a degenerative pathology and the occurrence of macular edema. OCT allows accurate analysis of the vitreoretinal surface and the retinal thickness.

Currently, the assessment of macular edema progression can be precisely done with OCT, although fluorescein angiography continues to be very useful in cases of unknown etiology.

Treatments

At present, drug therapy is the primary treatment modality for CME in patients with RP. Systemic carbonic anhydrase inhibitors, such as oral acetazolamide (Diamox) or topical dorzolamide, still are the mainstay of initial therapy. If CME is refractory to acetazolamide, intravitreal corticosteroid injections (i.e., triamcinolone acetonide) could be administered.

Intravitreal anti-vascular endothelial growth factor therapy has also been used in cases of CME persistence after oral acetazolamide therapy (Melo et al., 2007; Yuzbasioglu et al., 2009)[14,15], though with uncertain results. In cases of chronic and/or refractory CME despite oral and intravitreal therapies, vitrectomy can also be proposed, but its role is not yet clear.

The most effective current therapies are described below.

Oral Acetazolamide

Oral acetazolamide is considered the drug of first choice for treatment of CME in RP (Fishman et al., 1989; Chen et al., 1990; Orzalesi et al., 1993; Apushkin et al., 2007)[16–19]. Different dosing regimens have been suggested, the usual recommended dosage ranging from 250 to 500 mg per day.

Daily oral acetazolamide decreases the central macular thickness and allows CME regression that can be seen on OCT imaging 7–15 days after the introduction of the treatment. If there is no decrease in the retinal thickness after 2 weeks, the patient has to be considered nonresponsive to acetazolamide and the treatment can be discontinued. VA improvement and disappearance of metamorphopsias, together with normal foveal profile, can be noted in patients who respond to oral acetazolamide.

There is no correlation between functional improvement and angiographic modifications. A rebound of CME has often been described, despite the continuity in the treatment with oral acetazolamide (Apushkin et al., 2007)[19]. The mechanisms by which acetazolamide exerts its effects in CME remain uncertain (Cox et al., 1988)[13].

Topical carbonic anhydrase inhibitors have also been used in patients with RP, with a lower rate of systemic side effects than oral acetazolamide but also with lower effect. One study has shown a functional improvement in 20% of the patients treated with topical acetazolamide and a rebound effect in 30% of the patients during the treatment (Grover et al., 1997)[20].

Intravitreal Triamcinolone Acetonide Injection

Intravitreal triamcinolone injection is another therapeutic option for management of CME in RP patients. The therapeutic effect is fast and manifests with improvement in VA and normalization of the macular thickness profile (Sallum et al., 2003; Saraiva et al., 2003; Ozdemir et al., 2005; Scorolli et al., 2007)[21–24]. This therapeutic modality is used in patients that do not or only partially respond to oral acetazolamide, and in cases of rebound.

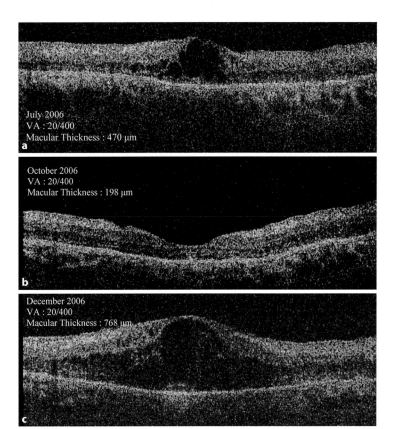

Fig. 1. OCT examination. Patient with macular edema secondary to RP. Before (**a**) and after (**b**) intravitreal triamcinolone acetonide. Five months after the injection a rebound effect was observed (**c**).

July 2006
VA : 20/400
Macular Thickness : 470 µm
a

October 2006
VA : 20/400
Macular Thickness : 198 µm
b

December 2006
VA : 20/400
Macular Thickness : 768 µm
c

The effect of intravitreal triamcinolone is often transient and may result in rebounds that sometimes lead to VA levels lower than those before treatment (fig. 1). Other disadvantages include possible reiterative injections (when necessary), cataract progression or development, and elevated intraocular pressure.

Vitreoretinal Surgery

Only one study has described vitreoretinal surgery with internal limiting membrane peeling in RP-associated CME nonresponding to acetazolamide. Twelve eyes with RP were operated using indocyanine green staining for internal limiting membrane peeling. The results after a 6-month follow-up showed a VA improvement (mean preoperative best-corrected VA: 20/115; mean postoperative best-corrected VA: 20/45) and a macular thickness decrease (mean preoperative foveal thickness: 477 µm; mean postoperative foveal thickness: 260 µm). Mechanisms of therapeutic action have not been discussed (Garcia-Arumi et al., 2003)[25].

Our personal experience with vitreoretinal surgery performing internal limiting membrane peeling without staining in patients that no longer responded to the above-described therapies suggests that improvement in VA and reduction in macular thickness can be obtained in all patients (fig. 2). Significant adherences of the internal limiting membrane to the neuroretinal tissue were noted during surgery in all cases. Surprisingly, although some patients presented a macular edema recurrence, the fovea was spared. Such experience cannot

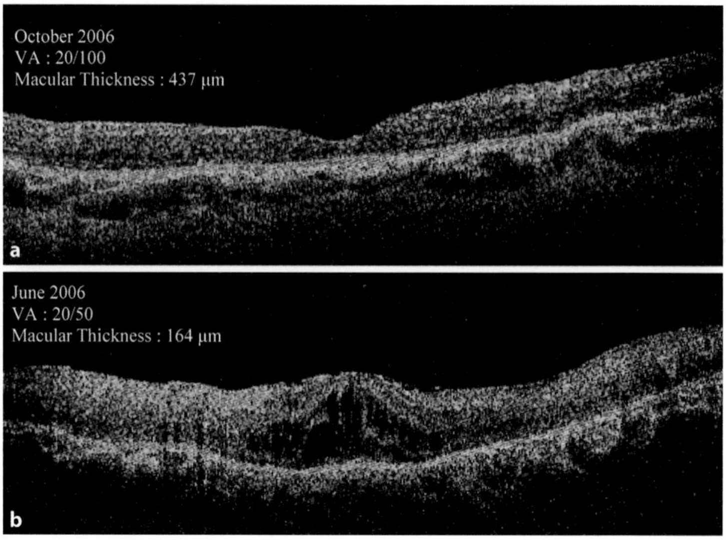

Fig. 2. OCT examination. Patient with macular edema secondary to RP. Before (**a**) and after (**b**) vitreoretinal surgery with limiting membrane peeling oral acetazolamide and intravitreal triamcinolone were used with rebound effects. Improvement in VA and reduction in macular thickness were observed during 2 years after surgery without additional treatment.

be considered as evidence for efficiency until comparative studies are conducted on larger series.

How to Treat and When

The management of CME in RP patients may differ depending on the clinical presentation. Not all CME need to be treated. For instance, CME without clinical manifestations (but OCT-detectable) needs only follow-up but no treatment. It is important to keep in mind that there is not always a correlation between retinal thickness and VA. The existence of a macular syndrome accompanied by a VA decrease is a prerequisite for proposing a therapeutic approach.

Oral acetazolamide at a dose of 250 mg per day is recommended as a first-line therapy. OCT should be performed 2 weeks after the introduction of the treatment. If there is no retinal thickness reduction, the patient can be considered a nonresponder to carbonic anhydrase inhibitors, and a dose of 500 mg a day can be used. In most cases, however, the therapeutic effect does not change. When oral acetazolamide is contraindicated, topical administration of dorzolamide can be considered.

As a second option, only when the VA is significantly decreased, sub-Tenon triamcinolone acetonide injection can be proposed. The results can be satisfactory in some cases, but if not, an intravitreal injection would be advised.

Intravitreal triamcinolone injection has a faster effect and restores ad integrum the foveal profile in most cases. The possibility of a rebound effect, which frequently takes place approximately 3 months after the injection, needs special attention. In addition, intraocular pressure follow-up has to be performed in those patients who usually respond after repeated injections of steroids. Furthermore, more frequent injections may be required as the efficacy and duration of the steroid therapy effect tend to reduce.

As a third line of therapy in patients with a significant functional deterioration, vitreoretinal surgery with internal limiting membrane peeling might be proposed. Surgery might be difficult to perform as the internal limiting membrane is very adherent. It should be kept as short as possible in order to avoid phototraumatism. Long-term efficacy of this surgical approach remains unknown.

Cataract Surgery and Macular Edema in RP
Posterior subcapsular cataract is typically associated with RP (Eshaghian et al., 1980)[26], and surgery improves the VA in patients with persistent visual field. Capsular opacification rate is higher than in normal patients and anterior capsular contraction can occur.

The rate of occurrence or aggravation of CME after cataract surgery (comparing the preoperative and postoperative macular profile) has not yet been studied (Jackson et al., 2001)[27].

Melanoma and Cancer-Associated Retinopathy

The autoimmune retinopathies (AIRs) are a group of diseases characterized by acute or subacute progressive vision loss, and are thought to be mediated by autoantibodies specific to retinal antigens (Adamus, 2000; Heckenlively et al., 2000)[28,29]. The prevalence of AIRs is unknown, although it is believed to be relatively uncommon. They are characterized by abnormal findings on electroretinogram (ERG) (either rod-cone or cone-rod patterns). The AIRs encompass the better-studied paraneoplastic syndromes, such as cancer-associated retinopathy and melanoma-associated retinopathy, and a larger group of AIRs that have similar clinical and immunological findings but without underlying malignancy.

This latter group is called *nonparaneoplastic autoimmune retinopathy* (npAIR). It has previously been called recoverin-associated retinopathy (Whitcup et al., 1998)[30] or autoimmune retinopathy in the absence of cancer (Mizener et al., 1997)[31]. Some npAIRs have CME as a prominent feature that appears to be a distinguishing factor (npAIR/CME).

Cancer-associated retinopathy, melanoma-associated retinopathy, npAIR, and npAIR/CME tend to have common clinical features despite the fact that no uniform set of antiretinal antibodies has been found in these patients (Hooks et al.,

2001; Chan, 2003)[32,33]. Patients may have a variety of antibody activity, sometimes multiple.

RP and AIRs share similar clinical features and many AIR patients may be referred with a diagnosis of RP. The figure is complicated by the fact that some cases of RP may develop secondary AIR with rapid visual field loss and severe CME (Hajali et al., 2009; Heckenlively et al., 1985; Heckenlively et al., 1999)[11,34,35]. Ninety percent of patients with RP and cysts do have circulating antiretinal antibodies by means of Western blot analysis, compared with 13% of patients with RP without macular cysts, and 6% of controls (Chant et al., 1985)[36]. However, it remains to be determined whether the presence of antiretinal antibodies is a direct cause of worsening of RP.

Common features of the presentation of patients with AIR include a rapid onset of photopsia, followed by night blindness, scotomata, and visual field loss. Some patients also develop diminished central vision. Frequently npAIR patients have CME as a prominent feature. The presentation may be asymmetrical between the eyes. Patients often reveal they have autoimmune family histories.

A standardized ERG will show abnormal responses. Some cases have negative waveforms, consisting of an a-wave that does not return to the isoelectric point on dark-adapted bright-flash ERG test. Kinetic visual fields are better at measuring peripheral losses or scotomata, blind spot enlargement, or pericentral losses.

Although OCT demonstrates intraretinal cystic spaces or schisis-like spaces, many of these cases do not have leakage on fluorescence angiography, and the AIR macular changes may be a form of degenerative schisis.

The rarity of AIRs, and the difficulty in firmly establishing the diagnosis, has limited therapeutic investigations. No specific treatment regimens for autoimmune retinopathies have emerged during the past decade. Immunosuppression with oral or intravenous corticosteroids has shown mixed results. Generally, short courses of steroids are ineffective. In a series of 30 patients, Ferreyra et al. reported their experience using immunosuppression to treat AIR. Long-term treatment with immunosuppression resulted in clinical improvement in all subgroups of AIR. The most responsive group was cancer-associated retinopathy, the last was npAIR. Sub-Tenon periocular injections of methylprednisolone have also been proposed (Ferreyra et al., 2009)[37].

References

1 Sahel JA, Mohand-Said S, Leveillard T, Hicks D, Picaud S, Dreyfus H: Rod-cone interdependence: implications for therapy of photoreceptor cell diseases. Prog Brain Res 2001;131:649–661.

2 Travis GH: Mechanisms of cell death in the inherited retinal degenerations. Am J Hum Genet 1998;62:503–508.

3 Mohand-Said S, Hicks D, Dreyfus H, Sahel JA: Selective transplantation of rods delays cone loss in a retinitis pigmentosa model. Arch Ophthalmol 2000;118:807–811.

4 Leveillard T, Mohand-Said S, Lorentz O, Hicks D, Fintz AC, Clerin E, et al: Identification and characterization of rod-derived cone viability factor. Nat Genet 2004;36:755–759.

5 Fishman GA, Fishman M, Maggiano J: Macular lesions associated with retinitis pigmentosa. Arch Ophthalmol 1977;95:798–803.

6 Pruett RC: Retinitis pigmentosa: clinical observations and correlations. Trans Am Ophthalmol Soc 1983;81:693–735.

7 Heckenlively JR: RP cone-rod degeneration. Trans Am Ophthalmol Soc 1987;85:438–470.

8 Hirakawa H, Iijima H, Gohdo T, Tsukahara S: Optical coherence tomography of cystoid macular edema associated with retinitis pigmentosa. Am J Ophthalmol 1999;128:185–191.

9 Adackapara CA, Sunness JS, Dibernardo CW, Melia BM, Dagnelie G: Prevalence of cystoid macular edema and stability in OCT retinal thickness in eyes with retinitis pigmentosa during a 48-week lutein trial. Retina 2008;28:103–110.

10 Hajali M, Fishman GA, Anderson RJ: The prevalence of cystoid macular oedema in retinitis pigmentosa patients determined by optical coherence tomography. Br J Ophthalmol 2008;92:1065–1068.

11 Hajali M, Fishman GA: The prevalence of cystoid macular oedema on optical coherence tomography in retinitis pigmentosa patients without cystic changes on fundus examination. Eye 2009;23:915–919.

12 Heckenlively JR, Aptsiauri N, Nusinowitz S, Peng C, Hargrave PA: Investigations of antiretinal antibodies in pigmentary retinopathy and other retinal degenerations. Trans Am Ophthalmol Soc 1996;94:179–200, discussion 200–206.

13 Cox SN, Hay E, Bird AC: Treatment of chronic macular edema with acetazolamide. Arch Ophthalmol 1988;106:1190–1195.

14 Melo GB, Farah ME, Aggio FB: Intravitreal injection of bevacizumab for cystoid macular edema in retinitis pigmentosa. Acta Ophthalmol Scand 2007;85:461–463.

15 Yuzbasioglu E, Artunay O, Rasier R, Sengul A, Bahcecioglu H: Intravitreal bevacizumab (Avastin) injection in retinitis pigmentosa. Curr Eye Res 2009;34:231–237.

16 Fishman GA, Gilbert LD, Fiscella RG, Kimura AE, Jampol LM: Acetazolamide for treatment of chronic macular edema in retinitis pigmentosa. Arch Ophthalmol 1989;107:1445–1452.

17 Chen JC, Fitzke FW, Bird AC: Long-term effect of acetazolamide in a patient with retinitis pigmentosa. Invest Ophthalmol Vis Sci 1990;31:1914–1918.

18 Orzalesi N, Pierrottet C, Porta A, Aschero M: Long-term treatment of retinitis pigmentosa with acetazolamide. A pilot study. Graefes Arch Clin Exp Ophthalmol 1993;231:254–256.

19 Apushkin MA, Fishman GA, Grover S, Janowicz MJ: Rebound of cystoid macular edema with continued use of acetazolamide in patients with retinitis pigmentosa. Retina 2007;27:1112–1118.

20 Grover S, Fishman GA, Fiscella RG, Adelman AE: Efficacy of dorzolamide hydrochloride in the management of chronic cystoid macular edema in patients with retinitis pigmentosa. Retina 1997;17:222–231.

21 Sallum JM, Farah ME, Saraiva VS: Treatment of cystoid macular edema related to retinitis pigmentosa with intravitreal triamcinolone acetonide: case report. Adv Exp Med Biol 2003;533:79–81.

22 Saraiva VS, Sallum JM, Farah ME: Treatment of cystoid macular edema related to retinitis pigmentosa with intravitreal triamcinolone acetonide. Ophthalmic Surg Lasers Imaging 2003;34:398–400.

23 Ozdemir H, Karacorlu M, Karacorlu S: Intravitreal triamcinolone acetonide for treatment of cystoid macular oedema in patients with retinitis pigmentosa. Acta Ophthalmol Scand 2005;83:248–251.

24 Scorolli L, Morara M, Meduri A, Reggiani LB, Ferreri G, Scalinci SZ, et al: Treatment of cystoid macular edema in retinitis pigmentosa with intravitreal triamcinolone. Arch Ophthalmol 2007;125:759–764.

25 Garcia-Arumi J, Martinez V, Sararols L, Corcostegui B: Vitreoretinal surgery for cystoid macular edema associated with retinitis pigmentosa. Ophthalmology 2003;110:1164–1169.

26 Eshaghian J, Rafferty NS, Goossens W: Ultrastructure of human cataract in retinitis pigmentosa. Arch Ophthalmol 1980;98:2227–2230.

27 Jackson H, Garway-Heath D, Rosen P, Bird AC, Tuft SJ: Outcome of cataract surgery in patients with retinitis pigmentosa. Br J Ophthalmol 2001;85:936–938.

28 Adamus G: Antirecoverin antibodies and autoimmune retinopathy. Arch Ophthalmol 2000;118:1577–1578.

29 Heckenlively JR, Fawzi AA, Oversier J, Jordan BL, Aptsiauri N: Autoimmune retinopathy: patients with antirecoverin immunoreactivity and panretinal degeneration. Arch Ophthalmol 2000;118:1525–1533.

30 Whitcup SM, Vistica BP, Milam AH, Nussenblatt RB, Gery I: Recoverin-associated retinopathy: a clinically and immunologically distinctive disease. Am J Ophthalmol 1998;126:230–237.

31 Mizener JB, Kimura AE, Adamus G, Thirkill CE, Goeken JA, Kardon RH: Autoimmune retinopathy in the absence of cancer. Am J Ophthalmol 1997;123:607–618.

32 Hooks JJ, Tso MO, Detrick B: Retinopathies associated with antiretinal antibodies. Clin Diagn Lab Immunol 2001;8:853–858.

33 Chan JW: Paraneoplastic retinopathies and optic neuropathies. Surv Ophthalmol 2003;48:12–38.

34 Heckenlively JR, Solish AM, Chant SM, Meyers-Elliott RH: Autoimmunity in hereditary retinal degenerations. 2. Clinical studies: antiretinal antibodies and fluorescein angiogram findings. Br J Ophthalmol 1985;69:758–764.

35 Heckenlively JR, Jordan BL, Aptsiauri N: Association of antiretinal antibodies and cystoid macular edema in patients with retinitis pigmentosa. Am J Ophthalmol 1999;127:565–573.

36 Chant SM, Heckenlively J, Meyers-Elliott RH: Autoimmunity in hereditary retinal degeneration. 1. Basic studies. Br J Ophthalmol 1985;69:19–24.

37 Ferreyra HA, Jayasundera T, Khan NW, He S, Lu Y, Heckenlively JR: Management of autoimmune retinopathies with immunosuppression. Arch Ophthalmol 2009;127:390–397.

Prof. Michel Paques
Quinze-Vingts Hospital and Vision Institute
Paris 6 University
28 rue de Charenton
FR - 75012 Paris (France)
E-Mail michel.paques@gmail.com

Coscas G (ed): Macular Edema.
Dev Ophthalmol. Basel, Karger, 2010, vol 47, pp 168–182

Macular Edema of Choroidal Origin

Gisèle Soubrane

Hôpital Intercommunal de Créteil, Service d'Ophthalmologie, Créteil, Paris, France

Abstract

Macular edema (ME) is most often clinically defined as an accumulation of serous fluid within the neurosensory retina with increased thickness of the central retina. In exudative age-related macular degeneration the leakage of fluid from the choroidal new vessels may be the origin of ME. Their abnormal permeability and the inflammatory reaction are mechanisms involved in this accumulation of fluid, which occurs in all layers. Cystoid ME is more often associated with subepithelial occult choroidal neovascularization (CNV) than it is with pre-epithelial classic CNV. The simultaneous presence of choroidal new vessels and ME implies a number of cellular dysfunctions and metabolic alternations. The leakage from the choroidal new vessels, predominantly VEGF-induced, may produce a large accumulation of fluid under the neurosensory retina. It is also likely that the key signalling steps occur prior to the upregulation of VEGF either initiated by, or facilitated by, cytokines, which act under normal basic conditions to counterbalance the integral VEGF effects and, in pathologic circumstances, may either counteract or serve to amplify the process.   Copyright © 2010 S. Karger AG, Basel

Definition

Age-related macular degeneration (AMD) is the result of an involvement of the choriocapillaris, retinal pigment epithelium (RPE), and photoreceptor layer triad. The neural retina is only partially involved, and additional pathways are required for the development of edema within the retina.

Age-related maculopathy is the initial clinical manifestation affecting the RPE and begins with drusen of various types and RPE mottling, clumping, or patches of atrophy. Age-related maculopathy can progress to an advanced stage, which is referred to as AMD. The atrophic or dry form of macular degeneration does not generally present with macular edema. The exudative form is due to choroidal neovascularization (CNV) that causes a serous detachment of the neurosensory retina resulting in a long-standing retinal detachment and possible development of cystoid macular edema.

Macular edema is most often clinically defined as an accumulation of serous fluid within the neurosensory retina with increased thickness of the central retina. In exudative AMD, the leakage of fluid from the choroidal new vessels may be the origin of macular edema. Their abnormal permeability and the associated inflammatory reaction are mechanisms involved in this accumulation of fluid.

The presence of cystoid macular edema is more likely if the retinal serous detachment is long-standing and if the choroidal neovascular membrane has involved most of the subfoveal region. In addition, after prolonged detachment, the retinal capillaries may become damaged and contribute to the leakage of dye into the extracellular compartment of the retina.

Pathophysiology: Theories of Macular Edema in Age-Related Macular Degeneration

CNV being of choroidal origin presents the same structure histologically as the choriocapillaris and thus, in pathological conditions, leads to an exudation within the subretinal space. The consequent damage of the outer retinal layers determines alterations of the overlying (and underlying) tissues. In addition, several inflammatory mediators and inflammatory cells, which secrete numerous cytokines such as vascular permeability factor, referred to as vascular endothelial growth factor (VEGF), are present at the site of the angiogenic stimulus and interact in a complex chain reaction, which is not yet completely understood.

Cellular Components

Choriocapillaris

The choriocapillaris is a key player in choroidal new vessel development and is implicated to a lesser degree in retinal vascular disease. Due to the presence of the fenestrations facing Bruch's membrane (Burns et al., 1986)[1], the capillaries leak more plasma components, even large proteins (Connolly et al., 1989)[2]. In addition, the high choroidal flow rate aids metabolic exchanges and maintains a high concentration gradient across the vessel walls.

With increasing age, there is a loss of choroidal vascular elements and a progressive decrease in the thickness of the choroid (from 200 μm at birth to 80 μm by the age of 90) (Ramrattan et al., 1994)[3]. Numerous publications have demonstrated an age-related decrease in the density and lumen diameter of the vessels of the choriocapillaris (Sarks, 1976; Bird et al., 1990; Olver et al., 1990)[4–6].

The decrease in the density and dimension of the choroidal capillary bed, and thus the blood flow, is likely to globally reduce the amount of fluid – as well as the potential for metabolic support – to the photoreceptors. Related to age, however, no change of the diffusion capability of the choriocapillaris has ever been described.

Bruch's Membrane

The overlying Bruch's membrane has a hydraulic conductivity that decreases with age (Fisher, 1987)[7], with the changes being more marked in

the macula than in the periphery (Moore et al., 1995)[8]. Deposition of material under the basal surface of the RPE resulting from the metabolic turnover of the polyunsaturated fatty acids from the photoreceptor outer segment membranes contributes to thickening of Bruch's membrane. With age, the amount of deposited lipids present increases exponentially. The change is more marked in the macula than in the periphery (Holtz et al., 1994)[9].

Although Bruch's membrane has been found to contain neutral fats (Sheraidah et al., 1993)[10], the predominant classes of lipids are phospholipids (Pauleikoff et al., 1992)[11]. The lipid deposition in Bruch's membrane will limit the diffusion of oxygen and metabolites.

The reduction of the hydraulic conductivity of Bruch's membrane may be implicated in fluid accumulation to form an RPE detachment. RPE cells normally pump fluid out toward the choroid through Bruch's membrane. In AMD, Bruch's membrane is made hydrophobic by the accumulation of lipids (Curcio et al., 2001)[12]. The trapped fluid will spread within the neurosensory retina and collect in cystic spaces. Impedance of metabolic exchange between the choroid and RPE across Bruch's membrane (Löffler and Lee, 1986)[13] may also compromise photoreceptor function and eventually lead to cell death.

Photoreceptors

Photoreceptors are dependent on the RPE for renewal of spent outer segments and on the choriocapillaris for nutrients and elimination of waste products. An age-related decrease in delivery or diffusion of oxygen or metabolites to the photoreceptors of the macula region has been theorized as the key event in the initiation of a compensatory mechanism, which ultimately leads to the formation of new vessels in AMD.

Among retinal cells, photoreceptors are most exposed to light stress and are the most fragile cells in the face of environmental or genetic stress. Conversely, photoreceptors have developed strong mechanisms of protection. Rods are more vulnerable than cones to senescence.

The external limiting membrane (ELM) is not a true membrane but composed of junctional complexes linking Müller cells to the photoreceptor inner segments. This barrier can partially limit the movement of large molecules and retain the proteins in the extracellular space.

Outer Retinal Barrier; Retinal Pigment Epithelium
The physiological roles of the RPE are numerous.

Fluid Movement
The RPE cells are joined near the apical side by tight junctions (formed by transmembrane molecules). This outer part of the retinal barrier blocks the free passage of water, ions, and proteins in normal conditions and regulates the environment of the retinal cells. The ability of the RPE to transport water by active mechanisms is very powerful. The healthy RPE transports proteins and resorbs fluid.

Passive mechanisms such as hydrostatic and osmotic pressure also work to drive water out of the subretinal space into the choroid. In AMD, a large amount of protein extravagates through the immature new vessels. This increases the oncotic pressure in the tissues, impedes the resorption of fluid from the tissue to the plasmatic compartment, and results in water accumulation in the surrounding extracellular space, which causes extracellular edema.

The proteins that have diffused into the retinal tissue will remain there and only diffuse in a limited amount into the vitreous cavity or subretinal space. Nevertheless, this amount of protein will be replaced by the constant leakage coming from the choroidal new vessels and be responsible for possible development of macular edema. In addition, the protein retained in the retina will also be retained by osmosis. This mechanism then aggravates the macular edema due to the breakdown of the outer retinal barrier.

Extracellular matrix changes affect the formation of macular edema. Matrix metalloproteinases cause a degradation and modulation of the extracellular matrix. The breakdown and the dysfunction of the blood-retinal barrier cause changes of the endothelial cell resistance. The fluid movement is thus profoundly disturbed in neovascular AMD.

Metabolism of the Retinal Pigment Epithelium Cells
The enzymatic machinery of the RPE assumes a large number of functions including membrane transport, waste product digestion, and elaboration of growth factors. The RPE assumes photoreceptor outer segment renewal. This phagocytosis process is involved in residual bodies within the cell and deposition of lipids in Bruch's membrane.

The RPE constitutively expresses VEGF to maintain the choriocapillaris. VEGF is also the major mediator of AMD related to CNV (Lopez et al., 1996)[14]. The RPE also produces neuronal traffic, neuronal protective and anti-angiogenic factor (pigment epithelium-derived factor) (Imai et al., 2005)[15]. The presence of macrophages in Bruch's membrane has also been implicated in the synthesis of VEGF since activated macrophages have long been recognized as stimulating blood vessel growth (Killingsworth et al., 1990)[16].

Vitreous
The development of macular edema may correlate with the presence of an attached posterior hyaloid as suggested in a number of publications about diabetic edema. Similarly the traction of the posterior hyaloid has been implicated in the increase and possibly occurrence of CNV (Robison et al., 2009)[17] and subsequent macular edema. Vitreomacular traction resulting from an incomplete or anomalous posterior vitreous detachment is suspected to play a role in the pathogenesis of different forms of exudative AMD along with other mechanisms.

It is probable that the fundamental pathomechanisms of AMD formation have already begun by the time tractional forces lead to a change. Hyaloid adhesion to the macula is associated with AMD and frequently causes vitreomacular traction in eyes with CNV. As shown on optical coherence tomography (OCT), there is a clinically high co-incidence of vitreomacular traction and CNV in a number of eyes. The area of hyaloid adhesion is claimed to be concentric to the area of CNV complex in such eyes (Mojana et al., 2008; Lee et al., 2009)[18, 19]. In addition, vitreomacular traction seems to be associated with the severity of AMD.

The concept of the pathogenesis of AMD should be extended to include the influence of the vitreous (Schulze et al., 2008)[20]. Persistent attachment of the posterior vitreous cortex to the macula may be a risk factor for the development of exudative AMD (Lee et al., 2009)[19] via vitreoretinal traction inducing chronic low-grade inflammation, by maintaining macular exposure to cytokines or free radicals in the vitreous gel, or by interfering in transvitreous oxygenation and nutrition of the macula (Krebs et al., 2007)[21].

Vascular Endothelial Growth Factor
VEGF is an important mediator of CNV by a selective mitogenic activity, but it is also a survival factor for endothelial cells and vessel maintenance. VEGF is involved in ocular pathologic processes such as new vessel formation and is implicated as well in the development of macular edema.

VEGF is primarily expressed in endothelial cells as well as in pericytes, monocytes, and neural cells. Its effects are launched when VEGF binds to its receptors on vessel endothelial cells. Basic and clinical studies have shown expression of VEGF on choroidal endothelial cells of new vessels and synthesis of VEGF in RPE cells (Lopez et al., 1996)[14].

Furthermore, eyes with AMD also showed VEGF expression in photoreceptors overlying CNV. In experimentally induced CNV, increased expression of VEGF was detected in infiltrating macrophages in RPE cells and Müller cells (Kliffen et al., 1997)[22]. In vitro RPE expressing VEGF promotes experimental choroidal angiogenesis.

Vascular ischemia is one of the major mechanisms inducing VEGF synthesis and release. Increased expression of VEGF in CNV supports the controversial hypothesis that tissue hypoxia may be a factor for this disorder since hypoxia stimulates VEGF expression in the RPE.

It has been theorized that age-related changes in Bruch's membrane may also limit the diffusion of oxygen and therefore create an ischemic environment. The RPE cells on top of drusen were thought to be particularly ischemic (Pauleikhoff et al., 1999)[23]. The ordinary daily exposure of the lipids in the photoreceptor outer segments helps to maintain the constitutive secretion of VEGF by the RPE cells.

This raises the possibility that excessive exposure to oxidative damage may lead the RPE cells to secrete excessive VEGF. The reactive oxygen species and peroxidized lipids increase the production of VEGF (Monte et al., 1997; Kuroki et al., 1996)[24, 25], which is involved in supporting vascular endothelial cells.

VEGF causes vascular hyperpermeability that is leukocyte-mediated. This results in an opening of interendothelial junctions. Elevated oxidative stress levels will induce tissue inflammation. Inflammation induces breakdown of the VEGF-mediated blood-retinal barrier via leukocyte binding and by inducing their recruitment to the site of inflammation. The cells involved in the pathogenesis of AMD and macular edema are macrophages and leukocytes that present VEGF receptors. These inflammatory cells can also produce and release cytokines (Penfold et al., 1986)[26].

Clinical Findings

The accumulation of serous fluid within the retina occurs in all layers: under the RPE as a pigment epithelial detachment (PED); under the neurosensory retina as subretinal fluid or a serous retinal detachment; within the retina, between the inner limiting membrane and the RPE band, either as diffuse fluid leakage or organized as cysts of various locations, importance, and size. These changes are easily identifiable and quantifiable on OCT.

Cystoid macular edema is more often associated with subepithelial occult CNV than it is with pre-epithelial classic CNV. The occurrence of macular edema is probably related to the slow growth rate of these new vessels, the constant leakage through their fenestrations, and their usual subfoveal location. The serous fluid originating from the choriocapillaris, the choroidal new vessels and in some cases from the deep plexus of the retinal capillaries spreads posteriorly and laterally where it accumulates within the inner nuclear and outer plexiform layers. The extension of the large cellular space available in the outer plexiform layer of Henle causes the typical biomicroscopic and angiographic picture of cystoid macular edema (Gass, 1997)[27].

The functional consequences of macular edema associated with CNV have never been precisely evaluated. It is quite challenging to attempt to do so, as the location, the extent, and the activity of the foveal CNV are predominantly responsible for the visual degradation. Controversy still exists regarding the timing of the occurrence of this cystoid macular edema: early (Soubrane et al., 1988)[28], or late (Bressler et al., 1991)[29].

Biomicroscopy
Biomicroscopic examination with a contact lens is the only way to clinically identify the optically empty clear spaces located within the shallow neurosensory retina elevation overlying a deep gray-green mound. The use of a slit lamp with a 10° angle best provides visualization. Subepithelial occult CNV is usually associated with an RPE detachment and in some instances may be surrounded by hard exudates.

Fluorescein Angiography
Fluorescein angiography is the method most used to identify macular edema despite the fact that it does not always clearly contrast the hyperfluorescence of the basic disease (fig. 1). Thus all frames used provide some information on the existence of macular edema.

The pre-injection fluorescein frames are helpful, especially in blue light, as it enables visualization of the cysts encroaching upon the xanthophyll pigment. The central cysts compress the foveal center, especially the Henle fibers, which contain a high concentration of yellow xanthophyll enhanced by the complementary wavelength.

Pre-epithelial classic CNV manifests as a discrete, well-demarcated focal area of hyperfluorescence that can sometimes be discerned in the early phases of the angiogram (Fine et al., 1986; Coscas, 1991; Soubrane, 2007)[30–32]. Fluorescein can occasionally perfuse in the early phase a deep capillary network of CNV that is not needed to diagnose pre-epithelial CNV. Through the mid and late phase, the hyperfluorescence in the initial area increases in intensity and extends beyond the boundaries due to leakage. The hallmark of pre-epithelial CNV is the fluorescein leakage in the late phases of the angiogram beyond the boundaries of the hyperfluorescence noted in earlier phases (Bressler et al., 2006)[33]. Fluorescein may pool in the subsensory retinal fluid overlying the new vessels, which is best seen on stereoscopic images.

Subepithelial occult CNV (formerly named 'late leakage of undetermined source') refers to late choroidal-based leakage in which there are no clearly identifiable vessels. This pattern can appear as speckled hyperfluorescence with pooling of dye in the subretinal space overlying the lesion. Usually the boundaries of this type of CNV cannot be determined precisely and are poorly demarcated. This ill-defined area of hyperfluorescence at the level of the RPE is later followed by pinpoints of leakage (ooze). Little or absence of early hyperfluorescence will progressively be replaced by leakage emanating from poorly defined areas and

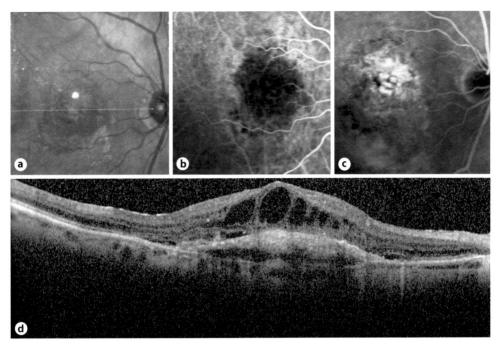

Fig. 1. Cystoid macular edema in a case of advanced subepithelial occult CNV. **a** Monochromatic green light. **b** Fluorescein angiography, early phase: 3 DD central area is dark. **c** Fluorescein angiography, late phase: the central area became heavily hyperfluorescent with at least 4 large macular cysts, distinctly visible. **d** SD-OCT (Spectralis): extensive multiple cysts occupying the complete thickness of the neurosensory retina. Some remaining Müller cell pillars. The retinal outer layers are modified by a hyperreflective dense spindle corresponding to a fibrovascular membrane. The ELM and the IS/OS interface are unrecognizable. Note the fibrovasculair PED partially organized.

become visible in the late frame of the angiogram (Soubrane et al., 1990; Bressler et al., 1992)[34, 35]. The angiographic appearance of the subepithelial CNV depends on the location, the density, and the maturity of the new vessels as well as the associated vascularized PED (Coscas, 2009)[36].

A second pattern of subepithelial occult CNV previously separated is fibrovascular PED (Macular Photocoagulation Study Group, 1991)[37]. Due to the progress of imaging it has been identified as an advanced stage in the natural history of subepithelial occult CNV (Soubrane, 2007)[32].

In the late phase, the hyperfluorescence of the cystoid spaces superimposes on the deep uneven fluorescence of the CNV. A careful analysis of the

mid and late phase is necessary in order to delineate each component. The cysts are usually encroaching the central avascular zone but may be difficult to identify in these instances. A large central cyst might be the cause of a hypofluorescent area seen on angiography if the RPE is not altered.

In addition, a PED can be clinically evident in the cleavage site created by the subepithelial occult CNV (Gass, 1997)[27].

The intraretinal collection of fluid caused by macular edema alters the structure of the macula and affects its function. The breakdown of the inner blood-retinal barrier gives rise to fluorescein leakage from the choroidal circulation and the choroidal new vessels. But the retinal vasculature

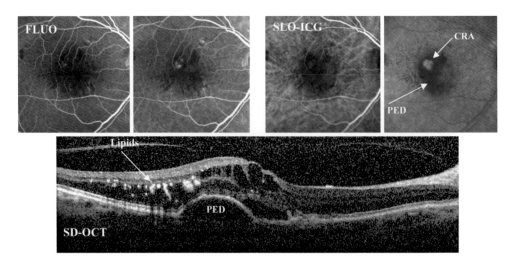

Fig. 2. Chorioretinal anastomoses. SD-OCT horizontal section (Spectralis), associated with fluorescein angiography (early and late stage) and SLO-ICG (early and late stage). Note the hyperfluorescent leakage on the late stage of the ICG-A contrasting in the dark area of the PED. Also note the extensive and accentuated intraretinal accumulation of fluid with large cystic spaces.

may also be involved in exudative AMD and contribute to macular edema. The retinal capillaries may become damaged, develop microaneurysms, and contribute to the leakage of dye into the extracellular compartment of the retina after a prolonged retinal detachment.

Extension of a choroidal neovascular membrane in the capillary-free zone, as is the rule in subepithelial occult CNV, may destroy the ELM and facilitate the collection of fluid in cystic spaces. The predisposition for the spaces to be located in the capillary-free zone may be related to structural weakness of the ELM where Müller cell processes are reduced in number as to the paucity of retinal vessels to enable drainage of the extracellular fluid in the intravascular compartment.

Indocyanine Green Angiography
Indocyanine green (ICG) angiography is able to confirm the fluorescein angiography appearance of pre-epithelial classic CNV (Hayashi and De Laey, 1986)[38]. With the improvement of the instruments, especially the scanning laser ophthalmoscope

(SLO), ICG angiography was shown to be very useful in the conversion of subepithelial CNV into well-delimited network (Yannuzzi et al., 1992)[39]. Further studies have demonstrated a variety of patterns of subepithelial occult CNV in ICG angiography (Soubrane, 1995)[40].

Areas of CNV that appear poorly defined on fluorescein angiography can be well defined on ICG angiography. Most subepithelial occult CNV is revealed as a visible clearly delineated network at the early phase contrasting on a larger hypofluorescent macular area. At the late phase, some subepithelial occult CNV may present as relatively large, well-defined staining plaques whereas others, active lesions, present an early washout. This difference might be related to the development stage of the lesion. ICG angiography is useful in identifying CNV with and without PED (Scheider and Schroedel, 1989)[41]. SLO-ICG angiography will be particularly helpful in chorioretinal anastomosis demonstrating anastomosis in the area of a uniformly dark and hypofluorescent PED and late intraretinal leakage (fig. 2).

ICG angiography is essential for imaging sub-epithelial occult CNV and the associated PED (Coscas, 2005)[42]. Thus, the best imaging strategy is to perform both fluorescein angiography and ICG angiography to detect CNV (Bressler et al., 2006)[33]. In rare cases, mainly at the inversion (late) phase, cystoid spaces might fill with ICG dye. ICG angiography is designed to reveal choroidal abnormalities and not associated retinal disturbances.

Optical Coherence Tomography
OCT is the easiest means to identify cystoid macular edema overlying the choroidal new vessels, as the imaging is quite obvious and allows both qualitative and quantitative evaluation. Following its variation and the correlations with the angiography, during the natural history or after treatment, is of primary interest and may provide additional prognostic clues (fig. 1d) (Coscas, 2009)[36].

Neurosensory Retina
The presence and accumulation of serous fluid in the neurosensory retina manifests either within the retinal tissue (as diffuse infiltration) or is collected in intraretinal cysts. The association of both patterns induces an increase in the retinal thickness and an attenuation of the foveal depression.

Fluid. The diffuse infiltration of fluid (associated or not associated with cystoid spaces) results in a significant increase in thickness of the central retina in about half of the eyes with retinal detachment. The fluid accumulation probably induces a swelling of Müller cells, which consequently may distort the photoreceptor segments and alter the ELM. This accumulation of fluid is usually associated with an inflammatory reaction that might account for the intraretinal hyperreflective dots (Coscas, 2009)[36]. The increase in fluid and inflammatory reaction may subsequently be revealed as a dense, uneven hyperreflectivity in the disorganized photoreceptor layer.

Cysts. The cysts are spaces, which are optically empty, homogenous and thus dark, in the neurosensory retina. The size of the cysts is variable according to the stage of the disease. They might be mostly small (70%) or tightly packed and confluent (30%). They are more or less extensive in the advanced stage. Their distribution in one layer (42%) or in two (58%) is of similar frequency. The swelling of the retina induces the loss of the foveal depression that is occupied early by 3–4 large cysts or by a single huge cyst, which is sometimes prolonged by a row of smaller cysts (fig. 3, 4).

In a series of 150 consecutive cases of exudative AMD, the cystoid spaces were present in nearly half of the eyes (41%), often multiple (97%), rarely isolated and centrally located (3%). These cysts are present in recent or active lesions with hyper-reflective dots and areas of intraretinal densification. During treatment, improvement or degradation parallels with the importance of the cysts. For example, after 3 intravitreous injections of anti-VEGF, the cysts are still present in 35% of the treated eyes. They vanish relatively slowly when compared with the functional improvement. The recurrence of the leakage will manifest with the reemergence of the cysts (Coscas, 2009)[36].

On the other hand, in the advanced form, the cysts are associated with various amounts of fibrosis. The persistence of the cysts in 30% of the eyes where no leakage is present means an irreversible degeneration of the neural tissue with a severe vision decrease (Coscas, 2009)[36].

Central Thickness
The central retinal thickness is often used in clinical studies. The thickness of the central retina is between 180 and 360 μm according to the OCT instrument used. The OCT may or may not include the RPE partially or totally, which is the reason for the variation of the measurement. The central retinal thickness helps to determine the indication for treatment or retreatment as well as the prognosis and the follow-up of exudative AMD. This criterion of central thickness is quite easy to use but is obviously insufficient for a precise

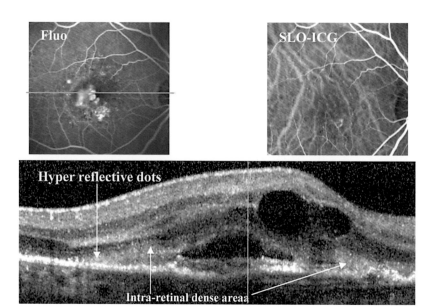

Fig. 3. Active CNV in AMD: SD-OCT horizontal section (Spectralis), associated with fluorescein and SLO-ICG angiography. Increased retinal thickness, intraretinal large cysts, hyperreflective dots, intraretinal dense area. Disorganization of the outer retinal layers [courtesy of Coscas (2009)[36]].

justification for retreatment due to the polymorphism of the disease.

Retinal Pigment Epithelium

The RPE layer is the indicator for why macular edema occurred. CNV proliferation is manifested either as a pre-RPE zone of hyperreflectivity (pre-epithelial classic CNV) or as an irregular thickening of the RPE (subepithelial occult CNV). It is then associated with the RPE elevation, which is ascertained by the visibility of Bruch's membrane. A large, prominent bullous PED with numerous packed cystic spaces in elevated retina is almost pathognomonic of anastomoses between retinal and choroidal vessels (Coscas et al., 2007)[43].

In total, the accumulation of intraretinal and subretinal fluid and the intraretinal cysts progress in parallel with the underlying disease but, until now, at an unpredictable speed that is sometimes delayed or sometimes rapid. The problem most difficult to predict is which residual lesion is likely to vanish and which cyst confirms an irreversible alteration of the retinal tissue. Review of the different OCT sections and correlations with the angiographic examinations are therefore of major value.

The determinant mechanism of intraretinal macular edema is yet unknown. One of the hypotheses implies the breakdown of the outer retinal barrier, which would allow the influx of exudation towards the central avascular zone (Gass, 1997)[27]. An alternative hypothesis suggests the possibility of an intracellular edema of the Müller cells (Yannoff et al., 1984)[44]. The role of vitreous traction in AMD is still debated: is it an initiating mechanism or, on the contrary, an aggravation for the development of CNV and of the macular edema? The choroidal new vessels are the determinant factor in the occurrence of macular edema;

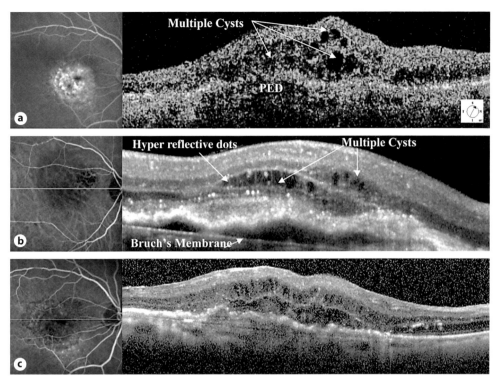

Fig. 4. Multiple intraretinal cysts and increased retinal thickness: OCT horizontal section, associated with fluorescein angiograph. **a** Advanced multiple chorioretinal anastomosis: multiple confluent cysts. **b** Persistent vascularized PED: presence of many hyperreflective dots and intraretinal dense area. Disorganization of the outer retinal layers. **c** Late advanced lesion not responding to treatment. Visual acuity: 20/800. Large number of cysts in the inner nuclear layer and between the outer plexiform layer and the outer nuclear layer [courtesy of Coscas (2009)[36]].

the initiating mechanism of which, however, remains to be clarified.

Treatment Approaches

The exudative form of AMD accounts for a disproportionate degree of legal blindness and efforts have been expended on the development of drugs to address this (Ambati et al., 2003)[45]. Visual loss occurs from the proliferation of new capillaries accompanied by exudation, bleeding and secondary fibrosis with disorganization of the RPE and outer retina. Further, secondary alterations in both the subretinal and retinal capillaries and in pigment epithelial permeability lead to the accumulation of fluid beneath the RPE, the neurosensory retina, and within the retina itself and induce more visual dysfunction. The treatment action thus may share a common goal in reducing the accumulation of intraretinal fluid.

Laser Treatment
Destruction and occlusion of the CNV will resolve leakage from the abnormal new capillaries and thus induce reduction of the macular edema. However, it will also destroy the neurosensory retina and the pigment epithelium in the area of laser burns.

Photocoagulation

If precisely performed, the heat produced by this direct laser treatment technique will occlude and destroy the new vessels causing the new vessel leakage to disappear. As a result, the cystoid macular edema will resolve. A side effect of the treatment, however, includes the occurrence of a definitive localized scotoma due to the destruction of the complete thickness of the neurosensory retina.

Photodynamic Therapy

Another means of neovascular occlusion is using a pharmacologic photosynthesizer (Verteporfin). The product injected into the veins has to be activated by the adapted wavelength. The healing process involves the formation of a glial scar. Clinical trial results are very encouraging regarding stabilization of visual acuity. Unfortunately the generation of free radicals necessary for the photothrombotic effect may also serve as a proangiogenic stimulus, possibly accounting for the apparent benefit associated with concomitant administration of steroids (Rudolf et al., 2004)[46].

Pharmacotherapy

Anti-Vascular Endothelial Growth Factor

VEGF produces an important increase in hydrolytic conductivity and is the central player of leakage both in choroidal new vessels and in macular edema. A variety of methods are available to directly block the VEGF165 molecule and its various other isoforms. Presently ranibizumab (Lucentis®) is a monoclonal antibody directed at all isoforms, which results in a decrease in leakage clearly visible on fluorescein angiography and OCT.

The results of the randomized clinical trials, which included pre-epithelial CNV or subepithelial occult CNV, have clearly demonstrated that visual acuity is stabilized and even increased in about 40% of the eyes. However, the decreased leakage of the choroidal new vessels, despite their continuing growth, requires a monthly injection of the antibody and regular follow-up for a period of 24 months or more.

A number of attempts have been made to decrease the frequency of injections. Most were able to stabilize visual acuity but no attempt resulted in a functional improvement as was obtained by the monthly injections. Thus one can suggest that a decrease in leakage from the choroidal vessels and also from the altered blood-retinal barrier is necessary in order to obtain such a positive result. In the eyes in which the treatment failed, one of the most prominent features is the persistence of cystic spaces. In addition, chronic degenerative cysts may be disseminated in the inner retina, which will not resorb despite treatment.

Direct and Indirect Vascular Endothelial Growth Factor Modulators

Cytokines may be divided into 2 classes: those that upregulate VEGF or VEGF-associated effects and those that act in an inhibitory capacity. Naturally occurring inhibitory factors include interferon-α, thrombospondin, angiostatin, endostatin, and metalloproteinases. Intracellular adhesion molecules (ICAM-1) mediate leukocyte adhesion and transmigration. They are expressed on the RPE and choroidal vascular endothelial cell surfaces and mediate extravasation from retinal and choroidal capillaries in response to inflammation. Naturally occurring downregulators include pigment epithelial-derived growth factor secreted by the RPE. Because VEGF is thought to initiate a cascade of intracellular signals followed by subsequent extracellular events, it is possible to inhibit VEGF effects either through prevention of secretion of the molecule, direct inhibition of the molecule in the extracellular space, blockade of the receptors, or through interruption in the downstream intracellular signaling pathway leading to both an intracellular and extracellular event (Campochiaro, 2004)[47].

A large body of evidence exists to support the critical and probably rate-limiting role of VEGF in the neovascular form of AMD (Ambati et al.,

2003; Grossniklaus et al., 2002)[45, 48]. Additionally, there are strong indicators that elevated levels of VEGF are the proximal causes for the hyperpermeability seen in eyes with subsensory and intraretinal fluid associated with CNV. These alterations are able to be either reversed by direct blockade of VEGF receptors or by using an NOS knockout model (Senger et al., 1983; Fukumura et al., 2001; Sennlaub et al., 2002)[49–51]. Inactivation of soluble VEGF by monoclonal antibodies directed against it or inhibition of ICAM also appears to be effective.

Other methods of direct inhibition of VEGF include inhibition of its tyrosine kinase receptors (VEGF-1 and VEGF-2) either by systemic administration or gene transfer. The VEGF inhibitors share an attempt to mitigate the proliferative and permeability effect of VEGF on normal and neovascular tissue. It remains unclear and the point of some debate as to the relative desirability and safety of a complete blockade of all major VEGF isoforms compared to exclusively VEGF165. Similarly, it is undetermined if the global blockade would stop all leakage from the retinal capillaries and restore the blood-retinal barrier in its integrity.

Steroids and Other Immunomodulators

Steroids have been associated with neovascularization reduction by mechanisms that are not clearly understood. The anti-angiogenic effect of steroids could be divided into 2 categories (Folkman and Ingber, 1987)[52]: (1) those related to anti-inflammatory effects paralleling conventional glucocorticoid and mineral corticoid activity, and (2) a separate structure configuration of the pregnan nucleus conferring distinct anti-angiogenic capabilities (Folkman et al., 1989)[53].

Clinical studies using conventional steroids alone have shown relatively unimpressive effects on the progression of AMD (Ranson et al., 2002)[54]. In one randomized clinical trial, a single 4-mg dose of intravitreal triamcinolone was administered to 73 eyes in the treatment group receiving laser. They were matched with 70 eyes in the

control group and were followed for 1 year (Ghazi et al., 2001)[55]. The change in size of the neovascular membrane was significantly less in the treated eyes, but there were no significant differences in the visual acuity outcomes between the 2 groups.

The use of conventional steroids with glucocorticoid and mineralcorticoid activity, including triamcinolone, has an inhibitory effect on ICAM and thus they inhibit VEGF.

Recently, a number of steroids have come on the market for the treatment of macular edema due to central retinal vein occlusion (CRVO) and branch retinal vein occlusion (BRVO). The triamcinolone steroid without preservative was used in the SCORE study, and the dexamethasone steroid in the GENEVA study using a biodegradable implant.

Both studies demonstrated a best corrected visual acuity improvement of ≥15 letters from baseline at month 12. The repeated intravitreal injections in the SCORE study (4 mg triamcinolone) resulted in an improvement in 27.2% of BRVO patients and in 25.6% of CRVO patients versus laser or observation, respectively. An increase in visual acuity was experienced in 29.3% of patients in a 2-month period and in 21.8% of patients in a 3-month period over the 12-month follow-up in the GENEVA study.

The adverse event rate, however, was quite important: 36% of patients with BRVO and 26 or 15.7% of patients with CRVO had an intraocular pressure (IOP) increase >10 mm Hg above baseline and 10 and 9%, or 3.7%, respectively, had an IOP >35 mm Hg at 2 or 12 months. Thus over 12 months, fewer patients treated with dexamethasone (23%) required IOP-lowering medication versus 35–41% of patients treated with triamcinolone. The major advantage of the implant versus repeated injections was a prolonged effect over 6 months despite a slow decrease in activity after 4 months. A nonbiodegradable implant containing fluocinolone was recently announced to be efficient in the same vascular pathology.

In these studies, the results can be attributed, at least in part, to the effect on macular edema of retinal vascular origin. None of the eyes presented with choroidal new vessels. The suggestion to use intravitreal triamcinolone for CNV has been generally greeted with enthusiasm, but the association with conventional photodynamic therapy has been disappointing. However, the effect of steroids on the inflammatory component of retinal vascular permeability may possibly suggest that a similar effect can be expected on the inflammatory component of choroidal new vessels in AMD either alone or in association with ranibizumab (study in progress).

Vitrectomy

In cystoid macular edema, there are 3 ways in which the vitreous contributes to macular edema. First, vitreoretinal traction via the internal limiting membrane leads directly to vessel distortion and damage causing them to leak (Schepens et al., 1984)[56]. The second role of the vitreous is to sequester cytokines and alter the pathways of their removal (Sebag and Balazs, 1984)[57]. Finally, it is thought that traction may contribute to the release of the cytokines via direct action on neuroretinal cells (Lewis, 2001)[58]. Thus, this traction can lead to vascular leakage both directly and through the release of cytokines that might be relieved by surgical vitrectomy (Aylward, 1999)[59]. There is a rationale for surgery that aims to relieve vitreomacular traction and remove the cytokine-laden vitreous.

Pharmacologic vitreolysis may improve vitreoretinal surgery and, ultimately, prevent disease by mitigating the contribution of the vitreous to retinopathy. Enzymatic-assisted posterior vitreous detachment with microplasmin increases vitreal O_2 levels and increases the rate of O_2 exchange within the porcine vitreous cavity (Quiram et al., 2007)[60]. Despite the fact that AMD formation has already begun before the persistent attachment of the posterior vitreous to the macula, it may be a risk factor for the development of exudative AMD (Lee et al., 2009)[19]. In addition to vitrectomy, vitreolysis is presently being evaluated in a phase II study in order to determine if the injection of

microplasmin, inducing a vitreous detachment, would decrease the CNV proliferation and possibly the persistence of CME.

Conclusion

The simultaneous presence of choroidal new vessels and macular edema imply a number of cellular dysfunctions and metabolic alterations. The implication of both circulations, retinal associated with choroidal, is not mandatory. The leakage from the choroidal new vessels, predominantly VEGF-induced, may produce a large accumulation of fluid under the neurosensory retina.

Without the participation of the retinal circulation, a major disturbance of 3 barriers must have taken place: the outer retinal barrier and the blood-retinal barrier both presented tight junctions that failed and the outer limiting membrane loosened. The shift of the RPE pump and the oncotic pressure are additional forces providing the opportunity for fluid invasion of the whole retina.

Also, the contribution of the retinal circulation as observed in chorioretinal anastomosis results in the maximum influx of fluid further depending upon VEGF-induced inflammation.

Finally, the mechanic traction of the vitreous delimiting the pocket described by Worst may constitute a cytokine reservoir. VEGF is, in all likelihood, the rate-limiting step rather than the initiating step in AMD.

It is also likely that the key signaling steps occur prior to the upregulation of VEGF either initiated by, or facilitated by, cytokines, which act under normal basic conditions to counterbalance the integral VEGF effects and, in pathologic circumstances, may either counteract or serve to amplify the process. The major factors implied in this complex construction are the cytokines under the control of inflammation that upregulate or downregulate a large number of mechanisms. The initiating mechanisms still remain to be identified.

References

1 Burns MS, Bellhorn RW, Korte GE, Heriot WJ: Plasticity of the retinal vasculature; in Osborne N, Chader G (eds): Progress in Retinal Research. Oxford, Pergamon Press, 1986, pp 253–308.

2 Connolly DT, Heuvelman DM, Nelson R, Olander JV, Eppley BL, Delfino JJ, Siegel NR, Leimgruber RM, Feder J: Tumor vascular permeability factor stimulates endothelial cell growth and angiogenesis. J Clin Invest 1989;84:1470–1478.

3 Ramrattan RS, van der Schaft TL, Mooy CM, de Bruijn WC, Mulder PG, de Jong PT: Morphometric analysis of Bruch's membrane, the choriocapillaris, and the choroid in aging. Invest Ophthalmol Vis Sci 1994;35:2857–2864.

4 Sarks SH: Ageing and degeneration in the macular region: a clinico-pathological study. Br J Ophthalmol 1976;60:324–341.

5 Bird AC, Pauleikhoff D, Olver J, Maguire J, Sheraidah G, Marshall J: The correlation of choriocapillaris and Bruch membrane changes in ageing. Invest Ophthalmol Vis Sci 1990;31:228.

6 Olver J, Pauleikhoff D, Bird AC: Morphometric analysis of age changes in the choriocapillaris. Invest Ophthalmol Vis Sci 1990;31:229.

7 Fisher RF: The influence of age on some ocular basement membranes. Eye 1987;1:184–189.

8 Moore DJ, Hussain AA, Marshall J: Age-related variation in the hydraulic conductivity of Bruch's membrane. Invest Ophthalmol Vis Sci 1995;36:1290–1297.

9 Holz FG, Sheraidah G, Pauleikhoff D, Bird AC: Analysis of lipid deposits extracted from human macular and peripheral Bruch's membrane. Arch Ophthalmol 1994;112:402–406.

10 Sheraidah G, Steinmetz R, Maguire J, Pauleikhoff D, Marshall J, Bird AC: Correlation between lipids extracted from Bruch's membrane and age. Ophthalmology 1993;100:47–51.

11 Pauleikhoff D, Zuels S, Sheraidah GS, Marshall J, Wessing A, Bird AC: Correlation between biochemical composition and fluorescein binding of deposits in Bruch's membrane. Ophthalmology 1992;99:1548–1553.

12 Curcio CA, Millican CL, Bailey T, Kruth HS: Accumulation of cholesterol with age in human Bruch's membrane. Invest Ophthalmol Vis Sci 2001;42:265–274.

13 Löffler KU, Lee WR: Basal linear deposit in the human macula. Graefes Arch Clin Exp Ophthalmol 1986;224:493–501.

14 Lopez PF, Sippy BD, Lambert HM, Thach AB, Hinton DR: Transdifferentiated retinal pigment epithelial cells are immunoreactive for vascular endothelial growth factor in surgically excised age-related macular degeneration-related choroidal neovascular membranes. Invest Ophthalmol Vis Sci 1996;37:855–868.

15 Imai D, Yoneya S, Gehlbach PL, Wei LL, Mori K: Intraocular gene transfer of pigment epithelium-derived factor rescues photoreceptors from light-induced cell death. J Cell Physiol 2005;202:570–578.

16 Killingsworth MC, Sarks JP, Sarks SH: Macrophages related to Bruch's membrane in age-related macular degeneration. Eye 1990;4:613–621.

17 Robison CD, Krebs I, Binder S, Barbazetto IA, Kotsolis AI, Yannuzzi LA, Sadun AA, Sebag J: Vitreomacular adhesion in active and end-stage age-related macular degeneration. Am J Ophthalmol 2009;148:79–82.

18 Mojana F, Cheng L, Bartsch DU, Silva GA, Kozak I, Nigam N, Freeman WR: The role of abnormal vitreomacular adhesion in age-related macular degeneration: spectral optical coherence tomography and surgical results. Am J Ophthalmol 2008;146:218–227.

19 Lee SJ, Lee CS, Koh HJ: Posterior vitreomacular adhesion and risk of exudative age-related macular degeneration: paired eye study. Am J Ophthalmol 2009;147:621–626.

20 Schulze S, Hoerle S, Mennel S, Kroll P: Vitreomacular traction and exudative age-related macular degeneration. Acta Ophthalmol 2008;86:470–481.

21 Krebs I, Brannath W, Glittenberg C, Zeiler F, Sebag J, Binder S: Posterior vitreomacular adhesion: a potential risk factor for exudative age-related macular degeneration? Am J Ophthalmol 2007;144:741–746.

22 Kliffen M, Sharma HS, Mooy CM, Kerkvliet S, de Jong PT: Increased expression of angiogenic growth factors in age-related maculopathy. Br J Ophthalmol 1997;8:154–162.

23 Pauleikhoff D, Spital G, Radermacher M, Brumm GA, Lommatzsch A, Bird AC: A fluorescein and indocyanine green angiographic study of choriocapillaris in age-related macular disease. Arch Ophthalmol 1999;117:1353–1358.

24 Monte M, Davel LE, Sacerdote de Lustig E: Hydrogen peroxide is involved in lymphocyte activation mechanisms to induce angiogenesis. Eur J Cancer 1997;33:676–682.

25 Kuroki M, Voest EE, Amano S, Beerepoot LV, Takashima S, Tolentino M, Kim RY, Rohan RM, Colby KA, Yeo KT, Adamis AP: Reactive oxygen intermediates increase vascular endothelial growth factor expression in vitro and in vivo. J Clin Invest 1996;98:1667–1675.

26 Penfold PL, Killingsworth MC, Sarks SH: Senile macular degeneration. The involvement of giant cells in atrophy of the retinal pigment epithelium. Invest Ophthalmol Vis Sci 1986;27:364–371.

27 Gass JDM: Stereoscopic Atlas of Macular Diseases. Diagnosis and Treatment, ed 4. Saint Louis, Mosby, 1997.

28 Soubrane G, Coscas G, Larcheveque F: Macular degeneration related to age and cystoid macular edema. Apropos of 95 cases (100 eyes). J Fr Ophtalmol 1988;11:711–720.

29 Bressler NM, Bressler SB, Alexander J, Javornik N, Fine SL, Murphy RP: Loculated fluid. A previously undescribed fluorescein angiographic finding in choroidal neovascularization associated with macular degeneration. Macular Photocoagulation Study Reading Center. Arch Ophthalmol 1991;109:211–215.

30 Fine AM, Elman MJ, Ebert JE, Prestia PA, Starr JS, Fine SL: Earliest symptoms caused by neovascular membranes in the macula. Arch Ophthalmol 1986;104:513–514.

31 Coscas G: Dégénérescences maculaires acquises liées à l'âge et néovaisseaux sous-rétiniens. Paris, Masson, 1991, pp 213–258.

32 Soubrane G: Les DMLA(s). Paris, Masson, 2007, pp 253–266.

33 Bressler N, Bressler S, Fine SL: Neovascular (exudative) age-related macular degeneration; in Ryan SJ (ed): Retina. Philadelphia, Mosby, 2006, pp 1075–1113.

34 Soubrane G, Coscas G, Français C, Koenig F: Occult subretinal new vessels in age-related macular degeneration. Natural History and early laser treatment. Ophthalmology 1990;97:649–657.

35 Bressler SB, Silva JC, Bressler NM, Alexander J, Green WR: Clinicopathologic correlation of occult choroidal neovascularization in age-related macular degeneration. Arch Ophthalmol 1992;110: 827–832.

36 Coscas G: Optical Coherence Tomography in Age-Related Macular Degeneration (OCT in AMD). Heidelberg, Springer, 2009, pp 1–389.

37 Macular Photocoagulation Study Group: Subfoveal neovascular lesions in age-related macular degeneration. Guidelines for evaluation and treatment in the macular photocoagulation study. Arch Ophthalmol 1991;109:1109–1114.

38 Hayashi K, De Laey JJ: Indocyanine green angiography of neovascular membranes. Ophthalmologica 1985;190:30–39.

39 Yannuzzi LA, Slakter JS, Sorenson JA, Guyer DR, Orlock DA: Digital indocyanine green videoangiography and choroidal neovascularization. Retina 1992;12:191–223.

40 Soubrane G: Affections acquises de la rétine et de l'épithélium pigmentaire rétinien. Bull Soc Ophtalmol Fr 1995;324–327.

41 Scheider A, Schroedel C: High resolution indocyanine green angiography with a scanning laser ophthalmoscope. Am J Ophthalmol 1989;108:458–459.

42 Coscas G: Atlas of Indocyanine Green Angiography. Paris, Elsevier, 2005, pp 1–383.

43 Coscas F, Coscas G, Souied E, Ticks S, Soubrane G: Optical coherence tomography identification of occult choroidal neovascularization in age related macular degeneration. Am J Ophthalmol 2007;144:592–599.

44 Yanoff M, Fine BS, Brucker AJ, Eagle RC Jr: Pathology of human cystoid macular edema. Surv Ophthalmol 1984; 28(suppl):505–511.

45 Ambati J, Ambati BK, Yoo SH, Ianchulev S, Adamis AP: Age-related macular degeneration: etiology, pathogenesis, and therapeutic strategies. Surv Ophthalmol 2003;48:257–293.

46 Rudolf M, Michels S, Schlötzer-Schrehardt U, Schmidt-Erfurth U: Expression of angiogenic factors by photodynamic therapy. Klin Monbl Augenheilkd 2004;221:1026–1032.

47 Campochiaro PA: Ocular neovascularisation and excessive vascular permeability. Expert Opin Biol Ther 2004;4:1395–1402.

48 Grossniklaus HE, Ling JX, Wallace TM, Dithmar S, Lawson DH, Cohen C, Elner VM, Elner SG, Sternberg P Jr: Macrophage and retinal pigment epithelium expression of angiogenic cytokines in choroidal neovascularization. Mol Vis 2002;8:119–126.

49 Senger DR, Galli SJ, Dvorak AM, Perruzzi CA, Harvey VS, Dvorak HF: Tumor cells secrete a vascular permeability factor that promotes accumulation of ascites fluid. Science 1983;219:983–985.

50 Fukumura D, Gohongi T, Kadambi A, Izumi Y, Ang J, Yun CO, Buerk DG, Huang PL, Jain RK: Predominant role of endothelial nitric oxide synthase in vascular endothelial growth factor-induced angiogenesis and vascular permeability. Proc Natl Acad Sci USA 2001;98:2604–2609.

51 Sennlaub F, Courtois Y, Goureau O: Inducible nitric oxide synthase mediates retinal apoptosis in ischemic proliferative retinopathy. J Neurosci 2002; 22:3987–3993.

52 Folkman J, Ingber DE: Angiostatic steroids. Method of discovery and mechanism of action. Ann Surg 1987;206:374–383.

53 Folkman J, Weisz PB, Joullié MM, Li WW, Ewing WR: Control of angiogenesis with synthetic heparin substitutes. Science 1989;243:1490–1493.

54 Ranson NT, Danis RP, Ciulla TA, Pratt L: Intravitreal triamcinolone in subfoveal recurrence of choroidal neovascularisation after laser treatment in macular degeneration. Br J Ophthalmol 2002;86:527–529.

55 Ghazi NG, Jabbour NM, De La Cruz ZC, Green WR: Clinicopathologic studies of age-related macular degeneration with classic subfoveal choroidal neovascularization treated with photodynamic therapy. Retina 2001;21:478–486.

56 Schepens CL, Avila MP, Jalkh AE, Trempe CL: Role of the vitreous in cystoid macular edema. Surv Ophthalmol 1984;28 Suppl:499–504.

57 Sebag J, Balazs EA: Pathogenesis of cystoid macular edema: an anatomic consideration of vitreoretinal adhesions. Surv Ophthalmol 1984;28(suppl):493–498.

58 Lewis H: Macular translocation with chorioscleral outfolding: a pilot clinical study. Am J Ophthalmol 2001;132:156–163.

59 Aylward GW: The place of vitreoretinal surgery in the treatment of macular oedema. Doc Ophthalmol 1999;97:433–438.

60 Quiram PA, Leverenz VR, Baker RM, Dang L, Giblin FJ, Trese MT: Microplasmin-induced posterior vitreous detachment affects vitreous oxygen levels. Retina 2007;27:1090–1096.

Prof. Gisèle Soubrane
Hôpital Intercommunal de Créteil, Service d'Ophthalmologie
40, Avenue de Verdun
FR–94010 Créteil (France)
E-Mail gisele.soubrane@chicreteil.fr

Coscas G (ed): Macular Edema.
Dev Ophthalmol. Basel, Karger, 2010, vol 47, pp 183–198

Miscellaneous

Catherine Creuzot-Garcher[a] · Sebastian Wolf[b]

[a]Service d'Ophtalmologie, CHU Dijon, Dijon, France; [b]Universitätsklinik für Augenheilkunde, Inselspital, University of Bern, Bern, Switzerland

Abstract

This chapter provides the reader with practical information to be applied to the various remaining causes of macular edema. Some clinical cases of macular edema linked to ocular diseases like postradiotherapy for ocular melanomas remained of poor functional prognosis due to the primary disease. On the contrary, macular edema occurring after retinal detachment or after diverse systemic or local treatment use is often temporary. Macular edema associated with epiretinal membranes or vitreomacular traction is the main cause of poor functional recovery. In other cases, as in tractional myopic vitreoschisis, the delay to observe a significant improvement of the vision after surgery should be long. Finally, macular edema associated with hemangiomas or macroaneurysms should be treated, if symptomatic, using the same current treatment as in diabetic macular edema or exudative macular degeneration.

The miscellaneous chapter is always a challenging one, laden with two serious caveats: being too exhaustive or forgetting common circumstances. The authors have attempted to provide the reader with useful, practical information that can be applied to the various causes of macular edema.

Radiation Therapy

Radiation retinopathy is a sight-threatening complication that mainly occurs after irradiation for tumors involving the choroid, retina, orbit and paranasal sinuses (Finger, 1997)[1]. Theoretically, this complication can occur in industrial and military activities. Ionizing radiation leads to cell death related to cellular DNA damage and can take years to appear (Finger et al., 2009)[2].

Clinically, it is characterized by an aspect of ischemic vasculopathy with microaneurysms, vessel occlusion, and capillary dropout. It is generally associated with exudative signs with retinal hemorrhage, edema, and exudation, which fluorescein angiography visualizes as leakage (fig. 1).

Histopathology shows impaired vascular endothelial vessels and pericytes with progressive closure and thickening of tumor vessel walls (occurring as well in normal adjacent retina), but also thickening of normal retinal vessels in the targeted zone treated by the radioactive plaque.

Risk factors for radiation therapy are: the use of larger doses and more rapid dose rates delivering the effective dose, the potential radiation sensitizers used with the radiation treatment, as well

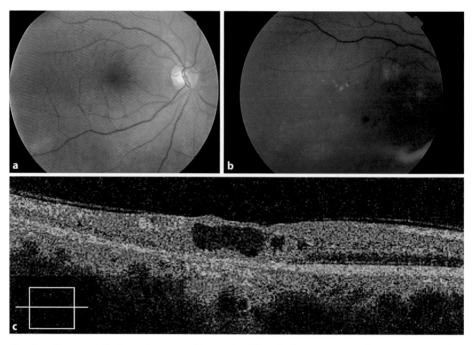

Fig. 1. **a** Temporoinferior melanoma with no visual loss, before treatment. **b** Same patient after treatment (1 year later), with macular edema. **c** OCT of the patient: increased macular thickness with visual loss.

as systemic risk factors such as diabetes, which potentiates the ischemic response (Finger, 2000)[3]. This progressive obliterative endarteritis can lead to progressive tissue ischemia with intraocular neovascularization.

In this disease, visual loss results from ischemic retinopathy with neovascularization and macular edema. Neovascular glaucoma is a frequent complication of neovascularization (Finger, 1997)[1].

To treat these severe complications, different treatments have been proposed:

Laser photocoagulation was reported by some authors to obliterate the irradiated zone surrounding the plaque (Hykin et al., 1998)[4]. While neovascular glaucoma can be prevented with panretinal photocoagulation, the efficacy of grid or focal laser in treating macular edema has remained only somewhat successful regarding visual acuity recovery. Improvement in visual acuity has been

reported in 70% of cases of radiation macular edema with a follow-up of 39 months (Kinyoun et al., 1995)[5]. The method for treating these edemas does not differ from the procedure used in macular edema found in diabetic retinopathy.

Intravitreal steroid use was reported to treat refractory macular edema in a 64-year-old woman with a parotid carcinoma (Sutter et al., 2003)[6]. This patient was treated with triamcinolone injection (4 mg) after long-lasting macular edema refractory to macular grid laser treatment. Clinical outcome showed visual acuity improvement and a decrease in macular thickness on optical coherence tomography (OCT). However, a relapse of macular edema 9 months later led to another intravitreal injection with the same efficacy but no recurrence during a 1-year follow-up. The pathophysiology of the mechanism of action remains unclear but is probably based on restoration of a compromised inner blood-retinal barrier (Gillies, 1999)[7].

Intravitreal antiangiogenic injection was reported in refractory macular edema caused by radiation therapy. The authors reported the results of intravitreal injections of bevacizumab in 6 patients suffering from macular edema stemming from ocular melanomas treated with plaque irradiation. They reported visual acuity improvement with reduced exudative signs documented on angiogram and OCT with no serious adverse events. The patients were treated with 2.8 injections (range, 1–4) with a mean follow-up of 4.7 months (range, 2–8 months). Interestingly, the delay between the plaque insertion and the onset of the radiation therapy ranged from 9 to 150 months (Finger et al., 2008)[8].

Macular Edema Resulting from Systemic or Topical Treatment

Prostaglandin Analogs

There have been a number of contradictory results suggesting the association between the development of anterior uveitis and cystoid macular edema (CME) and prostaglandin (PG) use. However, these cases were anecdotal without good evidence from controlled clinical trials. Indeed, in most cases a nonindependent risk factor for the development of uveitis such as previous ocular surgery, pseudophakia or aphakia, posterior capsule rupture, or past history of uveitis were associated (Hoyng et al., 1997; Schumer et al. 2000; Wand et al., 2002)[9–11].

The pathophysiology of this effect may be the proinflammatory action of PGs. However, PG analogs have a high affinity for the FP prostanoid receptor but a very low effect on vasoactive prostanoid receptors. Furthermore, experimental studies have failed to demonstrate a prochemotactic effect of PGs (Schumer et al. 2002)[12]. Additionally, no blood barrier breakdown should be observed in eyes treated for increased ocular pressure caused by PGs (Linden, 2001)[13].

A recent retrospective study demonstrated that PG analogs are not associated with increased risk of CME or anterior uveitis, although they can lead to substantially decreased intraocular pressure (Chang et al., 2008)[14]. In 163 eyes of 84 consecutive patients with uveitis, the authors compared the rate of uveitis and CME in eyes treated with PG and control eyes treated by non-PG-lowering treatment. They found no statistically significant difference between the two groups: neither patients with previous history of anterior uveitis or CME, nor patients with no CME history expressed significantly increased CME or uveitis once treated with PG in comparison with non-PG use.

Mitotic Inhibitors

Joshi and Garretson reported on cases of CME secondary to mitotic inhibitors: one was related to paclitaxel use in a patient suffering from a breast carcinoma (Joshi et al., 2007)[15]. This case was characterized by visual loss stemming from CME found on OCT with an increase in foveal thickness but no angiographic changes. Once discontinued, the CME disappeared with recovery of visual acuity 6 weeks after discontinuation.

The absence of angiographic signs remained unexplained but should be related to toxicity to Müller cells leading to an intracellular accumulation and subclinical leakage of extracellular fluid.

Glitazone Use

Glitazones belong to a class of drugs used to reduce insulin resistance in diabetic patients. These peroxisome proliferator-activated receptor γ activators were implicated in a potential induction of diabetic macular edema (DME) by a few reports in limited series (Colucciello, 2005; Ryan et al. 2006; Sivagnanam, 2006)[16–18].

The pathogenesis of this side effect remains unclear: mechanisms set off by increased plasma volume, sympathetic activation, protein kinase

C activation, or increased production of vascular endothelial growth factor remain speculative. Until now, there have been controversial results concerning this secondary macular edema. Shen et al. recently reported that rosiglitazone delayed the onset of proliferative diabetic retinopathy but did not increase the risk of macular edema (Shen et al., 2008)[19]. The authors emphasized that rosiglitazone has been demonstrated to have antiangiogenic properties in vivo and in animal models. These results are in contradiction with a large cohort study involving 17,000 glitazone users to evaluate the 1-year incidence of DME (Fong et al., 2009)[20]. The authors found that glitazone users were more likely to develop DME [odds ratio = 2.5 (2.4–3)], with an increased risk still present when adjusting for confounding factors [odds ratio = 1.6 (1.4–1.8)]. However, some confounding factors such as high blood pressure, renal status, and hyperlipidemia were not available in this electronically collected database study; nor was the diagnosis of macular edema, which was made upon computer data only, without assessed clinical data (fig. 2).

However, these controversial results clearly emphasize the need for large-scale studies to assess the risk-benefit ratio of these drugs. In all cases, the macular edema disappeared when the glitazone was stopped as long as no confounding factors such as poor diabetic balance or increased high blood pressure were associated (Colucciello, 2005)[16].

Epiretinal Membrane and Traction Syndrome

Epiretinal membrane (ERM) can be either idiopathic or associated with various conditions such as retinal breaks, diabetic retinopathy, branch retinal vein occlusion, inflammation, and exudative vitreoretinopathy. It also frequently appears after intraocular surgery, especially retinal detachment surgery (Margherio et al., 1985; Gaudric et al., 1993)[21,22].

In vitreomacular traction syndrome (VMTS), the presence of a persistent attachment of the vitreous to the macula with incomplete posterior vitreous detachment (PVD) is responsible for the thickening of the macular area (Smiddy et al. 1989)[23]. Many studies have found a clear visual improvement after vitreomacular traction removal (Smiddy et al., 1989; Smiddy et al., 1990; Rouhette et al., 2001)[23–25]. Histologic samples from VMTS found mainly fibrotic tissue with astrocytes, fibrocytes, and myofibrocytes (Shinoda et al., 2000)[26] (fig. 3).

The additional benefit of internal limiting membrane (ILM) peeling for VMTS remains unknown (Gandorfer et al., 2002)[27]. VMTS leads to a persistent traction of the macula, producing macular edema and visual loss. Idiopathic VMTS occurs without ERM or macular hole but most cases are secondary to ERM (Puliafito et al., 1995)[28].

The Role Played by OCT in the Surgical Decision: A Histologic-Like Assessment

OCT plays a major role in decision making in ERM and VMTS management (Do et al., 2007)[29]. Do et al. found that the diagnosis of macular edema was made in 67.9% of the cases by clinical examination in comparison with 83.3% with OCT. In contrast, OCT leads to fewer surgical decisions than does clinical examination (42.4 vs. 57.6%). In patients recommended for surgery, macular edema was more pronounced. Macular edema was thought to be associated with lower visual acuity (Gaudric et al., 1992)[30].

OCT has shown that it can take a long time to obtain complete resolution of macular changes. Subretinal fluid can persist as long as 1 year after surgery, the delay required for almost normal retinal tissue organization (Uchino et al., 2001)[31].

Recent OCT techniques have provided a better understanding of the relation between vitreous and retina in ERM and VMTS. In a recent study using spectral domain OCT with 3-dimensional images, Koizumi et al. clearly showed the potential overlap between ERM and VMTS (Koizumi et

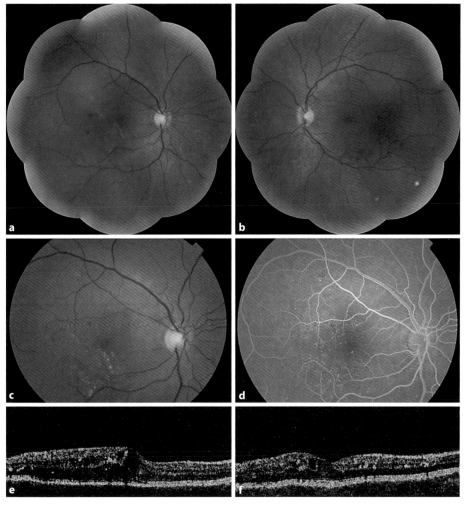

Fig. 2. a Patient treated with glitazone with focal macular edema (right eye). **b** Patient treated with glitazone with focal macular edema (left eye). **c** Patient with worsened focal macular edema in spite of grid treatment (right eye) – color retinophotography but good systemic diabetic control. **d** Patient with worsened focal macular edema in spite of grid treatment (right eye) – fluorescein angiogram. **e** Same patient, macula OCT, 3 months later with diffuse macular edema. **f** Same patient, 3 months later after glitazone was stopped.

al., 2008)[32]. Indeed, although a complete PVD was noted in the majority of ERM cases (30/36), some cases showed either an incomplete PVD with peripheral remnants or no PVD. Furthermore, in VMTS, the vitreous attachment was almost equally found as either broad (less than 1,500 μm) or diffuse (more than 1,500 μm). However, ERM was noted in almost all cases (Koizumi et al., 2008)[32].

The cells are present not only on the ERM, but also on the posterior hyaloid (Gastaud et al., 2000)[33]. Spectral domain OCT confirmed these findings with some hyperreflective placoid areas seen on the posterior hyaloid, probably due to this fibrotic proliferation.

The preoperative aspect revealed by OCT is important in VMTS, as demonstrated by Yamada et al. (Yamada et al., 2005)[34]. These authors reported two different aspects of PVD. One was an incomplete-shaped detachment, the other one only partial with remaining attached vitreous on the nasal part of the fovea. The former aspect was associated with a good visual outcome with a tomographic recovery within 4 months in almost all cases. In contrast, the latter was associated with greater preoperative macular thickness with a prominent CME in 3 out of 4 patients as well as an increased rate of postoperative complications (macular hole and macular atrophy). This complicated outcome resulted in decreased visual acuity (fig. 3).

Several authors have underlined poor visual outcome in VMTS (Smiddy et al., 1989; McDonald et al., 1994; Melberg et al., 1995)[23,35,36], but their observations of PVD status were mainly intraoperative. One of the main advantages of OCT is to detail PVD status as a histologic-like aspect.

Histologic analysis confirmed this hypothesis with two different features: (1) some samples collected during VMTS showed a single cell layer covering the vitreal side of the ILM and (2) a premacular fibrocellular tissue separated from the ILM by a native layer of collagen, as occurs with ERMs (Gandorfer et al., 2002)[27]. However, the cells differed from ERM with myofibroblasts as the predominant cells. The effects exerted by these cells should explain the high rate of CME and detachment of the macula observed in VMTS.

A variant of VMTS can be found with an incomplete PVD and a persistent central macular attachment. Spontaneous detachment can occur with more or less complete resolution of the clinical signs. These cases were identified by the absence of leakage with fluorescein. VMTS was associated with perifoveal hyaloidal detachment with a single adhesion in the center of the fovea leading to foveal thickening with cystoid spaces. The vitreous is firmly attached to the retina at the vitreous base, along temporal arcades and on papilla edges as well as the 500-μm central macular area. In contrast, the PVD initially begins at the periphery of the macula spreading progressively to the center (Uchino et al., 2001; Gaudric et al., 1999)[31,37]. Since the strength of the adhesion of the vitreous conditions the VMTS outcome, CME or macular hole occurrence strongly depends on this condition (Johnson et al., 2001)[38].

Is ILM Peeling Necessary to Avoid CME after ERM or VMTS?

The influence of ILM peeling on CME remains unclear. The ILM is the structural boundary between the retina and the vitreous. This 2.5-μm-thick membrane is closely associated with the plasma membrane of the Müller cells, suggesting that it derives from glial cells (Abdelkader et al., 2008)[39]. There is no general agreement on whether or not the ILM should be peeled during ERM removal. To ease ILM peeling, several dyes have been successively used with different histologic consequences (Haritoglou et al., 2003; Haritoglou et al., 2004)[40,41].

The histologic studies on ILM specimens have shown Müller cell plasma membranes and retinal elements on the retinal side of the indocyanine green-peeled ILM, suggesting that this dye alters the cleavage plane during ILM peeling (Haritoglou et al., 2004)[42] (fig. 4). Pathology studies have found cellular elements such as glial cells,

Fig. 3. a Tractional macular edema gives the typical aspect of honeycomb macular edema. It remains the only validated indication of ERM peeling in diabetic macular edema. **b** Vitreomacular traction in the nasal part of the fovea. Posterior hyaloid remains strongly attached. **c** VMTS with severe macular edema (preoperative aspect). **d** VMTS after ERM and ILM peeling. Macular thickness is strongly decreased with a partial recovery of normal macular profile on the OCT. **e** Macular edema secondary to a thick macular ERM (preoperative aspect). **f** Same patient. Postoperative (after 6 months) aspect. The macula remained thickened without normal macular profile. **g** ERM with macular edema (preoperative). Triamcinolone was injected during surgery. **h** Same patient, 1 month postoperatively: complete recovery of normal macular thickness with a partial recovery of visual acuity (20/80). **i** Same patient. Macular edema recurrence, 1 year later without recovery of visual acuity (20/80).

Creuzot-Garcher · Wolf

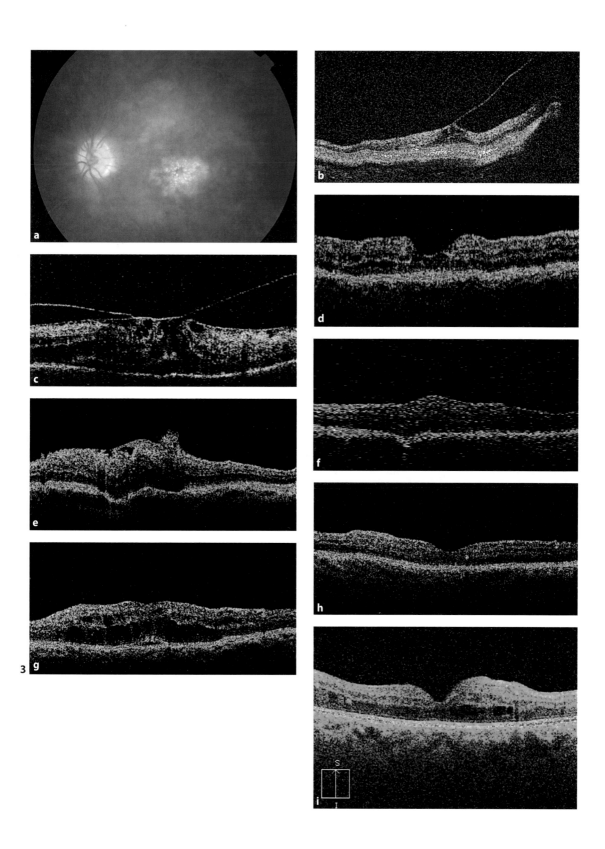

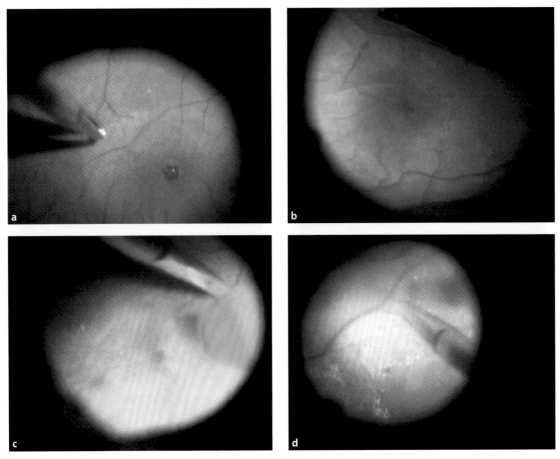

Fig. 4. a ILM peeling without any dye: the whitening of the retina clearly shows the limits where ILM was removed. **b** ILM peeling with indocyanine green: the dye strongly facilitates ILM removal but should not be advised due to its potential toxicity. **c** ILM peeling with brilliant blue peel: the dye seems to stain exclusively ILM without any retinal toxicity. **d** Vitreous removal can be facilitated by triamcinolone use: the crystals are trapped in the vitreous gel and improve vitreous visualization.

fibroblasts, macrophages, and collagen fibers, suggesting a multifactorial aspect combining inflammation, proliferation, and fibrosis (Kampik et al., 1980)[43]. ILM associated with ERM probably acts as a scaffold for cell proliferation and the authors suggested removing the ILM during epiretinal peeling to decrease the recurrence rate (Park et al., 2003; Sakamoto et al., 2003)[44,45]. The presence of a thin layer of collagen between the ILM and ERM found by Haritoglou et al. strongly suggested that

ILM removal should decrease the risk of recurrence by this means. Several case-control studies or case series showed that combined ILM and epiretinal peeling does not seem to alter the outcome after surgery.

However, as ILM peeling is a difficult technical procedure, the need for ILM peeling has to be confirmed. This remains unclear given the controversial results: some authors found the ILM remnants on epiretinal specimens were associated with better visual outcomes (Bovey et al., 2004)[46], whereas others have found the opposite (Sivalingam et al., 1990)[47].

The value of ILM peeling in CME combined with ERM was studied by Geerts et al. (Geerts et al., 2004)[48]. They showed that when they compared the outcome of CME in patients, the relief was better in patients with ILM removal than in patients without. However, these were diabetic patients, which could bias the results. Indeed, there have been many studies suggesting a potential role of vitrectomy and ILM peeling in the outcome of CME during diabetes, but to date no studies have clearly demonstrated the benefit of a surgical approach to CME during diabetes except for tractional macular edema. The arguments in favor of performing a vitrectomy for DME were both to decrease the vascular permeability by removing growth factors and to improve the oxygenation of the retina, which in turn decreases vasodilatation. Increased perifoveal blood flow velocity after pars plana vitrectomy has been found (Kadonosono et al., 1999)[49]. However, although a lower recurrence of ERM was found after ILM peeling (Gandorfer et al., 2000; Kuhn et al., 2004; Kimura et al., 2005)[50–52], some studies have reported controversial results regarding the outcome of CME with positive results (Tachi et al.,1996; Stolba et al., 2005)[53,54] and negative results (Thomas et al., 2005)[55].

Retinal Detachment

Many studies have focused on the postoperative analysis of the macula by OCT after retinal detachment. A study by Kiss et al. investigated the aspect of the macula after complicated retinal detachment with proliferative vitreoretinopathy (Kiss et al., 2007)[56]. They found that the macula remained normal in only 12.8% of cases and 17.1% of patients presented with macular edema (fig. 5). This rate was lower than that reported by Bonnet who found a 51.7% rate in 1994 (Bonnet,

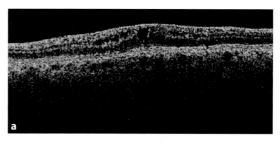
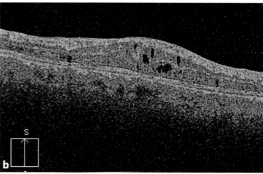

Fig. 5. Macular edema after a retinal detachment. **a** Six months after retinal detachment. **b** Same patient, 4 years later.

1994)[57], but the surgical technique was probably different. Macular edema can be present alone or combined with subretinal fluid (Benson et al., 2006)[58]. In about one third of patients, macular disease is eligible for treatment, namely in the cases of macular pucker or macular edema.

Ultrahigh-resolution OCT provides a very precise assessment of the vitreoretinal interface. Schocket et al. studied the microstructural changes in the retina in patients suffering from poor recovery after retinal detachment surgery (Schocket et al., 2006)[59]. They found an isolated macular edema in 12% of their patients and an ERM in 59% of the cases. Sophisticated OCT techniques are useful to distinguish the untreatable changes (distortion of the inner/outer junction) from the etiologies eligible for treatment.

However, today no validated treatment can be proposed to treat isolated macular edema secondary to retinal detachment. The use of anti-VEGF treatment or triamcinolone acetonide, already used in inflammatory macular edema resulting from uveitis, remains to be evaluated.

Tractional Myopic Vitreoschisis

Macular schisis is a vitreoretinal disease caused by splitting of the macular area. This condition is not really macular edema but corresponds to a thickening of the macular area and can be difficult to distinguish from macular edema in myopic patients.

OCT provides a very precise comprehensive mechanism. The usual presentation is an outer schisis where the retina is split into the outer retinal layers with a thick inner layer. In contrast, inner schisis involves the inner layers leading to a thick outer layer. This condition can be stable: Gaucher et al. reported a progression in 20 eyes of 29 patients with a follow-up of 31 months (Gaucher et al., 2007)[60]. Premacular structure (44.8%), foveal detachment (34.5%), and lamellar macular hole (20.7%) were the most common OCT findings. Visual acuity can be preserved even with severe macular thickening (fig. 6). The authors found that hyperreflective premacular structure and foveal detachment were associated with a worse outcome. Vitrectomy with cortex removal, with or without ILM peeling, and internal tamponade can be useful to treat the cases with impaired visual acuity (Ikuno et al., 2004; Kwok et al., 2005)[61,62], with some risk of postoperative macular hole.

Choroidal Hemangioma

Choroidal hemangioma is a rare benign vascular tumor that occurs in two circumstances: either in its diffuse form associated with Sturge-Weber syndrome or in its circumscribed form [circumscribed choroidal hemangioma (CCH)], usually sporadic without any systemic manifestations.

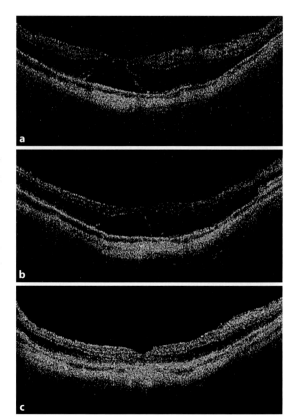

Fig. 6. Vitreofoveal schisis in a myopic patient with visual loss. The delay to recover a normal aspect is very long (sometimes 1 year). **a** Preoperative. **b** One month later. **c** Six months later.

These orange-red, smooth lesions can be discovered incidentally but can lead to severe loss of vision especially in cases of exudative detachment and CME. The diagnosis is made by angiography. Fluorescein angiography only shows an early and then persisting hyperfluorescence but indocyanine green angiography shows the typical 'wash-out' phenomenon, characteristic for CCH (with an early hyperfluorescence in the early frame followed by a relative hypofluorescence in the 15-min late frame) (fig. 7).

A long-term report of CCH concluded that about 50% of patients will suffer from a visual loss

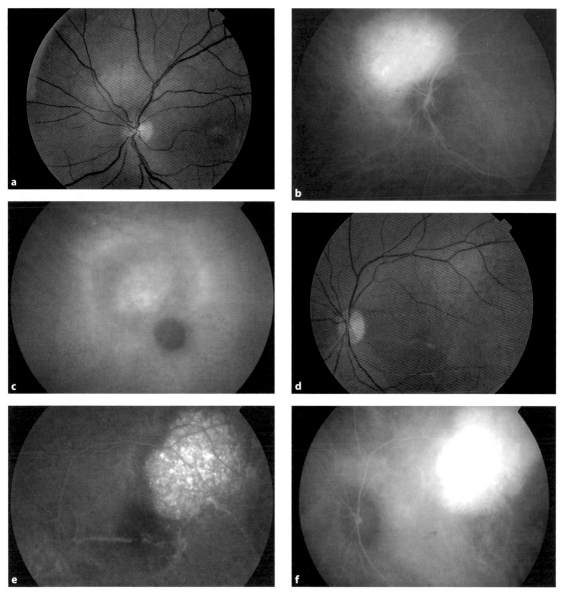

Fig. 7. Choroidal hemangioma. **a–c** Color images, fluorescein and indocyanine green angiogram with a washout of the indocyanine green in the late frame. **a** Hemangioma located in the superior part of the optic nerve head. **b** Hemangioma early frame. **c** Hemangioma late frame. **d–g** Patients operated for retinal detachment with subretinal folds. During the follow-up, the remaining subretinal fluid was in fact due to a temporal choroidal hemangioma. **d** Hemangioma, color image. **e** Hemangioma fluorescein angiogram. **f** Hemangioma, indocyanine green, early frame.

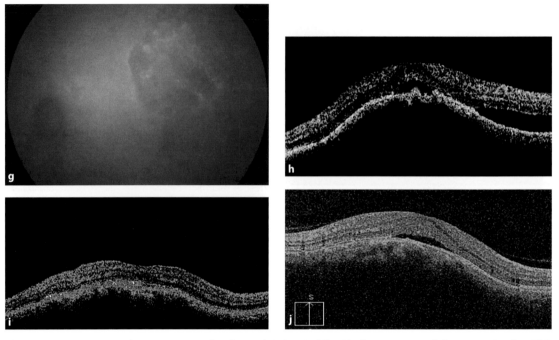

Fig. 7. **g** Hemangioma, indocyanine green, late frame. **h** Subretinal fluid before treatment. **i** Three months after PDT. **j** Recurrence of subretinal fluid, 9 months after initial treatment.

<20/200 due to a chronic macular edema (Shields et al., 2001)[63].

Asymptomatic CCHs not causing visual loss are usually not treated and only need periodical observation. By contrast, symptomatic CCHs require treatment (Gunduz, 2004)[64]. Treatment options have varied during the last decade: initial treatments were based mainly on laser photocoagulation but led to nerve fiber layer consequences and did not lead to regression of the tumor. Radiation therapy and transpupillary thermotherapy were also used and led to a good control of the tumor, but all these techniques have limited efficacy with common recurrences. Recent studies underlined the interest in photodynamic therapy (PDT). PDT allows a selective photochemical injury to the vascular endothelial cells but the protocols (mean radiation exposure between 50 and 100 J/cm²) and exposure time (between 83 and 186 s) used in the literature remain a matter of debate. Authors reported on treatments with a number of sessions ranging between 1 and 5 with intervals from 6 to 12 weeks. The aim of the treatment remained the elimination of subretinal fluid and not the tumor regression although PDT can lead to a decrease in CCH thickness.

CME regressed in almost all the cases after PDT and subretinal fluid disappeared with a single treatment only in most cases (Boixadera et al., 2009)[65].

Retinal Macroaneurysm

Retinal arterial macroaneurysm (MA) is an acquired dilation of a retinal artery occurring usually in the elderly. It is marked by a strong female predominance in a context of systemic hypertension

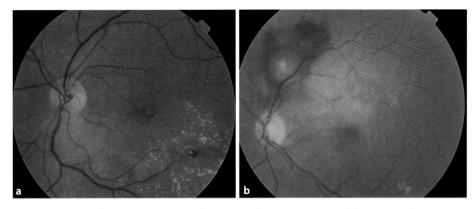

Fig. 8. a Temporal MA with exudative deposits in the temporal part of the fovea. **b** Superior MA with hemorrhage and macular edema.

and arteriosclerosis with a lesion present in one eye only in the majority of cases.

Although the most common presenting symptom remains the loss of vision, MAs should remain asymptomatic with a diagnosis found incidentally during a routine exam. MA usually involves the temporal arcade arteries. The vision loss depends on the involvement of the macula and should be progressive in case of exudation and edema or more sudden and severe in case of hemorrhage.

Hemorrhages can reach all retinal layers from the subretinal space to the subhyaloidal layer and can be associated with a vitreous hemorrhage in 10% of the cases. Exudative retinopathy looks like a circinate pattern around the MA and neurosensory retinal detachment can be associated with edema, hemorrhage or exudate. However, some MAs exhibit severe exudative changes.

The usual outcome of MA follows a course from thrombosis, fibrosis to spontaneous involution. This is the reason why, in most cases, it does not exhibit any macular leakage after hemorrhage disappearance (Rabb et al., 1988)[66]. Indeed, once the aneurysm ruptures, it usually spontaneously regresses (fig. 8).

Initially, if present, macular edema usually involves the outer layer. Most MAs exhibit vascular leakage leading to macular edema with secondary lipid deposits. Macular edema and its consequences are considered as the main cause of vision loss as it occurs in about 1/3 of patients. Chronic macular edema will cause destruction of the foveal outer photoreceptor layer responsible for a poor vision (Tsujikawa et al., 2009)[67].

As the majority of MAs resolve spontaneously with good vision, the indications of laser photocoagulation are recommended only in case of severe macular edema with exudates lasting for more than 3 months or in case of recurrent bleeding with vitreous hemorrhage. This situation remained rare as bleeding leads most often to a spontaneous thrombosis with secondary involution. In few cases, a photocoagulation therapy should be used with either direct treatment of the MA or an indirect treatment of the surrounding retina.

In eyes with exudative change, laser photocoagulation usually leads to a flattening of the fovea. However, after hemorrhage resolution, retinal structure and outer layers are usually impaired even if minimal hemorrhagic complications were found initially. The prognosis after laser photocoagulation of the MA depends on the amount of lipid deposits in the macular area and of the (irreversible) changes of the outer layers which could prevent from a good visual acuity recovery.

Recently, authors reported one case treated with bevacizumab for macular edema secondary to a retinal MA. Good visual acuity recovery was observed with 2 injections with subsequent complete resolution of macular edema on OCT (Chanana et al., 2009)[68]. This new proposal needs further investigation.

Conclusions

Macular edema remains a common clinical situation. Diabetes and vein occlusion still remain the main causes of macular edema. However, some circumstances should be associated with these diseases like ERM. Moreover, macular edema linked to topical or systemic treatment should be found in some diabetic or in uveitic patients. The learning from clinical trials for DME will provide us with very interesting results to be used in other circumstances like hemangioma or MA as these situations are not supposed to benefit from large-scale studies.

Finally, the more precise analysis of the foveal region and especially of the consequences of macular edema with new-generation OCT will probably enable us to better define the surgical indication and outcome of ERM and VMTS.

References

1 Finger PT: Radiation therapy for choroidal melanoma. Surv Ophthalmol 1997;42:215–232.
2 Finger PT, Chin KJ, et al: Palladium-103 ophthalmic plaque radiation therapy for choroidal melanoma: 400 treated patients. Ophthalmology 2009;116:790–796, 796e1.
3 Finger PT: Tumour location affects the incidence of cataract and retinopathy after ophthalmic plaque radiation therapy. Br J Ophthalmol 2000;84:1068–1070.
4 Hykin PG, Shields CL, et al: The efficacy of focal laser therapy in radiation-induced macular edema. Ophthalmology 1998;105:1425–1429.
5 Kinyoun JL, Zamber RW, et al: Photocoagulation treatment for clinically significant radiation macular oedema. Br J Ophthalmol 1995;79:144–149.
6 Sutter FK, Gillies MC: Intravitreal triamcinolone for radiation-induced macular edema. Arch Ophthalmol 2003;121:1491–1493.
7 Gillies MC: Regulators of vascular permeability: potential sites for intervention in the treatment of macular edema. Doc Ophthalmol 1999;97:251–260.

8 Finger RP, Charbel Issa P, et al: Intravitreal bevacizumab for choroidal neovascularisation associated with pseudoxanthoma elasticum. Br J Ophthalmol 2008;92:483–487.
9 Hoyng PF, Rulo AH, et al: Fluorescein angiographic evaluation of the effect of latanoprost treatment on blood-retinal barrier integrity: a review of studies conducted on pseudophakic glaucoma patients and on phakic and aphakic monkeys. Surv Ophthalmol 1997;41(suppl 2):S83–S88.
10 Schumer RA, Camras CB, et al: Latanoprost and cystoid macular edema: is there a causal relation? Curr Opin Ophthalmol 2000;11:94–100.
11 Wand M, Gaudio AR: Cystoid macular edema associated with ocular hypotensive lipids. Am J Ophthalmol 2002;133:403–405.
12 Schumer RA, Camras CB, et al: Putative side effects of prostaglandin analogs. Surv Ophthalmol 2002;47(suppl 1): S219.
13 Linden C: Therapeutic potential of prostaglandin analogues in glaucoma. Expert Opin Investig Drugs 2001;10:679–694.

14 Chang JH, McCluskey P, et al: Use of ocular hypotensive prostaglandin analogues in patients with uveitis: does their use increase anterior uveitis and cystoid macular oedema? Br J Ophthalmol 2008;92:916–921.
15 Joshi MM, Garretson BR: Paclitaxel maculopathy. Arch Ophthalmol 2007;125:709–710.
16 Colucciello M: Vision loss due to macular edema induced by rosiglitazone treatment of diabetes mellitus. Arch Ophthalmol 2005;123:1273–1275.
17 Ryan EH Jr, Han DP, et al: Diabetic macular edema associated with glitazone use. Retina 2006;26:562–570.
18 Sivagnanam G: Rosiglitazone and macular edema. CMAJ 2006;175:276.
19 Shen LQ, Child A, et al: Rosiglitazone and delayed onset of proliferative diabetic retinopathy. Arch Ophthalmol 2008;126:793–799.
20 Fong DS, Contreras R: Glitazone use associated with diabetic macular edema. Am J Ophthalmol 2009;147:583–586e1.
21 Margherio RR, Cox MS Jr, et al: Removal of epimacular membranes. Ophthalmology 1985;92:1075–1083.

22 Gaudric A, Fardeau C, et al: Ablation of the internal limiting membrane, macular unfolding and visual outcome in surgery of idiopathic epimacular membranes. J Fr Ophtalmol 1993;16:571–576.

23 Smiddy WE, Green WR, et al: Ultrastructural studies of vitreomacular traction syndrome. Am J Ophthalmol 1989;107:177–185.

24 Smiddy WE, Michels RG, et al: Morphology, pathology, and surgery of idiopathic vitreoretinal macular disorders. A review. Retina 1990;10:288–296.

25 Rouhette H, Gastaud P: Idiopathic vitreomacular traction syndrome. Vitrectomy results. J Fr Ophtalmol 2001;24:496–504.

26 Shinoda K, Hirakata A, et al: Ultrastructural and immunohistochemical findings in five patients with vitreomacular traction syndrome. Retina 2000;20:289–293.

27 Gandorfer A, Rohleder M, et al: Epiretinal pathology of vitreomacular traction syndrome. Br J Ophthalmol 2002;86:902–909.

28 Puliafito CA, Hee MR, et al: Imaging of macular diseases with optical coherence tomography. Ophthalmology 1995;102:217–229.

29 Do DV, Cho M, et al: Impact of optical coherence tomography on surgical decision making for epiretinal membranes and vitreomacular traction. Retina 2007;27:552–556.

30 Gaudric A, Cohen D: Surgery of idiopathic epimacular membranes. Prognostic factors. J Fr Ophtalmol 1992;15:657–668.

31 Uchino E, Uemura A, et al: Postsurgical evaluation of idiopathic vitreomacular traction syndrome by optical coherence tomography. Am J Ophthalmol 2001;132:122–123.

32 Koizumi H, Spaide RF, et al: Three-dimensional evaluation of vitreomacular traction and epiretinal membrane using spectral-domain optical coherence tomography. Am J Ophthalmol 2008;145:509–517.

33 Gastaud P, Betis F, et al: Ultrastructural findings of epimacular membrane and detached posterior hyaloid in vitreomacular traction syndrome. J Fr Ophtalmol 2000;23:587–593.

34 Yamada N, Kishi S: Tomographic features and surgical outcomes of vitreomacular traction syndrome. Am J Ophthalmol 2005;139:112–117.

35 McDonald HR, Johnson RN, et al: Surgical results in the vitreomacular traction syndrome. Ophthalmology 1994;101:1397–1402, discussion 1403.

36 Melberg NS, Williams DF, et al: Vitrectomy for vitreomacular traction syndrome with macular detachment. Retina 1995;15:192–197.

37 Gaudric A, Haouchine B, et al: Macular hole formation: new data provided by optical coherence tomography. Arch Ophthalmol 1999;117:744–751.

38 Johnson MW, Van Newkirk MR, et al: Perifoveal vitreous detachment is the primary pathogenic event in idiopathic macular hole formation. Arch Ophthalmol 2001;119:215–222.

39 Abdelkader E, Lois N: Internal limiting membrane peeling in vitreo-retinal surgery. Surv Ophthalmol 2008;53:368–396.

40 Haritoglou C, Gandorfer A, et al: The effect of indocyanine-green on functional outcome of macular pucker surgery. Am J Ophthalmol 2003;135:328–337.

41 Haritoglou C, Eibl K, et al: Functional outcome after trypan blue-assisted vitrectomy for macular pucker: a prospective, randomized, comparative trial. Am J Ophthalmol 2004;138:1–5.

42 Haritoglou C, Gandorfer A, et al: Anatomic and visual outcomes after indocyanine green-assisted peeling of the retinal internal limiting membrane in idiopathic macular hole surgery. Am J Ophthalmol 2004;138:691–692, author reply 692.

43 Kampik A, Green WR, et al: Ultrastructural features of progressive idiopathic epiretinal membrane removed by vitreous surgery. Am J Ophthalmol 1980;90:797–809.

44 Park DW, Dugel PU, et al: Macular pucker removal with and without internal limiting membrane peeling: pilot study. Ophthalmology 2003;110:62–64.

45 Sakamoto H, Yamanaka I, et al: Indocyanine green-assisted peeling of the epiretinal membrane in proliferative vitreoretinopathy. Graefes Arch Clin Exp Ophthalmol 2003;241:204–207.

46 Bovey EH, Uffer S, et al: Surgery for epimacular membrane: impact of retinal internal limiting membrane removal on functional outcome. Retina 2004;24:728–735.

47 Sivalingam A, Eagle RC Jr, et al: Visual prognosis correlated with the presence of internal-limiting membrane in histopathologic specimens obtained from epiretinal membrane surgery. Ophthalmology 1990;97:1549–1552.

48 Geerts L, Pertile G, et al: Vitrectomy for epiretinal membranes: visual outcome and prognostic criteria. Bull Soc Belge Ophtalmol 2004;293:7–15.

49 Kadonosono K, Itoh N, et al: Capillary blood flow velocity in patients with idiopathic epiretinal membranes. Retina 1999;19:536–539.

50 Gandorfer A, Messmer EM, et al: Resolution of diabetic macular edema after surgical removal of the posterior hyaloid and the inner limiting membrane. Retina 2000;20:126–133.

51 Kuhn F, Kiss G, et al: Vitrectomy with internal limiting membrane removal for clinically significant macular oedema. Graefes Arch Clin Exp Ophthalmol 2004;242:402–408.

52 Kimura T, Kiryu J, et al: Efficacy of surgical removal of the internal limiting membrane in diabetic cystoid macular edema. Retina 2005;25:454–461.

53 Tachi N, Ogino N: Vitrectomy for diffuse macular edema in cases of diabetic retinopathy. Am J Ophthalmol 1996;122:258–260.

54 Stolba U, Binder S, et al: Vitrectomy for persistent diffuse diabetic macular edema. Am J Ophthalmol 2005;140:295–301.

55 Thomas D, Bunce C, et al: A randomised controlled feasibility trial of vitrectomy versus laser for diabetic macular oedema. Br J Ophthalmol 2005;89:81–86.

56 Kiss CG, Richter-Muksch S, et al: Anatomy and function of the macula after surgery for retinal detachment complicated by proliferative vitreoretinopathy. Am J Ophthalmol 2007;144:872–877.

57 Bonnet M: Macular changes and fluorescein angiographic findings after repair of proliferative vitreoretinopathy. Retina 1994;14:404–410.

58 Benson SE, Schlottmann PG, et al: Optical coherence tomography analysis of the macula after vitrectomy surgery for retinal detachment. Ophthalmology 2006;113:1179–1183.

59 Schocket LS, Witkin AJ, et al: Ultrahigh-resolution optical coherence tomography in patients with decreased visual acuity after retinal detachment repair. Ophthalmology 2006;113:666–672.

60 Gaucher D, Haouchine B, et al: Long-term follow-up of high myopic foveoschisis: natural course and surgical outcome. Am J Ophthalmol 2007;143:455–462.

61 Ikuno Y, Sayanagi K, et al: Vitrectomy and internal limiting membrane peeling for myopic foveoschisis. Am J Ophthalmol 2004;137:719–724.

62 Kwok AK, Lai TY, et al: Vitrectomy and gas tamponade without internal limiting membrane peeling for myopic foveoschisis. Br J Ophthalmol 2005;89:1180–1183.

63 Shields CL, Honavar SG, et al: Circumscribed choroidal hemangioma: clinical manifestations and factors predictive of visual outcome in 200 consecutive cases. Ophthalmology 2001;108:2237–2248.

64 Gunduz K: Transpupillary thermotherapy in the management of circumscribed choroidal hemangioma. Surv Ophthalmol 2004;49:316–327.

65 Boixadera A, Arumi JG, et al: Prospective clinical trial evaluating the efficacy of photodynamic therapy for symptomatic circumscribed choroidal hemangioma. Ophthalmology 2009;116:100–105e1.

66 Rabb MF, Gagliano DA, et al: Retinal arterial macroaneurysms. Surv Ophthalmol 1988;33:73–96.

67 Tsujikawa A, Sakamoto A, et al: Retinal structural changes associated with retinal arterial macroaneurysm examined with optical coherence tomography. Retina 2009;29:782–792.

68 Chanana B; Azad RV: Intravitreal bevacizumab for macular edema secondary to retinal macroaneurysm. Eye 2009;23:493–494.

Prof. Catherine Creuzot-Garcher
Service d'Ophtalmologie, CHU Dijon
FR–21000 Dijon (France)
E-Mail catherine.creuzot-garcher@chu-dijon.fr

Author Index

Subject Index